Case Files™:
Internal Medicine

NOTICE

Case Files™: Internal Medicine

EUGENE C. TOY, MD
THE JOHN S. DUNN, SR. ACADEMIC CHAIR AND PROGRAM DIRECTOR
CHRISTUS ST. JOSEPH HOSPITAL OBSTETRICS AND GYNECOLOGY RESIDENCY PROGRAM
HOUSTON, TEXAS
CLERKSHIP DIRECTOR, ASSISTANT CLINICAL PROFESSOR
DEPARTMENT OF OBSTETRICS/GYNECOLOGY
UNIVERSITY OF TEXAS-HOUSTON MEDICAL SCHOOL
HOUSTON, TEXAS

JOHN T. PATLAN, JR., MD
ASSISTANT PROFESSOR OF MEDICINE AND PEDIATRICS
DEPARTMENT OF INTERNAL MEDICINE
UNIVERSITY OF TEXAS-HOUSTON MEDICAL SCHOOL
HOUSTON, TEXAS

S. ELIZABETH CRUSE, MD
ASSISTANT PROFESSOR OF MEDICINE AND PEDIATRICS
DEPARTMENT OF INTERNAL MEDICINE
UNIVERSITY OF TEXAS-HOUSTON MEDICAL SCHOOL
HOUSTON, TEXAS

FABRIZIA FAUSTINELLA, MD, PHD
ASSISTANT PROFESSOR, DIVISION OF GENERAL MEDICINE
DEPARTMENT OF INTERNAL MEDICINE
UNIVERSITY OF TEXAS-HOUSTON MEDICAL SCHOOL
HOUSTON, TEXAS

Lange Medical Books/McGraw-Hill

MEDICAL PUBLISHING DIVISION

New York Chicago San Francisco
Lisbon London Madrid Mexico City
Milan New Delhi San Juan Seoul
Singapore Sydney Toronto

The McGraw-Hill Companies

Case Files™: Internal Medicine

4567890 DOC/DOC 098765

ISBN: 0-07-142191-2

This book was set in Times New Roman by McGraw-Hill Desktop.
The editors were Catherine A. Johnson and Karen G. Edmonson.
The production supervisor was Catherine H. Saggese.
The cover designer was Aimee Nordin.
The index was prepared by Pamela J. Edwards.
RR Donnelly was printer and binder.

This book is printed on acid-free paper.

Library of Congress Cataloging-in-Publication Data

Case files™ : Internal medicine / [edited by] Eugene C. Toy.
p. ; cm.
Includes bibliographical references and index.
ISBN 0-07-142191-2
1. Internal medicine—Case studies. I.Title: Internal medicine. II.Toy, Eugene C.
[DNLM: 1. Internal medicine—Case Reports. 2. Internal medicine—Problems and Exercises.
3. Diagnosis Differential—Case Report. 4. Diagnosis Differential—Problems and Exercises.
5. Medical History Taking—Case Report. 6. Medical History Taking—Problems and Exercises.
7. Physical Examination—Case Report. 8. Physical Examination—Problems and Exercises.
WB 18.2 C3365 2004]
RC66.C36 2004
616′.09—dc22

2003066549

To our coach Victor, and our father–son teammates Bob & Jackson, Steve & Weston, Ron & Wesley, and Dan & Joel. At the inspirational JH Ranch Father–Son Retreat, all of us, including my loving son Andy, arrived as strangers, but in 6 days, we left as lifelong friends.

— ECT

To my parents who instilled an early love of learning and of the written word, and who continue to serve as role models for life.

To my beautiful wife Elsa and children Sarah and Sean, for their patience and understanding, as precious family time was devoted to the completion of "the book."

To all my teachers, particularly Drs. Carlos Pestaña, Robert Nolan, Herbert Fred, and Cheves Smythe, who make the complex understandable, and who have dedicated their lives to the education of physicians, and served as role models of healers.

To the medical students and residents at the University of Texas–Houston Medical School whose enthusiasm, curiosity, and pursuit of excellent and compassionate care provide a constant source of stimulation, joy, and pride.

To all readers of this book everywhere in the hopes that it might help them to grow in wisdom and understanding, and to provide better care for their patients who look to them for comfort and relief of suffering.

And to the Creator of all things, Who is the source of all knowledge and healing power, may this book serve as an instrument of His will.

— JTP

CONTENTS

CONTRIBUTORS

Rajiv Agarwal, MD
Cardiology Fellow
University of Texas–Houston Medical School
Houston, Texas
Congestive Heart Failure
Atrial Fibrillation

Firas Al-kassab, MD
Internal Medicine Resident
University of Texas–Houston Medical School
Houston, Texas
Diverticulitis

Roberto Andrade, MD
Fellow, Infectious Diseases
University of Texas–Houston Medical School
Houston, Texas
Neutropenic Fever

Ana Arango, MD
Internal Medicine Resident
University of Texas–Houston Medical School
Houston, Texas
Acute Monarticular Arthritis

Eugene Boisaubin, MD
Professor, Division of General Medicine
University of Texas–Houston Medical School
Houston, Texas
Headache

Thi Cao, MD
Chief Medical Resident
University of Texas–Houston Medical School
Houston, Texas
Pulmonary Tuberculosis

Lara Colton, MD
Internal Medicine Resident
University of Texas–Houston Medical School
Houston, Texas
Pulmonary Embolism

Holly Dluzniewski, MD
Medicine-Pediatrics Resident
University of Texas–Houston Medical School
Houston, Texas
Urinary Tract Infection

Saadia Faiz, MD
Fellow, Pulmonary and Critical Care Medicine
University of Texas–Houston Medical School
Houston, Texas
Chronic Obstructive Pulmonary Disease
Chronic Cough

Kevin Finkel, MD
Associate Professor, Division of Renal Diseases
University of Texas–Houston Medical School
Houston, Texas
Acute Renal Failure

Dipak Ghelani, MD
Internal Medicine Resident
University of Texas–Houston Medical School
Houston, Texas
Transfusion Reaction

Shefali Goel, MD
Internal Medicine Resident
University of Texas–Houston Medical School
Houston, Texas
Acute Myocardial Infarction

Jaime Gomez, MD
Cardiology Fellow
University of Texas–Houston Medical School
Houston, Texas
Aortic Dissection

Khawar Gul, MD
Internal Medicine Resident
University of Texas–Houston Medical School
Houston, Texas
Limb Ischemia

Aditya Gupta, MD
Internal Medicine Resident
University of Texas–Houston Medical School
Houston, Texas
Acute Pancreatitis

Michael Hepfer, MD
Medicine-Pediatrics Resident
University of Texas–Houston Medical School
Houston, Texas
Acute Hepatitis

Trieu Ho, MD
Internal Medicine Resident
University of Texas–Houston Medical School
Houston, Texas
Pericarditis

Charles Hu, MD
Medicine-Pediatrics Resident
University of Texas–Houston Medical School
Houston, Texas
Syncope

Philip Johnson, MD
Professor
Director, Division of General Medicine
University of Texas–Houston Medical School
Houston, Texas
HIV with Fever

Andrew Jorgensen, MD
Medicine-Pediatrics Resident
University of Texas–Houston Medical School
Houston, Texas
Sickle Cell Crisis

Sona Kashyap, MD
Fellow, Endocrinology
University of Texas–Houston Medical School
Houston, Texas
Adrenal Insufficiency
Diabetic Ketoacidosis

Clair Lakkis, MD
Internal Medicine Resident
University of Texas–Houston Medical School
Houston, Texas
Fever and Rash

Esteban Lopez, MD
Medicine-Pediatrics Resident
University of Texas–Houston Medical School
Houston, Texas
Oligomenorrhea

Thomas Lux, MD
Assistant Professor, Division of General Medicine
University of Texas–Houston Medical School
Houston, Texas
Osteoarthritis

Ruckshanda Majid, MD
Internal Medicine Resident
University of Texas–Houston Medical School
Houston, Texas
Pleural Effusion

Apurva Modi, MD
Internal Medicine Resident
University of Texas–Houston Medical School
Houston, Texas
Chronic Liver Disease

Seema Modi, MD
Medicine-Pediatrics Resident
University of Texas– Houston Medical School
Houston, Texas
Nephrotic Syndrome

Philip Orlander, MD
Professor
Director, Division of Endocrinology
University of Texas–Houston Medical School
Houston, Texas
Adrenal Insufficiency
Thyrotoxicosis

Bhairav Patel, MD
Internal Medicine Resident
University of Texas–Houston Medical School
Houston, Texas
Carotid Stenosis

Annie Philip, MD
Fellow, Infectious Diseases
University of Texas–Houston Medical School
Houston, Texas
Infective Endocarditis

Michalis Picolos, MD
Fellow, Endocrinology
University of Texas–Houston Medical School
Houston, Texas
Thyrotoxicosis

Alberto Puig, MD, PhD
Assistant Professor, Division of General Medicine
University of Texas–Houston Medical School
Houston, Texas
Acute Glomerulonephritis

Michael Rupp, MD
Medicine-Pediatrics Resident
University of Texas–Houston Medical School
Houston, Texas
Anaphylaxis

Ibrahim Saeed, MD
Chief Medical Resident
University of Texas–Houston Medical School
Houston, Texas
Hypertensive Encephalopathy

Amber D. Shamburger, MS4
Senior Medical Student
University of Texas–Houston Medical School
Houston, TX
Approach to Acute Pericarditis
Approach to Lung Cancer

Charles Sims, MD
Internal Medicine Resident
University of Texas–Houston Medical School
Houston, Texas
Jaundice

Cheves McCord Smythe, MD
Professor, Division of General Medicine
University of Texas–Houston Medical School
Houston, Texas
Acute Delirium

Adam Weinstein, MD
Internal Medicine Resident
University of Texas–Houston Medical School
Houston, Texas
Inflammatory Bowel Disease

INTRODUCTION

Mastering the cognitive knowledge within a field such as internal medicine is a formidable task. It is even more difficult to draw on that knowledge, procure and filter through the clinical and laboratory data, develop a differential diagnosis, and, finally, to make a rational treatment plan. To gain these skills, the student learns best at the bedside, guided and instructed by experienced teachers, and inspired toward self-directed, diligent reading. Clearly, there is no replacement for education at the bedside. Unfortunately, clinical situations usually do not encompass the breadth of the specialty. Perhaps the best alternative is a carefully crafted patient case designed to stimulate the clinical approach and the decision-making process. In an attempt to achieve that goal, we have constructed a collection of clinical vignettes to teach diagnostic or therapeutic approaches relevant to internal medicine.

Most importantly, the explanations for the cases emphasize the mechanisms and underlying principles, rather than merely rote questions and answers. This book is organized for versatility: it allows the student "in a rush" to go quickly through the scenarios and check the corresponding answers, and it allows the student who wants thought-provoking explanations to obtain them. The answers are arranged from simple to complex: the bare answers, an analysis of the case, an approach to the pertinent topic, a comprehension test at the end, clinical pearls for emphasis, and a list of references for further reading. The clinical vignettes are purposely placed in random order to simulate the way that real patients present to the practitioner. A listing of cases is included in Section III to aid the student who desires to test his/her knowledge of a certain area, or to review a topic, including basic definitions. Finally, we intentionally did not use a multiple choice question format in the case scenarios, because clues (or distractions) are not available in the real world.

ACKNOWLEDGMENTS

The curriculum that evolved into the ideas for this series was inspired by Philbert Yau and Chuck Rosipal, two talented and forthright students, who have since graduated from medical school. It has been a tremendous joy to work with my excellent coauthors, especially Dr. John Patlan, who exemplifies the qualities of the ideal physician- caring, empathetic, and avid teacher, and who is intellectually unparalleled. Likewise, I appreciate the help from the many outstanding contributors. I am greatly indebted to my editor, Catherine Johnson, whose exuberance, experience, and vision helped to shape this series. I appreciate McGraw-Hill's believing in the concept of teaching through clinical cases, and I would like to especially acknowledge Karen Edmonson for her editing expertise. At CHRISTUS St. Joseph Hospital, I applaud the finest administrators I have encountered—Jeff Webster, Mark Mullarkey, and Dr. Benton Baker, III—for their commitment to medical education, and Dorothy Mersinger for her sage advice and support. I am extremely grateful to fourth-year medical student Amber Shamburger for her critique on the content. Without my dear colleagues, Drs.Weilie Tjoa, John Pappadas, Nicolas Stephanou, and Vincente Zapata, this book could not have been written. Most of all, I appreciate my ever-loving wife Terri, and our four wonderful children, Andy, Michael, Allison, and Christina, for their patience and understanding.

Eugene C. Toy

SECTION I

How to Approach Clinical Problems

PART 1. APPROACHING THE PATIENT

The transition from the textbook or journal article to the clinical situation is one the most challenging tasks in medicine. Retention of information is difficult; organization of the facts and recall of a myriad of data in precise application to the patient is crucial. The purpose of this text is to facilitate in this process. The first step is gathering information, also known as establishing the database. This includes taking the history (asking questions), performing the physical examination, and obtaining selective laboratory and/or imaging tests. Of these, the historical examination is the most important and useful. Sensitivity and respect should always be exercised during the interview of patients.

> **CLINICAL PEARL**
>
> ❖ The history is the single most important tool in obtaining a diagnosis. All physical findings, laboratory and imaging studies are first obtained, and then interpreted, in the light of the pertinent history.

History

1. Basic information:
   a. Age, gender, and ethnicity must be recorded because some conditions are more common at certain ages; for instance, pain on defecation and rectal bleeding in a 20-year-old may indicate inflammatory bowel disease, whereas the same symptoms in a 60-year-old would more likely suggest colon cancer.
2. Chief complaint: What is it that brought the patient into the hospital or office? Is it a scheduled appointment, or an unexpected symptom? The patient's own words should be used if possible, such as, "I feel like a ton of bricks are on my chest." The chief complaint, or real reason for seeking medical attention, may not be the first subject the patient talks about (in fact, it may be the last thing), particularly if the subject is embarrassing, such as a sexually transmitted disease, or highly emotional, such as depression. It is often useful to clarify exactly what is the patient's concern, for example, they may fear their headaches represent an underlying brain tumor.
3. History of present illness: This is the most crucial part of the entire database. The questions one asks are guided by the differential diagnosis one begins to consider the moment the patient identifies the chief complaint, as well as the clinician's knowledge of typical disease patterns and their natural history. The duration and character of the primary

complaint, associated symptoms, and exacerbating/relieving factors should be recorded. Sometimes, the history will be convoluted and lengthy, with multiple diagnostic or therapeutic interventions at different locations. For patients with chronic illnesses, obtaining prior medical records is invaluable. For example, when extensive evaluation of a complicated medical problem has been done elsewhere, it is usually better to first obtain those results than to repeat a "million-dollar workup." When reviewing prior records, it is often useful to review the primary data (e.g., biopsy reports, echocardiograms, serologic evaluations) rather than to rely upon a diagnostic label applied by someone else, which then gets replicated in medical records and by repetition, acquires the aura of truth, when it may not be fully supported by data. Some patients will be poor historians because of dementia, confusion, or language barriers; recognition of these situations and querying of family members is useful. When little or no history is available to guide a focused investigation, more extensive objective studies are often necessary to exclude potentially serious diagnoses.

4. Past history
   a. Any illnesses such as hypertension, hepatitis, diabetes mellitus, cancer, heart disease, pulmonary disease, and thyroid disease should be elicited. If an existing or prior diagnosis is not obvious, it is useful to ask exactly how it was diagnosed; that is, what investigations were performed. Duration, severity, and therapies should be included.
   b. Any hospitalizations and emergency room visits should be listed with the reason(s) for admission, the intervention, and the location of the hospital.
   c. Transfusions with any blood products should be listed, including any adverse reactions.
   d. Surgeries. The year and type of surgery should be elucidated and any complications documented. The type of incision and any untoward effects of the anesthesia or the surgery should be noted.

5. Allergies: Reactions to medications should be recorded, including severity and temporal relationship to the medication. An adverse effect (such as nausea) should be differentiated from a true allergic reaction.

6. Medications: Current and previous medications should be listed, including dosage, route, frequency, and duration of use. Prescription, over-the-counter, and herbal medications are all relevant. Patients often forget their complete medication list; thus, asking each patient to bring in all their medications—both prescribed and nonprescribed—allows for a complete inventory.

7. Family history: Many conditions are inherited, or are predisposed in family members. The age and health of siblings, parents, grandparents, and others can provide diagnostic clues. For instance, an individual with first-degree family members with early onset coronary heart disease is at risk for cardiovascular disease.

8. Social history: This is one of the most important parts of the history in that the patient's functional status at home, social and economic circumstances, and goals and aspirations for the future are often the critical determinant in what is the best way to manage a patient's medical problem. Living arrangements, economic situations, and religious affiliations may provide important clues for puzzling diagnostic cases, or suggest the acceptability of various diagnostic or therapeutic options. Marital status and habits such as alcohol, tobacco, or illicit drug use may be relevant as risk factors for disease.

9. Review of systems: A few questions about each major body system ensures that problems will not be overlooked. The clinician should avoid the mechanical "rapid-fire" questioning technique that discourages patients from answering truthfully because of fear of "annoying the doctor."

Physical Examination

The physical examination begins as one is taking the history, by observing the patient and beginning to consider a differential diagnosis. When performing the physical examination, one focuses on body systems suggested by the differential diagnosis, and performs tests or maneuvers with specific questions in mind; for example, does the patient with jaundice have ascites? When the physical examination is performed with potential diagnoses and expected physical findings in mind ("one sees what one looks for"), the utility of the examination in adding to diagnostic yield is greatly increased, as opposed to an unfocused "head-to-toe" physical.

1. General appearance: A great deal of information is gathered by observation, as one notes the patient's body habitus, state of grooming, nutritional status, level of anxiety (or perhaps inappropriate indifference), degree of pain or comfort, mental status, speech patterns, and use of language. This forms your impression of "who this patient is."

2. Vital signs: Temperature, blood pressure, heart rate, and respiratory rate. Height and weight are often placed here. Blood pressure can sometimes be different in the two arms; initially, it should be measured in both arms. In patients with suspected hypovolemia, pulse and blood pressure should be taken in lying and standing positions to look for orthostatic hypotension. It is quite useful to take the vital

signs oneself, rather than relying upon numbers gathered by ancillary personnel using automated equipment, because important decisions regarding patient care are often made using the vital signs as an important determining factor.

3. Head and neck examination: Facial or periorbital edema, pupillary responses should be noted. Funduscopic examination provides a way to visualize the effects of diseases such as diabetes on the microvasculature; papilledema can signify increased intracranial pressure. Estimation of jugular venous pressure is very useful to estimate volume status. The thyroid should be palpated for a goiter or nodule, and carotid arteries auscultated for bruits. Cervical (common) and supraclavicular (pathologic) nodes should be palpated.

4. Breast examination: Inspect for symmetry, skin or nipple retraction with the patient's hands on her hips (to accentuate the pectoral muscles), and also with arms raised. With the patient sitting and supine, the breasts should then be palpated systematically to assess for masses. The nipple should be assessed for discharge and the axillary and supraclavicular regions should be examined for adenopathy.

5. Cardiac examination: The point of maximal impulse (PMI) should be ascertained for size and location, and the heart auscultated at the apex of the heart as well as at the base. Heart sounds, murmurs, and clicks should be characterized. Murmurs should be classified according to intensity, duration, timing in the cardiac cycle, and changes with various maneuvers. Systolic murmurs are very common and often physiologic; diastolic murmurs are uncommon and usually pathologic.

6. Pulmonary examination: The lung fields should be examined systematically and thoroughly. Wheezes, rales, rhonchi, and bronchial breath sounds should be recorded. Percussion of the lung fields may be helpful in identifying the hyperresonance of tension pneumothorax, or the dullness of consolidated pneumonia or a pleural effusion.

7. Abdominal examination: The abdomen should be inspected for scars, distension, discoloration (such as the Grey-Turner sign of discoloration at the flank areas indicating intraabdominal or retroperitoneal hemorrhage). Auscultation of bowel sounds to identify normal versus high-pitched, and hyperactive versus hypoactive. The abdomen should be percussed, including the sizes of the liver and spleen, and for the presence of shifting dullness (indicating ascites). Careful palpation should begin initially away from the area of pain, involving one hand on top of the other, to assess for masses, tenderness, and peritoneal signs. Tenderness should be recorded on a scale (e.g., 1 to 4 where 4 is the most severe pain). Guarding, and whether it is voluntary or involuntary, should be noted.

8. Back and spine examination: The back should be assessed for symmetry, tenderness, and masses. The flank regions are particularly important to assess for pain on percussion, which might indicate renal disease.

9. Genitalia:
   a. Females: The pelvic examination should include an inspection of the external genitalia, and with the speculum, evaluation of the vagina and cervix. A pap smear and/or cervical cultures may be obtained. A bimanual examination to assess the size, shape, and tenderness of the uterus and adnexa is important.
   b. Males: An inspection of the penis and testes is performed. Evaluation for masses, tenderness, and lesions is important. Palpation for hernias in the inguinal region with the patient coughing to increase intraabdominal pressure is useful.

10. Rectal examination: A digital rectal examination is generally performed for those individuals with possible colorectal disease, or gastrointestinal bleeding. Masses should be assessed, and stool for occult blood should be tested. In men, the prostate gland can be assessed for enlargement and for nodules.

11. Extremities: An examination for joint effusions, tenderness, edema, and cyanosis may be helpful. Clubbing of the nails might indicate pulmonary diseases such as lung cancer or chronic cyanotic heart disease.

12. Neurological examination: Patients who present with neurological complaints usually require a thorough assessment, including the mental status, cranial nerves, motor strength, sensation, and reflexes.

13. The skin should be carefully examined for evidence of pigmented lesions (melanoma), cyanosis, or rashes that may indicate systemic disease (malar rash of systemic lupus erythematosus).

Laboratory and Imaging Assessment

1. Laboratory:
   a. CBC (complete blood count) to assess for anemia and thrombocytopenia.
   b. Chemistry panel is most commonly used to evaluate renal and liver function.
   c. Lipid panel is particularly relevant in cardiovascular diseases.
   d. Urinalysis is often referred to as a "liquid renal biopsy," because the presence of cells, casts, protein, or bacteria provides clues about underlying glomerular or tubular diseases.
   e. Gram stain and culture of urine, sputum, and cerebrospinal fluid, as well as blood cultures, are frequently useful to isolate the cause of infection.

2. Imaging procedures:
   a. Chest radiography is extremely useful in assessing cardiac size and contour, chamber enlargement, pulmonary vasculature and infiltrates, and the presence of pleural effusions.
   b. Ultrasonographic examination is useful for identifying fluid–solid interfaces, and for characterizing masses as cystic, solid, or complex. It is also very helpful in evaluating the biliary tree, kidney size, and evidence of ureteral obstruction, and can be combined with Doppler flow to identify deep venous thrombosis. Ultrasonography is noninvasive and has no radiation risk, but cannot be used to penetrate through bone or air, and is less useful in obese patients.

CLINICAL PEARL

❖ Ultrasonography is helpful in evaluating the biliary tree, looking for ureteral obstruction, and evaluating vascular structures, but has limited utility in obese patients.

   c. Computed tomography (CT) is helpful in possible intracranial bleeding, abdominal and/or pelvic masses, and pulmonary processes, and may help to delineate the lymph nodes and retroperitoneal disorders. CT exposes the patient to radiation and requires the patient to be immobilized during the procedure. Generally, CT requires administration of a radiocontrast dye, which can be nephrotoxic.
   d. Magnetic resonance imaging (MRI) identifies soft-tissue planes very well and provides the best imaging of the brain parenchyma. When used with gadolinium contrast (which is not nephrotoxic), MR angiography (MRA) is useful for delineating vascular structures. MRI does not use radiation, but the powerful magnetic field prohibits its use in patients with ferromagnetic metal in their bodies, for example, many prosthetic devices.
   e. Cardiac procedures:
      i. Echocardiography: Uses ultrasonography to delineate the cardiac size, function, ejection fraction, and presence of valvular dysfunction.
      ii. Angiography: Radiopaque dye is injected into various vessels and radiographs or fluoroscopic images are used to determine the vascular occlusion, cardiac function, or valvular integrity.
      iii. Stress treadmill tests: Individuals at risk for coronary heart disease are monitored for blood pressure, heart rate, chest

pain, and electrocardiogram (EKG) while increasing oxygen demands on the heart, such as running on a treadmill. Nuclear medicine imaging of the heart can be added to increase the sensitivity and specificity of the test. Individuals who cannot run on the treadmill (such as those with severe arthritis), may be given medications such as Persantine to "stress" the heart.

Interpretation of Test Results: Using Pretest Probability and Likelihood Ratio

Because no test is 100% accurate, it is essential when ordering them to have some knowledge of the test's characteristics, as well as how to apply the test results to an **individual patient's clinical situation**. Let us use the example of a patient with chest pain. The first diagnostic concern of most patients and physicians regarding chest pain is **angina pectoris**, that is, the pain of myocardial ischemia caused by coronary insufficiency. Distinguishing angina pectoris from other causes of chest pain relies upon two important factors: the clinical history, and an understanding of how to use objective testing. In making the diagnosis of angina pectoris, the clinician must establish whether the pain satisfies the **three criteria for typical anginal pain**: (a) retrosternal in location, (b) precipitated by exertion, and (c) relieved within minutes by rest or nitroglycerin. Then, the clinician considers other factors, such as patient age and other risk factors, to determine a **pretest probability** for angina pectoris.

After a pretest probability is estimated by applying some combination of statistical data, epidemiology of the disease, and clinical experience, the next decision is whether and how to use an objective test. **A test should only be ordered if the results would change the posttest probability high enough or low enough in either direction that it will affect the decision-making process**. For example, a 21-year-old woman with chest pain that is not exertional and not relieved by rest or nitroglycerin has a very low pretest probability of coronary artery disease, and any positive results on a cardiac stress test are very likely to be false positive. Any test result is unlikely to change her management; thus, the test should not be obtained. Similarly, a 69-year-old diabetic smoker with a recent coronary angioplasty who now has recurrent episodes of typical angina has a very high pretest probability that the pain is a result of myocardial ischemia. One could argue that a negative cardiac stress test is likely to be a falsely negative, and that the clinician should proceed directly to a coronary angiography to assess for a repeat angioplasty. **Diagnostic tests, therefore, are usually most useful for those patients in the midranges of pretest probabilities, in whom a positive or negative test will move the clinician past some decision threshold.**

In the case of diagnosing a patient with atherosclerotic coronary artery disease (CAD), one test that is frequently used is the exercise treadmill test. Patients are monitored on an electrocardiogram, while they perform graded exercise on a treadmill. A positive test is the development of ST-segment depression during the test; the greater the degree of ST depression, the more useful the test becomes in raising the posttest probability of CAD. In the example below, of a patient with pretest probability of 50%, the development of 2 mm of ST segment depression raised the posttest probability to 90%.

If one knows the sensitivity and specificity of the test used, one can calculate the **likelihood ratio** of the positive test as **sensitivity/1 – specificity**. Posttest probability is calculated by multiplying the positive likelihood ratio by the pretest probability, or plot the probabilities using a nomogram *(see Figure I-1)*.

Thus, knowing something about the characteristics of the test you are employing, and how to apply them to the patient at hand is essential in reach-

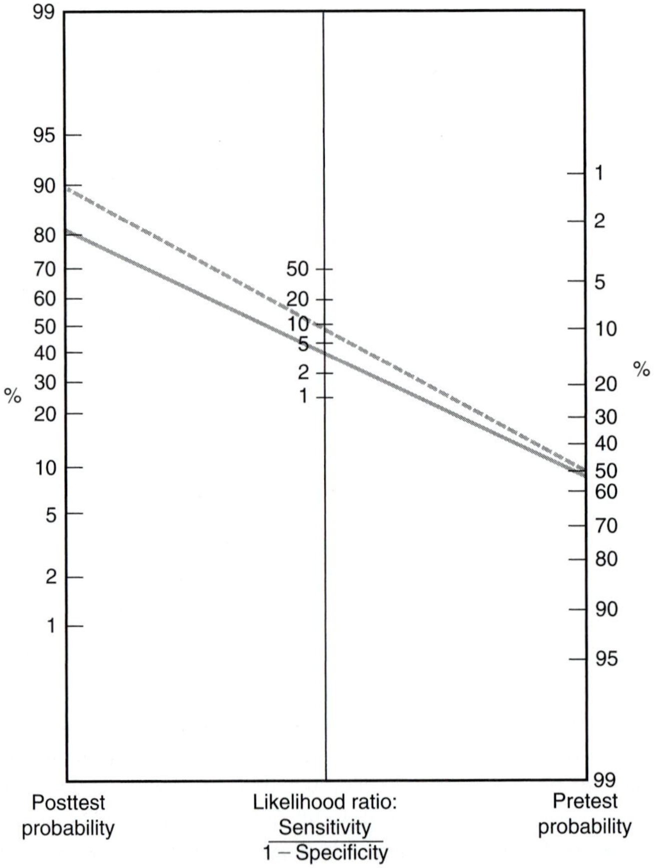

Figure 1-1. Nomogram illustrating the relationship between pretest probability, posttest probability, and likelihood ratio. (Reproduced with permission from Braunwald E, Fauci AS, Kasper KL, et al. Harrison's Principles of Internal Medicine, 15th Ed. New York: McGraw-Hill, 2001:12.)

ing a correct diagnosis and avoid falling into the common trap of "positive test = disease" and "negative test = no disease." Stated another way, **tests do not make diagnoses; doctors do, considering test results quantitatively in the context of their clinical assessment.**

> **CLINICAL PEARL**
>
> ❖ If Test Result is Positive,
>
> Posttest Probability = Pretest Probability × Likelihood Ratio
>
> Likelihood Ratio = Sensitivity / 1 – Specificity

PART 2. APPROACH TO CLINICAL PROBLEM SOLVING

There are typically four distinct steps to the systematic solving of clinical problems:

1. Making the diagnosis
2. Assessing the severity of the disease (stage)
3. Rendering a treatment based on the stage of the disease
4. Following the patient's response to the treatment

MAKING THE DIAGNOSIS

INTRODUCTION

There are two ways to make a diagnosis. Experienced clinicians often make a diagnosis very quickly using **pattern recognition**, that is, the features of the patient's illness match a scenario the physician has seen before. If it does not fit a readily recognized pattern, then one has to undertake several steps in diagnostic reasoning:

1. The first step is to **gather information with a differential diagnosis in mind**. The clinician should start considering diagnostic possibilities with initial contact with the patient, which are continually refined as information is gathered. Historical questions and physical examination tests and findings are all pursued tailored to the potential diagnoses one is considering. This is the principle that "you find what you are looking for." When one is trying to perform a thorough head-to-toe examination, for instance, without looking for anything in particular, one is much more likely to miss findings.
2. The next step is to try to move from subjective complaints or nonspecific symptoms to focus on objective abnormalities in an effort to

conceptualize the patient's objective problem with the greatest specificity one can achieve. For example, a patient may come to the physician complaining of pedal edema, a relatively common and nonspecific finding. Laboratory testing may reveal that the patient has renal failure, a more specific cause of the many causes of edema. Examination of the urine may then reveal red blood cell casts, indicating glomerulonephritis, which is even more specific as the cause of the renal failure. The patient's problem, then, described with the greatest degree of specificity, is glomerulonephritis. The clinician's task at this point is to consider the differential diagnosis of glomerulonephritis rather than that of pedal edema.

3. The last step is to **look for discriminating features** of the patient's illness. This means the features of the illness, which by their presence or their absence most narrow the differential diagnosis. This is often difficult for junior learners because it requires a well-developed knowledge base of the typical features of disease, so the diagnostician can judge how much weight to assign to the various clinical clues present. For example, in the diagnosis of a patient with a fever and productive cough, the finding by chest x-ray of bilateral apical infiltrates with cavitation is highly discriminatory. There are few illnesses besides tuberculosis that are likely to produce that radiographic pattern. A negatively predictive example is a patient with exudative pharyngitis who also has rhinorrhea and cough. The presence of these features makes the diagnosis of streptococcal infection unlikely as the cause of the pharyngitis. Once the differential diagnosis has been constructed, the clinician uses the presence of discriminating features, knowledge of patient risk factors, and the epidemiology of diseases to decide which potential diagnoses are most likely.

CLINICAL PEARL

❖ There are three steps in diagnostic reasoning:

1. Gathering information with a differential diagnosis in mind.
2. Identifying the objective abnormalities with the greatest specificity.
3. Looking for discriminating features to narrow the differential diagnosis.

Once the most specific problem has been identified, and a differential diagnosis of that problem is considered using discriminating features to order the possibilities, the next step is to consider using diagnostic testing, such as laboratory, radiologic, or pathologic data, to confirm the diagnosis. Quantitative reasoning in the use and interpretation of tests were discussed in the previous section. Clinically, the timing and effort with which one pursues a definitive diagnosis using objective data depends on several factors: the potential gravity of the diagnosis in question, the clinical state of the patient, the potential risks of diagnostic testing, and the potential benefits or harms of empiric treatment. For example, if a young man is admitted to the hospital with bilateral pulmonary nodules on chest x-ray, there are many possibilities including metastatic malignancy, and aggressive pursuit of a diagnosis is necessary, perhaps including a thoracotomy with an open-lung biopsy. The same radiographic findings in an elderly bed-bound woman with advanced Alzheimer dementia who would not be a good candidate for chemotherapy might be best left alone without any diagnostic testing. Decisions like this are difficult, require solid medical knowledge, as well as a thorough understanding of one's patient and the patient's background and inclinations, and constitute the art of medicine.

Assessing the Severity of the Disease

After ascertaining the diagnosis, the next step is to characterize the severity of the disease process; in other words, it is describing "how bad" a disease is. There is usually prognostic or treatment significance based on the stage.With malignancy, this is done formally by cancer staging. Most cancers are categorized from stage I (localized) to stage IV (widely metastatic). Some diseases, such as congestive heart failure, may be designated as mild, moderate, or severe based on the patient's functional status, that is, their ability to exercise before becoming dyspneic. With some infections, such as syphilis, the staging depends on the duration and extent of the infection, and follows along the natural history of the infection (i.e., primary syphilis, secondary, latent period, and tertiary/neurosyphilis).

Treating based on Stage

Many illnesses are stratified according to severity because prognosis and treatment often vary based on the severity. If neither the prognosis nor the treatment were affected by the stage of the disease process, there would not be a reason to subcategorize as to mild or severe. As an example, a man with mild chronic obstructive pulmonary disease (COPD) may be treated with inhaled bronchodilators as needed and advice for smoking cessation. However, an individual with severe COPD may need around-the-clock oxygen supplementation, scheduled bronchodilators, and possibly oral corticosteroid therapy.

The treatment should be tailored to the extent or "stage" of the disease.

In making decisions regarding treatment, it is also essential that the clinician identify the therapeutic objectives. When patients seek medical attention, it is generally because they are bothered by a symptom and want it to go away. When physicians institute therapy, they often have several other goals besides symptom relief, such as prevention of short- or long-term complications or a reduction in mortality. For example, patients with congestive heart failure are bothered by the symptoms of edema and dyspnea. Salt restriction, loop diuretics, and bedrest are effective at reducing these symptoms. However, heart failure is a progressive disease with a high mortality, so other treatments such as angiotensin-converting enzyme (ACE) inhibitors and some beta-blockers are also used to reduce mortality in this condition. It is essential that the clinician know what the therapeutic objective is, so that one can monitor and guide therapy.

CLINICAL PEARL

❖ The clinician needs to identify the objectives of therapy: symptom relief, prevention of complications, or reduction in mortality.

FOLLOWING THE RESPONSE TO TREATMENT

The final step in the approach to disease is to follow the patient's response to the therapy. The "measure" of response should be recorded and monitored. Some responses are clinical, such as the patient's abdominal pain, or temperature, or pulmonary examination. Obviously, the student must work on being more skilled in eliciting the data in an unbiased and standardized manner. Other responses may be followed by imaging tests, such as CT scan of a retroperitoneal node size in a patient receiving chemotherapy, or a tumor marker such as the prostate-specific antigen (PSA) level in a man receiving chemotherapy for prostatic cancer. For syphilis, it may be the nonspecific treponemal antibody test rapid plasma reagent (RPR) titer over time. The student must be prepared to know what to do if the measured marker does not respond according to what is expected. Is the next step to retreat, or to repeat the metastatic workup, or to followup with another more specific test?

PART 3. APPROACHING READING

The clinical problem-oriented approach to reading is different from the classic "systematic" research of a disease. Patients rarely present with a clear diagnosis; hence, the student must become skilled in applying the textbook information to the clinical setting. Furthermore, one retains more information when one reads with a purpose. In other words, the student should read with the goal of answering specific questions. There are several fundamental questions that facilitate **clinical thinking**. These questions are:

1. What is the most likely diagnosis?
2. What should be your next step?

3. What is the most likely mechanism for this process?
4. What are the risk factors for this condition?
5. What are the complications associated with the disease process?
6. What is the best therapy?
7. How would you confirm the diagnosis?

CLINICAL PEARL

❖ Reading with the purpose of answering the seven fundamental clinical questions improves retention of information and facilitates the application of "book knowledge" to "clinical knowledge."

What is the Most Likely Diagnosis?

The method of establishing the diagnosis was discussed in the previous section. One way of attacking this problem is to develop standard "approaches" to common clinical problems. It is helpful to understand the most common causes of various presentations, such as "the most common causes of pancreatitis are gallstones and alcohol." (See the *Clinical Pearls* at end of each case.)

The clinical scenario would entail something such as:

"A 28-year-old woman pregnant woman complains of severe epigastric pain radiating the back, nausea and vomiting, and an elevated serum amylase level. What is the most likely diagnosis?"

With no other information to go on, the student would note that this woman has a clinical diagnosis of pancreatitis. Using the "most common cause" information, the student would make an educated guess that the patient has gallstones, because being female and pregnant are risk factors. If, instead, cholelithiasis is removed from the equation of this scenario, a phrase may be added such as:

"The ultrasonogram of the gallbladder shows no stones."

CLINICAL PEARL

❖ The two most common causes of pancreatitis are gallstones and alcohol abuse.

Now, the student would use the phrase "patients without gallstones who have pancreatitis most likely abuse alcohol." Aside from these two causes, there are many other etiologies of pancreatitis.

What Should be Your Next Step?

This question is difficult because the next step may be more diagnostic information, or staging, or therapy. It may be more challenging than "the most likely diagnosis," because there may be insufficient information to make a diagnosis and the next step may be to pursue more diagnostic information. Another possibility is that there is enough information for a probable diagnosis, and the next step is the stage the disease. Finally, the most appropriate action may be to treat. Hence, from clinical data, a judgment needs to be rendered regarding how far along one is on the road of:

Make a Dx → Stage the disease → Treat based on stage → Follow response

Frequently, the student is "taught" to regurgitate the same information that someone has written about a particular disease, but is not skilled at giving the next step. This talent is learned optimally at the bedside, in a supportive environment, with freedom to make educated guesses, and with constructive feedback. A sample scenario may describe a student's thought process as follows.

1. *Make the diagnosis:* "Based on the information I have, I believe that Mr. Smith has stable angina *because* he has retrosternal chest pain when he walks three blocks, but it is relieved within minutes by rest and with sublingual nitroglycerin."
2. *Stage the disease:* "I don't believe that this is severe disease because he does not have pain lasting for more than 5 minutes, angina at rest, or congestive heart failure."
3. *Treat based on stage:* "Therefore, my next step is to treat with aspirin, beta-blockers, and sublingual nitroglycerin as needed, as well as lifestyle changes."
4. *Follow response:* "I want to follow the treatment by assessing his pain (I will ask him about the degree of exercise he is able to perform without chest pain), perform a cardiac stress test, and reassess him after the test is done."

In a similar patient, when the clinical presentation is unclear or more severe, perhaps the best "next step" may be diagnostic in nature such as thallium stress test, or even coronary angiography. The **next step** depends upon the **clinical state of the patient** (if unstable, the next step is therapeutic), the **potential severity** of the disease (the next step may be staging), or the **uncertainty of the diagnosis** (the next step is diagnostic).

Usually, the vague question, "What is your next step?" is the most difficult question, because the answer may be diagnostic, staging, or therapeutic.

What is the Likely Mechanism for This Process?

This question goes further than making the diagnosis, but also requires the student to understand the underlying mechanism for the process. For example, a clinical scenario may describe an "18-year-old woman who presents with several months of severe epistaxis, heavy menses, petechiae, and a normal CBC except for a platelet count of $15,000/mm^3$." Answers that a student may consider to explain this condition include immune-mediated platelet destruction, drug-induced thrombocytopenia, bone marrow suppression, and platelet sequestration as a result of hypersplenism.

The student is advised to learn the mechanisms for each disease process, and not merely memorize a constellation of symptoms. In other words, rather than solely committing to memory the classic presentation of idiopathic thrombocytopenic purpura (ITP) (isolated thrombocytopenia without lymphadenopathy or offending drugs), the student should understand that ITP is an autoimmune process whereby the body produces IgG antibodies against the platelets. The platelets-antibody complexes are then taken from the circulation in the spleen. Because the disease process is specific for platelets, the other two cell lines (erythrocytes and leukocytes) are normal. Also, because the thrombocytopenia is caused by excessive platelet peripheral destruction, the bone marrow will show increased megakaryocytes (platelet precursors). Hence, treatment for ITP includes oral corticosteroid agents to decrease the immune process of antiplatelet IgG production, and, if refractory, then splenectomy.

What are the Risk Factors for This Process?

Understanding the risk factors helps the practitioner to establish a diagnosis and to determine how to interpret tests. For example, understanding the risk factor analysis may help to manage a 45-year-old obese woman with sudden onset of dyspnea and pleuritic chest pain following an orthopedic surgery for a femur fracture. This patient has numerous risk factors for deep venous thrombosis and pulmonary embolism. The physician may want to pursue angiography even if the ventilation/perfusion scan result is low probability. Thus, the number of risk factors help to categorize the likelihood of a disease process.

CLINICAL PEARL

❖ When the pretest probability of a disease is high based on risk factors, even with a negative initial test, more definitive testing may be indicated.

What are the Complications to This Process?

A clinician must understand the complications of a disease so that one may monitor the patient. Sometimes the student has to make the diagnosis from clinical clues and then apply his/her knowledge of the sequelae of the pathological process. For example, the student should know that chronic hypertension may affect various end organs, such as the brain (encephalopathy or stroke), the eyes (vascular changes), the kidneys, and the heart. Understanding the types of consequences also helps the clinician to be aware of the dangers to a patient. The clinician is acutely aware of the need to monitor for the end-organ involvement and undertakes the appropriate intervention when involvement is present.

What is the Best Therapy?

To answer this question, the clinician needs to reach the correct diagnosis, assess the severity of the condition, and weigh the situation to reach the appropriate intervention. For the student, knowing exact dosages is not as important as understanding the best medication, the route of delivery, mechanism of action, and possible complications. It is important for the student to be able to verbalize the diagnosis and the rationale for the therapy. A common error is for the student to "jump to a treatment," like a random guess, and therefore is given "right or wrong" feedback. In fact, the student's guess may be correct, but for the wrong reason; conversely, the answer may be a very reasonable one, with only one small error in thinking. Instead, the student should verbalize the steps so that feedback may be given at every reasoning point.

For example, if the question is, "What is the best therapy for a 25-year-old man who complains of a nontender penile ulcer?," the incorrect manner of response is for the student to blurt out "azithromycin." Rather, the student should reason it out in a way similar to this: "The most common cause of a nontender infectious ulcer of the penis is syphilis. Nontender adenopathy is usually associated. Therefore, the best treatment for this man with probable syphilis is intramuscular penicillin (but I would want to confirm the diagnosis). His partner also needs treatment."

CLINICAL PEARL

❖ Therapy should be logical based on the severity of disease. Antibiotic therapy should be tailored for specific organisms.

How Would you Confirm the Diagnosis?

In the scenario above, the man with a nontender penile ulcer is likely to have syphilis. Confirmation may be achieved by serology (rapid plasma reagent [RPR] or Venereal Disease Research Laboratory [VDRL] test); however, there is a significant possibility that patients with primary syphilis may not have developed antibody response yet, and have negative serology. Thus, confirmation of the diagnosis is attained with darkfield microscopy. Knowing the limitations of diagnostic tests and the manifestations of disease aid in this area.

SUMMARY

1. There is no replacement for a careful history and physical examination.

2. There are four steps to the clinical approach to the patient: making the diagnosis, assessing severity, treating based on severity, and following response.
3. Assessment of pretest probability and knowledge of test characteristics are essential in the application of test results to the clinical situation.
4. There are seven questions that help to bridge the gap between the textbook and the clinical arena

REFERENCES

Bordages G. Elaborated knowledge: a key to successful diagnostic thinking. Acad Med 1994;69(11):883–5.

Bordages G. Why did I miss the diagnosis? Some cognitive explanations and educational implications. Acad Med 1999;74(10):138–43.

Gross R. Making medical decisions. Philadelphia, American College of Physicians, 1999.

Mark DB. Decision-Making in Clinical Medicine. In: Braunwald E, Fauci AS, Kasper KL, et al., (eds.). Harrison's Principles of Internal Medicine, 15th ed. New York: McGraw-Hill. 2001:8-14.

SECTION II

Clinical Cases

CASE 1

A 56-year-old man comes to the emergency department complaining of chest discomfort. He describes it as a severe, retrosternal pressure sensation, which woke him from sleep 3 hours earlier. He had previously been well, has a past medical history of hypercholesterolemia, and a 40-pack-year history of smoking. On examination, he appears uncomfortable and diaphoretic with a heart rate of 95 beats per minute, a blood pressure of 166/102 mmHg, and a respiratory rate of 22 breaths per minute with an oxygen saturation of 96% on room air. The jugular venous pressure appears normal. Auscultation of the chest reveals clear lung fields, and a regular heart rate with an S4 gallop and no murmurs or rubs. A chest radiograph shows clear lungs and a normal cardiac silhouette. The EKG is shown below in Figure 1–1.

- **What is the most likely diagnosis?**

- **What is the next step in therapy?**

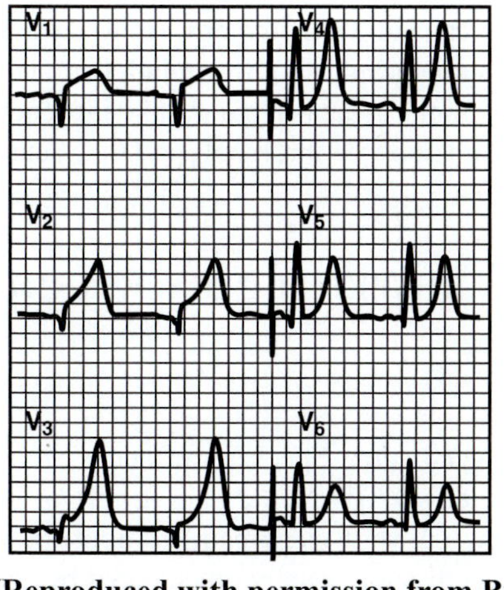

Figure 1–1. EKG. **(Reproduced with permission from Braunwald E, Fauci AS, Kasper KL, et al, (eds). Electrocardiography. Harrison's Principles of Internal Medicine, 15th ed. New York: McGraw-Hill. 2001:1268.**

ANSWERS TO CASE 1: Myocardial Infarction, Acute

Summary: This is a 56-year-old man with risk factors for coronary atherosclerosis (smoking and hypercholesterolemia) who has chest pain typical of cardiac ischemia; that is, retrosternal pressure sensation. The cardiac examination reveals an S4 gallop, which may be seen with myocardial ischemia because of relative noncompliance of the ischemic heart, as well as hypertension, tachycardia, and diaphoresis, which may all represent sympathetic activation. The duration of the pain and the EKG findings suggest an acute myocardial infarction.

- **Most likely diagnosis:** Acute ST-elevation myocardial infarction.
- **Next step in therapy:** Administer aspirin and a beta-blocker, and assess whether he would be a candidate for rapid reperfusion of the myocardium, i.e. thrombolytics or percutaneous angioplasty.

Analysis

Objectives

1. Know the diagnostic criteria for acute myocardial infarction (MI).
2. Know which patients should receive thrombolytics, and other therapies that may reduce mortality.
3. Be familiar with the complications of MI and their treatment options.
4. Understand post-MI risk stratification and secondary prevention strategies.

Considerations

The three most important issues for this patient are (a) the **suspicion of acute MI** based on the clinical and EKG findings, (b) to decide whether the patient has indications or contraindications for **thrombolytics**, and (c) to **exclude other diagnoses** that might mimic acute MI, but would not benefit or which might be worsened by anticoagulation or thrombolysis (e.g., acute pericarditis, aortic dissection).

APPROACH TO SUSPECTED MYOCARDIAL INFARCTION

Definitions

Acute coronary syndrome: Spectrum of acute cardiac ischemia ranging from **unstable angina** (ischemic pain at rest or at lower threshold of exertion or new onset of chest pain) to **acute myocardial infarction** (death of cardiac tissue), usually precipitated by thrombus formation in a coronary artery with an atherosclerotic plaque.

Acute myocardial infarction: Death of myocardial tissue due to inadequate blood flow.

Non-ST elevation MI: Myocardial infarction, but without ST elevation as defined below. May have other EKG changes, such as ST depression or T-wave inversion. Previously referred to as Non-Q wave or subendocardial myocardial infarction.

PTCA: Percutaneous coronary angioplasty.

ST elevation MI: MI as defined as above, with ST-segment elevation >0.1 mV in two or more contiguous leads. Previously referred to as Q-wave or transmural myocardial infarction

Thrombolytics: Drugs such as tissue plasminogen activator (tPA), streptokinase, and reteplase (rPA), which act to lyse fibrin thrombi in order to restore patency of the coronary artery.

Pathophysiology

Acute coronary syndromes, which exist on a continuum, ranging from **unstable angina** pectoris, to **non-ST elevation MI**, to **ST elevation MI,** are usually caused by **in situ thrombosis** at the site of a ruptured atherosclerotic plaque in a coronary artery. Occasionally, they may be caused by embolic occlusion, coronary vasospasm, vasculitis, aortic root or coronary artery dissection, or use of cocaine (which promotes both vasospasm and thrombosis). The resultant clinical syndrome is related to both the degree of atherosclerotic stenosis in the artery, and to the duration and extent of sudden thrombotic occlusion of the artery. If the occlusion is incomplete, or if the thrombus undergoes spontaneous lysis, unstable angina results; if the occlusion is complete and remains for more than 30 minutes infarction occurs. In contrast, the mechanism of chronic stable angina is usually a flow-limiting stenosis caused by atherosclerotic plaque that causes ischemia during exercise without acute thrombosis (see Table 1–1).

Diagnostic Criteria for Acute MI

History

Chest pain is the cardinal feature of myocardial infarction, even though it is not universally present. It is of the same character as angina pectoris; that is, described as heavy, squeezing, or crushing, and localized to the retrosternal area or epigastrium, sometimes with radiation to the arm, lower jaw, or neck. **In contrast to stable angina, however, it persists >30 minutes and is not relieved by rest.** The pain is often accompanied by sweating, nausea, vomiting, and/or the sense of impending doom. In an older patient > 70 years old or a diabetic, an acute MI may be painless or have only vague discomfort, and may be heralded by the sudden onset of dyspnea, pulmonary edema, or ventricular arrhythmias.

Table 1-1
CORONARY ARTERY AND CLINICAL MANIFESTATION

VESSEL ARCHITECTURE	BLOOD FLOW	CLINICAL MANIFESTATION
Normal	Unobstructed	Asymptomatic
Early Plaque	Unobstructed	Asymptomatic
Significant Plaque	Blood flow limited during exertion	Exertional Angina
Plaque Rupture	Platelet thrombus begins to form and spasm limit blood flow at rest	Unstable Angina
Platelet Thrombus on Ruptured Plaque	Transient complete vessel occlusion (lysis occurs)	Non-Q wave Myocardial Infarction
Platelet Thrombus on Ruptured Plaque	Complete Vessel Occlusion (no lysis)	Q wave Myocardial Infarction

Physical Findings

There are **no specific physical findings** in a patient with an acute MI. Many patients are anxious and diaphoretic. Cardiac auscultation may reveal an S4 gallop, reflecting myocardial noncompliance because of ischemia, an S3 gallop, representing severe systolic dysfuntion, or a new apical systolic murmur of mitral regurgitation caused by ischemic papillary muscle dysfunction.

EKG

The EKG is often critical in making the diagnosis of acute myocardial infarction, and in guiding therapy. There are a series of EKG changes that reflect the evolution of the infarction. (see Figure 1–2)

1. The earliest changes are tall, positive, **hyperacute T waves** in the ischemic vascular territory.
2. This is followed by **elevation of the ST segments** (the myocardial “injury pattern”).
3. Over hours to days, **T-wave inversion** frequently develops.
4. Finally, diminished R-wave amplitude or **Q waves** occur, representing significant myocardial necrosis and replacement by scar tissue, and is what one seeks to prevent in treating the acute MI (see Figure 1–3).

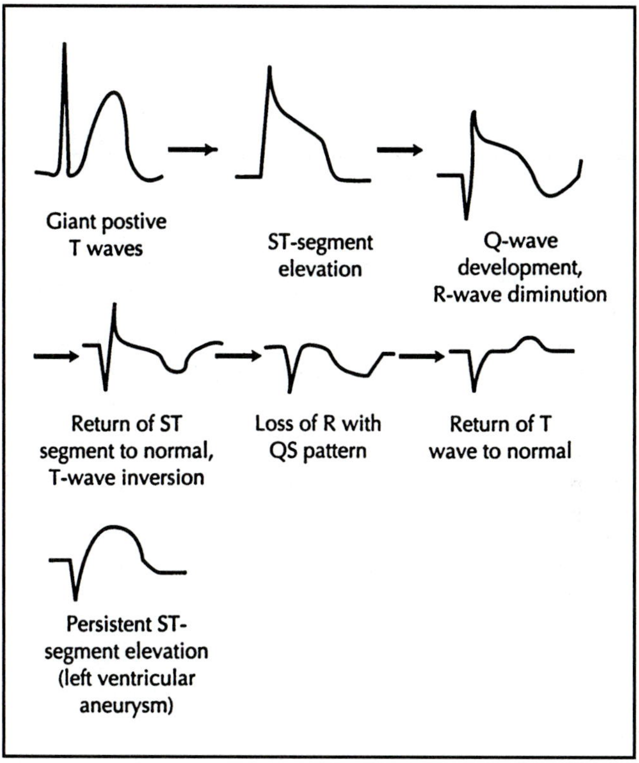

Figure 1–2. Temporal Evolution of EKG Changes in acute myocardial infarction: tall hyperacute T waves, loss of R-wave amplitude, followed by ST-segment elevation, T-wave inversion, and the development of Q waves. Persistent ST-segment elevation suggests left ventricular aneurysm. **(Reproduced with permission from Schroeder JS. Unstable Angina and Non-Q-Wave Myocardial Infarct. In: Alpert JS. Cardiology for the primary care physician, 2nd ed. Stamford: Appleton and Lange. 1998:168 pp 219-229.)**

Sometimes, when acute ischemia is limited to the **subendocardium, ST depression,** rather than ST elevation, develops. **ST elevation is typical of acute transmural ischemia**; that is, a greater degree of myocardial involvement than a non-ST elevation MI.

From the EKG we can localize the ischemia related to a vascular territory supplied by one of the three major coronary arteries. **ST elevation MI** is defined as ST-segment elevation >0.1 mV in two or more contiguous leads (i.e., in the same vascular territory) and/or a new left bundle-branch block (the LBBB obscures usual ST-segment analysis).

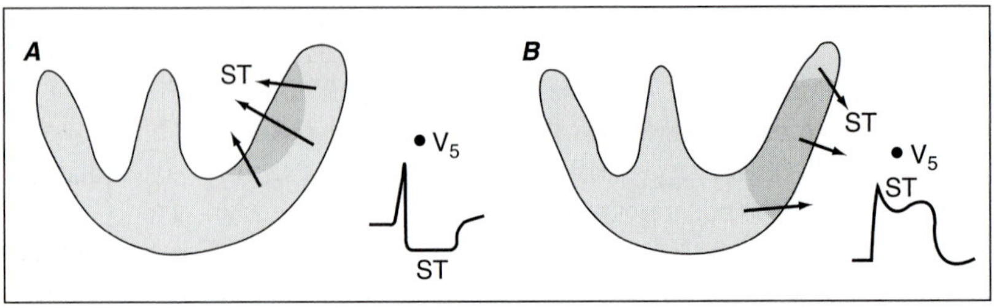

Figure 1–3. Subendocardial Infarction produces an inward ST vector, resulting in ST segment depression. Transmural infarction produces an outward ST vector, resulting in ST-segment elevation in the overlying leads. **(Reproduced with permission from Braunwald E, Fauci AS, Kasper KL, et al, eds. Harrison's, Principles of Internal Medicine, 15th ed. New York: McGraw-Hill, 2001: 1268.)**

Cardiac Enzymes

Certain proteins, referred to as cardiac enzymes, are released into blood from necrotic heart muscle after an acute MI. Creatine phosphokinase (CK) rises within 4–8 hours and returns to normal by 48–72 hours. CK is found in skeletal muscle and other tissues, but the CK-MB (creatine kinase myocardial band) isoenzyme is not found in significant amounts outside of heart muscle, so elevation of this fraction is more specific for myocardial injury. Cardiac-specific troponin I (cTnI) and troponin T (cTnT) are also specific to heart muscle. These enzymes rise at about 6 hours after infarct, and cTnI levels may remain elevated for 7–10 days and cTnT remain elevated for 10–14 days. They are very sensitive indicators of myocardial injury, and may be elevated with even small amounts of myocardial necrosis. Generally, two sets of normal troponin levels 4–6 hours apart exclude myocardial infarction.

The diagnosis of **acute MI** is made by finding **at least two of the following three features**: typical **chest pain persisting greater than 30 minutes**, typical **EKG findings**, and **elevated cardiac enzymes**. Because of the urgency in initiating treatment, diagnosis often rests upon the clinical history and the EKG findings, while cardiac enzymes are pending. During the initial evaluation, one must consider and exclude other diagnoses that typically present with chest pain, but would be worsened by the anticoagulation or thrombolysis usually employed to treat acute MI. **Aortic dissection** often presents with **unequal pulses or blood pressures in the arms**, a **new murmur of aortic insufficiency**, or a **widened mediastinum** on chest x-ray. Acute pericarditis often presents with chest pain and a pericardial friction rub, but the EKG findings show **diffuse ST elevation**, rather than those limited to a vascular territory.

Treatment of Acute MI

Once an acute MI has been diagnosed based on history, EKG, or cardiac enzymes, several therapies are initiated. Because the process is caused by acute thrombosis, antiplatelet agents such as **aspirin,** and anticoagulation with **heparin**, are used. To limit infarct size, **beta-blockers** are used to decrease myocardial oxygen demand, and **nitrates** given to increase coronary blood flow. All of these therapies appear to reduce mortality in acute MI. In addition, morphine may be given to reduce pain and the consequent tachycardia, and patients are placed on supplemental oxygen. (see Figure 1–4)

Next, a decision should be made whether the patient may benefit from rapid reperfusion of myocardium by either thrombolytics or primary angioplasty. **Individuals with ST-segment elevation MI benefit from thrombolytics, with a lower mortality, more preservation of myocardial function, and fewer complications**; patients without ST-segment elevation don't have the same mortality benefit. Because myocardium can be salvaged only before it is irreversibly injured ("time is muscle"), patients **benefit maximally** when the drug is given early, for example, **within 1–3 hours after the onset of chest pain**, and the relative benefits decline with time. Because systemic coagulopathy may develop, the **major risk of thrombolytics is bleeding**, which can be potentially disastrous, for example, intracranial hemorrhage. The risk of hemorrhage is relatively constant, so the risk begins to outweigh the benefit by 12 hours, at which time most infarctions are completed; that is, the at-risk myocardium is dead.

Thrombolytic therapy is indicated if each of the following criteria are met:

1. Clinical complaints are consistent with ischemic type chest pain.
2. ST elevation >1 mm in at least two anatomically contiguous leads.
3. There are no contraindications to thrombolytic therapy.
4. Patient is younger than 75 years of age (greater risk of hemorrhage).

Patients with ST-elevation MI should not receive thrombolytics if they have any of the absolute contraindications, such as recent major surgery or aortic dissection (Table 1–2).

Percutaneous Transluminal Coronary Angioplasty (PTCA) is also effective in restoring perfusion in acute MI, and may be used in an individual with a contraindication to thrombolytic therapy. It may also be used in patients who are hypotensive or in cardiogenic shock, in whom thrombolytics offer no survival benefit. This is accomplished by cardiac catheterization, during which a guidewire is inserted into the occluded coronary artery, over which a small balloon is threaded and inflated, in an attempt to open the blockage and restore blood flow. Sometimes intraluminal expandable stents are deployed which may improve vessel patency. The use of primary PTCA is limited by availability because of the facilities and personnel required to perform it in a timely fashion.

Complications of Acute MI

Mortality in acute MI is usually a result of either myocardial pump failure and resultant cardiogenic shock, or of ventricular arrhythmias.

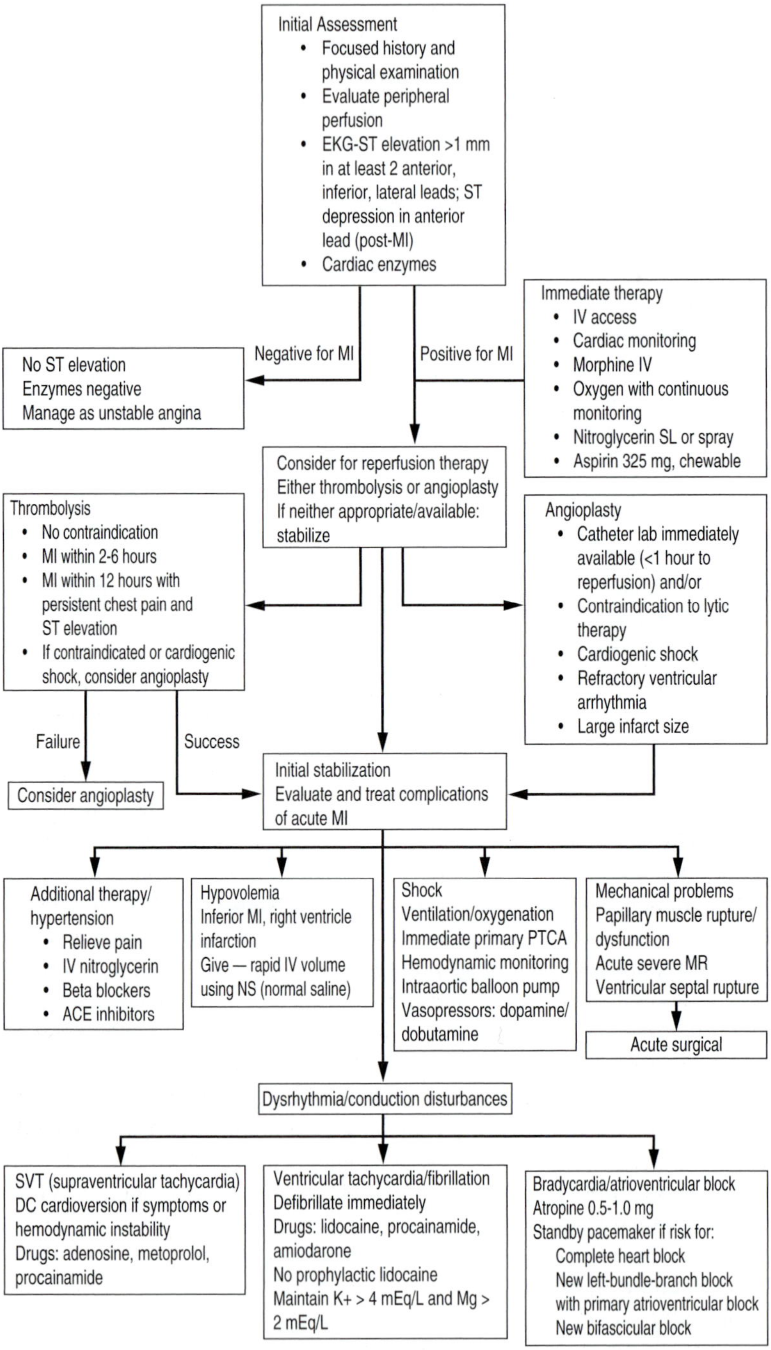

Figure 1–4. Suggested algorithm for assessment and treatment of chest pain.

Table 1–2
CONTRAINDICATIONS TO THROMBOLYTIC THERAPY

Absolute contraindications
- Major surgery/trauma within past 2 weeks
- Aortic dissection
- Active internal bleeding (excluding menses)
- Pericarditis
- History of cerebral tumor/hemorrhage/arteriovenous malformation
- Prolonged, traumatic cardiopulmonary resuscitation
- Bleeding diasthesis
- Allergy to agent/prior reaction
- Cerebrovascular accident known to be hemorrhage within past 12 months
- Pregnancy
- History of uncontrolled hypertension
- Recent hepatic/renal biopsy

Relative contraindications
- Blood pressure >180/110 mmHg on > 2 readings
- Bacterial endocarditis
- Diabetic retinopathy with recent bleed
- Severe renal/liver disease
- Chronic warfarin therapy
- Stroke/transient ischemic attack within past 12 months

Life-threatening **ventricular arrhythmias** such as **ventricular tachycardia (VT)** and **ventricular fibrillation (VF)** are common, especially in the first 24 hours. Historically, the majority of deaths from acute MI occurred in the first hour and were caused by VT/VF. This has diminished in recent years with earlier and more aggressive treatment of ischemia, and of arrhythmias. Premature ventricular contractions (PVCs) are very common, but generally are not treated with antiarrhythmic agents unless they are very frequent, sustained, or induce hemodynamic compromise. Sustained ventricular tachycardia (>30 seconds) or ventricular fibrillation are life-threatening, because they prevent coordinated ventricular contraction, and thus often cause pulselessness and cardiovascular collapse. They are treated with **DC cardioversion**, followed by infusion of intravenous antiarrhythmics such as **lidocaine** or **amiodarone**. Electrolyte deficiencies, such as hypokalemia or hypomagnesemia, which can potentiate ventricular arrhythmias, should be corrected. One benign ventricular arrhythmia that is generally not suppressed with antiarrhythmics is the **accelerated idioventricular rhythm**, which is a wide-complex escape rhythm between 60 and 110 beats per minute, and frequently accompanies reperfusion of the myocardium and causes no hemodynamic compromise.

Supraventricular or atrial tachyarrhythmias are much less common after acute MI, but can worsen ischemia and cause infarct extension as a consequence of the rate-related increase in myocardial oxygen demand. When they cause hemodynamic instability, they are also treated with immediate DC cardioversion. Another frequent rhythm disturbance are bradyarrhythmias. **Sinus bradycardia** is frequently seen in inferior MI because the right coronary artery supplies the sinoatrial node, but generally requires no treatment unless it causes hypotension. If the rate is slow enough to cause cardiac output and blood pressure to fall, intravenous **atropine** is usually administered. Bradyarrhythmias may also be caused by atrioventricular conduction disturbances. **First-degree atrioventricular (AV) block** (PR interval prolongation) and **Mobitz I second-degree AV block** (gradual prolongation of the PR interval before a nonconducted P wave) are often caused by AV nodal dysfunction, for example, nodal ischemia caused by inferior MI. If patients are symptomatic, they may be treated with **atropine.**

AV conduction disturbances may also be caused by dysfunction below the AV node, within the bundles of His, and typically produce a widened QRS complex. Examples include **Mobitz II second-degree AV block** (nonconducted P waves not preceded by PR prolongation), or **third-degree AV block** (complete atrioventricular dissociation with no P-wave conduction). Third-degree AV block can also be caused by AV nodal dysfunction. These are described more fully in Chapter 15. Other conduction disturbances caused by involvement of the bundles of His include **left bundle-branch block** or **right bundle-branch block with left anterior hemiblock.** All of these conduction disturbances have a worse prognosis than the AV nodal dysfunction because they are generally seen with anterior infarction in which a significant amount of myocardium is damaged. When these disturbances develop, they are best treated with external pacing or placement of a **temporary transvenous pacemaker**.

Cardiac Pump Failure and Cardiogenic Shock

Cardiogenic shock in acute MI is usually the most severe form of left ventricular pump failure. Ischemic reduction in ventricular diastolic compliance may lead to transient pulmonary congestion, associated with elevated left-sided filling pressures. Extensive myocardial necrosis and less contracting heart muscle may cause systolic failure and reduced cardiac output. Patients with hypotension frequently are evaluated by pulmonary artery (Swan-Ganz) catheterization to assess hemodynamic parameters. **Cardiogenic shock** is diagnosed when there is **hypotension** with systolic arterial pressure of <80 mm Hg, a **markedly reduced cardiac index <1.8 L/min/m^2**, and an **elevated left ventricular filling pressure** (measured indirectly with a pulmonary capillary wedge pressure >18 mmHg). Clinically, such patients would appear hypotensive, with cold extremities because of peripheral vasoconstriction, pulmonary edema, and elevated jugular venous pressure, reflecting high left- and right-sided filling pressures. Supportive treatment includes hemodynamic monitoring, adequate ventilation and oxygenation, and blood pressure support with vasopressors such as dobutamine and dopamine. They may also require mechanical assistance to augment blood pressure while providing afterload reduction, using intraaortic balloon counterpulsation. Cardiogenic shock may also require urgent revascularization with primary PTCA or coronary artery bypass surgery.

Hypotension may also be seen in patients with **right ventricular infarction**, which is a complication of right coronary artery occlusion and inferior infarction. In this case, left ventricular function is not impaired, but there is a dramatic reduction in filling of the left ventricle because of the right-sided ventricular failure (the left heart can only pump out what it receives from the right heart). These patients may be recognized clinically as hypotensive, with markedly elevated jugular venous pressure, but clear lung fields and no pulmonary edema radiographically (in contrast to the pulmonary edema seen in patients with hypotension to left ventricular [LV] failure described above), and confirmed by seeing ST elevation in a right-sided EKG. In this setting, right ventricular (RV) function is impaired and highly dependent on adequate preload, so it requires support with **volume replacement with saline** or colloid solution. Giving diuretics or nitrates that might lower the preload can be disastrous in these patients, causing complete cardiovascular collapse.

A number of mechanical problems can complicate acute MI, usually within the first week. The most common is **papillary muscle dysfunction** caused by left ventricular ischemia or infarction and leading to mitral regurgitation, which may or may not be hemodynamically significant. This is in contrast with **papillary muscle rupture**, which produces a flail mitral leaflet and acute mitral regurgitation with development of heart failure and cardiogenic shock. Development of acute heart failure and shock in association with a new holosystolic murmur may also signify **ventricular septal rupture.** Doppler echocardiography can be used to distinguish between these conditions. In all of them, stabilization of the cardiogenic shock is accomplished using afterload reduction with IV nitroglycerin or nitroprusside, and sometimes with aortic balloon counterpulsation, until definitive, urgent, surgical repair can be accomplished.

The most catastrophic mechanical complication is **rupture of the ventricular free wall**. As blood fills the pericardium, there is rapid development of cardiac tamponade with sudden pulselessness, hypotension, and loss of consciousness. This complication is nearly always fatal.

Late complications occurring several weeks after an acute MI include development of a **ventricular aneurysm**, which should be suspected if there is persistent ST elevation weeks after the event, as well as **Dressler syndrome**, an immune phenomenon characterized by pericarditis, pleuritis, and fever. Dressler syndrome may remit and relapse, and is treated with antiinflammatory drugs, including nonsteroidal antiinflammatory drugs (NSAIDs) and sometimes prednisone.

Post-MI Risk Stratification

The goal is to identify patients who are at high risk for subsequent cardiac events, who might benefit from revascularization. The initial evaluation involves the use of noninvasive testing. **Submaximal exercise stress testing** is generally performed in stable patients before hospital discharge to detect residual ischemia and ventricular ectopy and to provide a guideline for exercise in early recovery period. **Maximal exercise stress testing** is carried out 4–6 weeks after infarction. Evaluation of LV function at rest and during exercise is warranted. High-risk patients include those with impaired systolic function, large areas of ischemic myocardium on stress testing or postinfarction angina, and those with ventricular ectopy who might benefit from coronary angiography to evaluate for revascularization. Angioplasty can be performed to reduce anginal symptoms, and **coronary artery bypass surgery** should be considered for patients with **multivessel atherosclerotic stenosis** and **impaired systolic function**, because it may reduce symptoms and prolong survival.

Secondary Prevention of Ischemic Heart Disease

Medical therapy to reduce modifiable risk factors is the cornerstone of post-MI care. Besides the goal of symptoms relief, the major goal of medical therapy is to prevent cardiac events: fatal or nonfatal MI. By far, the **most important risk factor is smoking cessation**. Quitting tobacco use can reduce the risk of fatal or nonfatal cardiac events by >50%, more than any other medical or surgical therapy available. A number of other therapies reduce risk of recurrent cardiovascular events and prolong survival in patients with coronary artery disease: antiplatelet agents such as **aspirin** and **clopidogrel** reduce the risk of thrombus formation, **beta-blockers** reduce myocardial oxygen demand and may help suppress ventricular arrhythmias, and cholesterol-lowering agents such as **beta-hydroxy-beta-methylglutaryl-coenzyme A (HMG-CoA) reductase inhibitors** ("statins") reduce events and prolong survival. Patients with established coronary artery disease (CAD) should have a low-density lipoprotein (LDL)-cholesterol level of <100 mg/dL. **Angiotensin-converting enzyme (ACE) inhibitors** should be used in patients with clinically evident heart failure, and in asymptomatic patients with impaired systolic function (ejection fraction <40%), to prevent late ventricular remodeling and recurrent ischemic events. New data seem to suggest that **implantable defibrillators** in patients with poor systolic function after a myocardial infarction may improve survival.

Comprehension Questions

[1.1] A 36-year-old woman has severe burning chest pain that radiates to her neck particularly after meals, especially when she lies down, which is not precipitated by exertion. She is admitted for observation, and has a normal serial EKG and normal troponin I levels. Which of the following is the best next step?

A. Stress thallium treadmill test
B. Initiation of a proton pump inhibitor
C. Coronary angiography
D. Initiation of an antidepressant such as a serotonin-selective reuptake inhibitor
E. Referral to a psychiatrist

[1.2] A 56-year-old male is admitted to the hospital for chest pain for 2 hours. His heart rate is noted to be 42 beats per minute, with sinus bradycardia on EKG, as well as ST elevation in leads II, III, and aVF. Which of the following is the most likely diagnosis?

A. He is likely in good physical condition with increased vagal tone.
B. He likely has suffered an inferior wall MI.
C. He likely has a left ventricular aneurysm.
D. The low heart rate is a reflection of a good cardiac ejection fraction.

[1.3] A 59-year-old diabetic woman is noted to have suffered an acute anterior wall MI. Five days later, she gets into an argument with her husband, and she complains of chest pain. Her initial EKG shows no ischemic changes, but serum cardiac troponin I levels are drawn and return mildly elevated at this time. Which of the following is the best next step?

A. Thrombolytic therapy
B. Percutaneous coronary intervention
C. Coronary artery bypass
D. Perform serial EKGs and obtain CK-MB.
E. Prepare the patient for dialysis

[1.4] A 49-year-old male smoker complains of severe substernal squeezing chest pain for 30 minutes. The paramedics have given a sublingual nitroglycerin and oxygen by nasal cannula. His blood pressure is 110/70 mmHg and heart rate 90 bpm on arrival to the emergency room. The EKG is normal. Which of the following is the best next step?

A. Echocardiography
B. Thallium stress test
C. Aspirin
D. Coronary angiography
E. Coronary artery bypass

Answers

[1.1] **B.** This patient has classic symptoms of reflux esophagitis and is best treated with a proton pump inhibitor. If the chest pain has the characteristics of angina pectoris (substernal location, precipitated by exertion, relieved by rest or nitroglycerin) it should be investigated with a stress test or coronary angiography.

[1.2] **B.** Sinus bradycardia is often seen with inferior wall MI, because the right coronary artery supplies the inferior wall of the left ventricle and the sinoatrial node.

[1.3] **D.** Troponin levels often stay elevated for 7–10 days and should not be used to diagnose reinfarction, especially if they are trending downward. New EKG findings or rapidly rising markers such as serum myoglobin or CK-MB can be used in this setting.

[1.4] **C.** Aspirin is the first agent that should be used after oxygen and nitroglycerin. Aspirin use decreases mortality in the face of an acute coronary event. Initial EKGs and cardiac enzymes may be normal in acute MI, which is why serial studies are obtained. Clinical assessment to exclude other causes of chest pain should also be undertaken.

CLINICAL PEARLS

❖ Acute coronary syndromes (unstable angina or acute MI) occur when a thrombus forms at the site of rupture of an atherosclerotic plaque and acutely occludes a coronary artery.

❖ Acute myocardial infarction is diagnosed based on the presence of at least two of three criteria: typical symptoms, EKG findings, and cardiac enzymes. Initial EKG and enzymes may be normal, so serial studies are necessary.

❖ Early reperfusion with thrombolytics or PTCA reduces mortality and preserves ventricular function (time is muscle). Thrombolytics are reserved for patients who have ST elevation, no contraindications, and who receive treatment within the first 6–12 hours.

❖ The goal of secondary prevention after myocardial infarction is to prevent recurrent cardiac events or death. Smoking cessation, aspirin and clopidogrel, beta-blockers, and statins all reduce rate of events and reduce mortality.

❖ After myocardial infarction, angioplasty can be performed to reduce ischemia and anginal symptoms. Bypass surgery may be indicated for patients with multivessel stenosis and impaired systolic function to reduce symptoms, and prolong survival.

❖ The EKG can indicate the location of the ischemia or infarction: anterior (leads V_2-V_4), lateral (leads I, aV_L, V_5, V_6), inferior (leads II, III and aV_F) and posterior (R waves in leads V_1 and V_2).

REFERENCES

Alpert. JS, Cardiology for the primary care physician. Stamford: Appleton & Lange, 1998:168.

Antman EM, Braunwald E. Acute Myocardial Infarction. In: Braunwald E, Fauci AS, Kasper KL, et al., eds. Harrison's principles of internal medicine, 15th ed. New York: McGraw-Hill, 2001:1386-1399.

Selwyn AP, Braunwald E. Ischemic Heart Disease. In: Braunwald E, Fauci AS, Kasper KL, et al., eds. Harrison's principles of internal medicine, 15th ed. New York: McGraw-Hill, 2001:1399-1410.

CASE 2

A 72-year-old man presents to the office complaining of several weeks of worsening exertional dyspnea. Previously, he had been able to work in his garden and mow the lawn, but now he feels short of breath after walking 100 feet. He does not have chest pain when he walks, although in the past, he has had episodes of retrosternal chest pressure with strenuous exertion. Once he also felt lightheaded, as if he were about to faint while climbing a flight of stairs, but the symptom passed after he sat down. Recently, he also has been having some difficulty sleeping at night, and has to prop himself up with two pillows. Occasionally, he wakes up at night feeling quite short of breath, which is relieved within minutes by sitting upright and dangling his legs over the bed. He has also noticed that his feet have become swollen, especially by the end of the day. He denies any significant medical history, takes no medications, and prides himself on the face that he hasn't seen a doctor in years. He does not smoke or drink alcohol.

On physical examination, he is afebrile, with a heart rate of 86 bpm, a blood pressure of 115/92 mmHg, and a respiratory rate of 16 breaths per minute. Examination of the head and neck reveals pink mucosa without pallor, a normal thyroid gland, and distended neck veins. Bibasilar inspiratory crackles are heard on examination. On cardiac examination, his heart is regular with a normal S1 and a second heart sound that splits during expiration, an S4 at the apex, a nondisplaced apical impulse, and a late-peaking systolic murmur at the right upper sternal border that radiates to his carotids. The carotid upstrokes have diminished amplitude.

- **What is the most likely diagnosis?**
- **What test would confirm the diagnosis?**

ANSWERS TO CASE 2: Aortic Stenosis and Congestive Heart Failure

Summary: A 72-year-old man complains of several weeks of worsening exertional dyspnea. He has had angina-like chest pressure with strenuous exertion, near-syncope while climbing a flight of stairs, orthopnea, paroxysmal nocturnal dyspnea, and pedal edema. He does not smoke or drink alcohol. He is normotensive, has distended neck veins, and has diminished carotid upstrokes. Bibasilar inspiratory crackles are heard on examination. His heart is regular with a normal S1 and a second heart sound that paradoxically splits during expiration, an S4 at the apex, a nondisplaced apical impulse, and a late-peaking systolic murmur at the right upper sternal border that radiates to his carotids.

- **Most likely diagnosis:** Congestive heart failure, possibly as a result of aortic stenosis.

- **Diagnostic test:** Echocardiogram to assess aortic valve area.

Analysis

Objectives

1. Know the causes of chronic heart failure (such as ischemia, hypertension, valvular disease, alcohol abuse, cocaine, thyrotoxicosis).
2. Recognize impaired systolic function versus diastolic dysfunction.
3. Be familiar with the treatment of acute and chronic heart failure.
4. Know the complications of treatment: hypo- and hyperkalemia, renal failure, digoxin toxicity.
5. Be familiar with the evaluation of aortic stenosis and the indications for valve replacement.

Considerations

This is an elderly patient with symptoms and signs of aortic stenosis, based on the late systolic murmur radiating to the carotids. The valvular disorder has progressed to heart failure from previous angina and presyncopal symptoms, reflecting worsening severity of the stenosis and worsening prognosis for survival. This patient should have urgent evaluation of his aortic valve surface area and coronary artery status to assess the need for valve replacement.

APPROACH TO SUSPECTED HEART FAILURE

Definitions

Acute heart failure: Acute (hours, days) presentation of cardiac decompensation with pulmonary edema and low cardiac output, which may proceed to cardiogenic shock.

Chronic heart failure: Chronic (months, years) presence of cardiac dysfunction; symptoms may range from minimal to severe.

Diastolic dysfunction: Increased diastolic filling pressures caused by impaired diastolic relaxation and decreased ventricular compliance.

Systolic dysfunction: Low cardiac output caused by impaired systolic function (low ejection fraction).

Clinical Approach

Congestive heart failure (CHF) is a **clinical syndrome** that is produced when the heart is **unable to meet the metabolic needs of the body while maintaining normal ventricular filling pressures.** A series of **neurohumoral responses** develop, including activation of the renin–angiotensin–aldosterone axis and increased sympathetic activity, which may initially be compensatory, but ultimately cause further cardiac decompensation. Symptoms may be a result of **forward failure** (low cardiac output or systolic dysfunction) including **fatigue, lethargy, and even hypotension**, or **backward failure** (increased filling pressures or diastolic dysfunction) including **dyspnea, peripheral edema, and ascites**. Some patients have isolated diastolic dysfunction with a preserved left ventricular ejection fraction (LVEF >40–45%), most often as a consequence of hypertension or simply of aging. The majority of patients with CHF have impaired systolic dysfunction (LVEF <40–45%) with associated increased filling pressures. Some patients may have isolated right-sided heart failure (with elevated jugular venous pressure, hepatic congestion, peripheral edema but no pulmonary edema), but more commonly, there is left ventricular failure (with low cardiac output and pulmonary edema) that progresses to biventricular failure.

Heart failure is a **chronic and progressive disease** that can be assessed by following patients' exercise tolerance, such as the **New York Heart Association (NYHA) functional classification (see Table 2–1).** This functional classification carries prognostic significance. Individuals in class III who have low oxygen consumption during exercise have an annual mortality rate of 20%; in class IV, it is 60% annually. Patients with a low ejection fraction (LVEF <20%) also have very high mortality risks. Death associated with

Table 2–1

NYHA FUNCTIONAL CLASSIFICATION

Class I:	No limitation during ordinary physical activity.
Class II:	Slight limitation of physical activity. Develops fatigue or dyspnea with moderate exertion.
Class III:	Marked limitation of physical activity. Even light activity produces symptoms.
Class IV:	Symptoms at rest. Any activity causes worsening.

CHF may occur from the underlying disease process, cardiogenic shock, or sudden death as a result of ventricular arrhythmias.

Although there are many causes of heart failure (see Table 2–2), it is essential to try to identify underlying treatable or reversible causes of disease. For example, heart failure related to tachycardia, alcohol consumption, or viral myocarditis may be reversible with removal of the inciting factor. In patients with underlying multivessel atherosclerotic coronary disease and a low ejection fraction, revascularization with coronary artery bypass grafting improves cardiac function, and prolongs survival. For patients with heart failure, appropriate investigation is guided by the history, but may include echocardiography to assess ejection fraction and valvular function, cardiac stress testing or coronary angiography as indicated, and in some cases, endomyocardial biopsy.

The two major treatment goals for patients with chronic heart failure are relief of symptoms and a reduction in mortality risk. The heart failure symptoms, which are mainly caused by low cardiac output and fluid overload, are usually relieved with dietary sodium restriction, loop diuretics, and digoxin. Patients with acute pulmonary edema also benefit from the use of nitrates for preload reduction, and morphine for relief of dyspnea (also reduces preload). Because heart failure has such a substantial mortality, however, measures are necessary to try to halt or reverse disease progression. Reversible causes should be aggressively sought and treated. When no reversible causes can be found, use of **ACE inhibitors and some beta-blockers such as carvedilol or metoprolol reduce mortality in patients with impaired systolic function and moderate to severe symptoms.**

Table 2–2

SELECTED CAUSES OF CONGESTIVE HEART FAILURE

Myocardial Injury
- Adriamycin
- Alcohol use
- Cocaine
- Ischemic cardiomyopathy (atherosclerotic coronary artery disease)
- Rheumatic fever
- Viral myocarditis

Chronic pressure overload
- Aortic stenosis
- Hypertension

Chronic volume overload
- Mitral regurgiation

Infiltrative diseases
- Amyloidosis
- Hemochromatosis

Aortic Stenosis In the patient presented in the scenario, the history and physical findings suggest that his heart failure may be a result of aortic stenosis. This is the **most common valvular abnormality in adults**. The large majority of cases occur in men. The causes of the valvular stenosis varies depending on typical age of presentation: stenosis in patients **younger than 30 years old** is usually caused by a **congenital bicuspid valve**, in patients 30–70 years old, it is usually caused by congenital stenosis or acquired rheumatic heart disease, **after age 70 years, it is usually caused by senile calcific stenosis**.

Typical physical findings include a **narrow pulse pressure**, a **harsh late-peaking systolic murmur** heard best at the right second intercostal space with radiation to the carotid arteries, and a delayed slow-rising carotid upstroke (pulsus parvus et tardus). The EKG often shows left ventricular hypertrophy. Doppler echocardiography reveals a thickened, abnormal valve, and can define severity as assessed by the aortic valve area and by estimating the transvalvular pressure gradient. As the valve orifice narrows, the pressure gradient increases in an attempt to maintain cardiac output. Severe aortic stenosis often have valve areas <0.7 cm^2 and mean pressure gradients >50 mmHg.

Symptoms of aortic stenosis develop as a consequence of the left ventricular hypertrophy that results, as well as of the diminished cardiac output caused by the flow-limiting valvular stenosis. The first symptoms are typically **angina pectoris**; that is, retrosternal chest pain that is precipitated by exercise and relieved by rest. As the stenosis worsens and cardiac output falls, patients may experience **syncopal episodes**, typically precipitated by exertion. Finally, because of the low cardiac output and the high diastolic filling pressures, patients develop clinically apparent **heart failure** as described above. The prognosis for patients worsens as symptoms develop, with mean survival with angina, syncope, or heart failure of 5 years, 3 years, and 2 years, respectively.

Patients with severe stenosis and with symptoms should be considered for aortic valve replacement. Preoperative cardiac catheterization is routinely performed to provide definitive assessment of aortic valve area and the pressure gradient, as well as to assess the coronary arteries for significant stenosis. In patients who are not good candidates for valve replacement, the stenotic valve can be enlarged using balloon valvuloplasty , but this will provide only temporary relief of symptoms.

Comprehension Questions

[2.1] A 55-year-old American man is noted to have moderately severe CHF with impaired systolic function. Which of the following drugs would most likely lower his risk of mortality?

A. Angiotensin converting enzyme inhibitor and beta-blockers
B. Thiazide diuretics
C. Low-cholesterol diet
D. Daily aspirin

[2.2] Which of the following is most likely to have caused the CHF in question [2.1]?

A. Diabetes
B. Atherosclerosis
C. Alcohol
D. Rheumatic heart disease

[2.3] A 35-year-old woman is noted to have significant aortic stenosis. Which of following findings would be most important regarding this patient's mortality risk?

A. Systolic murmur
B. Angina
C. Syncope
D. Congestive heart failure

[2.4] A 55-year-old man is noted to have alcohol-induced cardiomyopathy and states that he becomes dyspneic even with walking to bathroom. Which of the following best describes his NYHA functional classification?

A. I
B. II
C. III
D. IV

Answers

[2.1] **A.** Angiotensin converting enzyme inhibitor and beta-blockers decrease the risk of mortality when used to treat CHF with impaired systolic function.

[2.2] **B.** In the United States, the most common cause of CHF associated with impaired systolic function is atherosclerosis.

[2.3] **D.** Aortic stenosis classically progresses through angina, syncope, and, finally, the last, congestive heart failure, has the worse prognosis.

[2.4] **C.** Symptoms with minimal exertion are indicative of a level III functional class. The worst class is level IV, symptoms at rest.

CLINICAL PEARLS

❖ Congestive heart failure is a clinical syndrome that is always caused by some underlying heart disease: most commonly ischemic cardiomyopathy as a result of atherosclerotic coronary disease or hypertension.

❖ Heart failure can be caused by an impaired systolic function (ejection fraction <40–45%) or by an impaired diastolic function (with preserved systolic ejection fraction).

- ❖ Chronic heart failure is a progressive disease with a high mortality. A patient's functional class, that is, their exercise tolerance, is the best predictor of mortality, and often guides therapy.
- ❖ The primary goals of therapy are to relieve congestive symptoms with salt restriction, diuretics, digoxin, and vasodilators, and to prolong survival with ACE inhibitors or certain beta-blockers.
- ❖ Aortic stenosis produces progressive symptoms such as angina, exertional syncope, and heart failure, with an increasingly higher risk of mortality. Valve replacement should be considered for patients with symptoms and severe aortic stenosis, for example, an aortic valve area $<0.7\ cm^2$.

REFERENCES

Asif M, Regan TJ. Congestive Cardiomyopathy. In: Alpert JS. Cardiology for the primary care physician, Stamford: Appleton and Lange, 1998: 2nd ed. pp 219-229

Antman EM, Braunwald E. Acute Myocardial Infarction. In: Braunwald E, Fauci AS, Kasper KL, et al., eds. Harrison's principles of internal medicine, 15th ed. New York: McGraw-Hill, 2001:1386-1399.

Selwyn AP, Braunwald E. Ischemic Heart Disease. In: Braunwald E, Fauci AS, Kasper KL, et al., eds. Harrison's principles of internal medicine, 15th ed. New York: McGraw-Hill, 2001:1399-1410.

Lejemtel TH, Sonnenblick EH, Frishman WH. Diagnosis and Mangement of Heart Failure. In: Fuster V, Alexander RX, O'Rourke RA, eds. Hurst's the heart, 10th ed. New York: McGraw-Hill, 2001:687-724.

CASE 3

A 26-year-old woman presents to the emergency room complaining of a sudden onset of palpitations and severe shortness of breath and coughing. She reports that she has had several episodes of palpitations in the past, often lasting a day or two, but never with dyspnea like this. She has a history of rheumatic fever at age 14 years. She is now 20 weeks pregnant with her first child and takes prenatal vitamins. She denies use of any other medications, tobacco, alcohol, or illicit drugs.

On examination, her heart rate is between 110 and 130 bpm and is irregularly irregular, with a blood pressure of 92/65 mmHg, and a respiratory rate of 24 breaths per minute with an oxygen saturation of 92% on room air. She appears uncomfortable with labored respirations. She is coughing, producing scant amounts of frothy sputum with a pinkish tint. She has ruddy cheeks and a normal jugular venous pressure. She has bilateral inspiratory crackles in the lower lung fields. On cardiac examination, her heart rate is irregularly irregular with a loud S1 and low-pitched diastolic murmur at the apex. Her apical impulse is nondisplaced. Her uterine fundus is palpable at the umbilicus, and she has no peripheral edema. An EKG is obtained. (Figure 3–1)

- **What is the most likely diagnosis?**
- **What is your next step?**

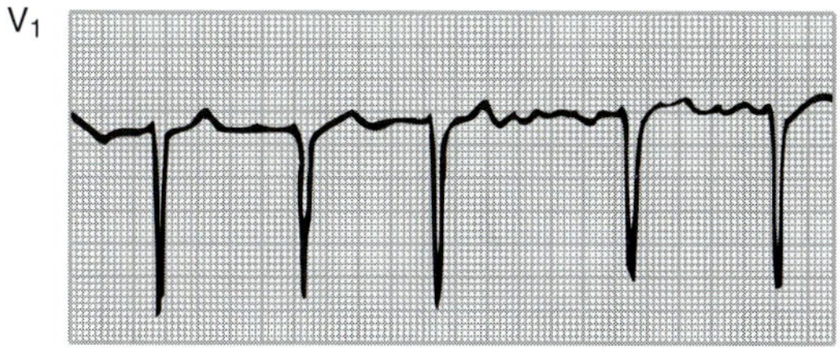

Figure 3–1. EKG. **(Reproduced with permission from Braunwald E, Fauci AS, Kasper KL, et al., eds. Harrison's principles of internal medicine, 15th ed. New York: McGraw-Hill, 2001:1296.)**

ANSWERS TO CASE 3: Atrial Fibrillation, Mitral Stenosis

Summary: This 26-year-old woman, with a history of rheumatic fever during adolescence, is now in the second trimester of pregnancy and presents with acute onset of palpitations. She is found to have atrial fibrillation with a rapid ventricular response. She has a diastolic rumble and "ruddy cheeks," both features of mitral stenosis, which is the likely cause of her atrial fibrillation as a result of left atrial enlargement. Because of the increased blood volume associated with pregnancy and the onset of tachycardia and loss of atrial contraction, the atrial fibrillation has caused her to develop pulmonary edema.

- **Most likely diagnosis:** Atrial fibrillation caused by rheumatic heart disease.

- **Next step:** Cardiac rate control with intravenous beta-blockers.

Analysis

Objectives

1. Know the causes of atrial fibrillation.
2. Understand the management of acute atrial fibrillation with rapid ventricular response.
3. Understand the rationale for anticoagulation in chronic atrial fibrillation.
4. Know the typical cardiac lesions of rheumatic heart disease and the physical findings in mitral stenosis.
5. Understand the physiologic basis of Wolff-Parkinson-White syndrome and the special considerations in atrial fibrillation.

Clinical Approach

Atrial fibrillation (AF) is the most common arrhythmia for which patients seek treatment; it occurs in acute, paroxysmal, and chronic forms. During AF, disordered atrial depolarization, often at rates exceeding 300–400 bpm, produces an irregular ventricular response, depending on the number of impulses that are conducted through the atrioventricular (AV) node. The electrocardiogram is characterized by **absence of discrete P waves** and an **irregularly irregular ventricular response**. The incidence of AF increases with age, affecting 10% of patients older than 75 years of age. Although many patients can maintain a normal activity level and remain essentially asymptomatic with chronic AF, there are several causes of morbidity from this arrhythmia: it may trigger a rapid ventricular rate leading to myocardial ischemia or exacerbation of heart failure in patients with heart disease, and **thrombus formation** in the noncontractile atria can lead to systemic embolization (AF is a common cause of stroke).

Anything that causes atrial dilatation or excessive sympathetic tone can lead to atrial fibrillation, but the **two most common causes** of AF are **hypertension**

and coronary atherosclerosis. The **causes of AF** can be remembered with the **mnemonic "I SMART CHAP"** (Table 3–1).

Acute atrial fibrillation with rapid ventricular response must be addressed quickly. The four major goals are (a) stabilization, (b) rate control, (c) conversion to sinus rhythm, and (d) anticoagulation. If a patient is **hemodynamically unstable** (hypotensive, angina pectoris, pulmonary edema), **urgent DC cardioversion** is indicated. If the patient is hemodynamically stable, **ventricular rate control** can generally be achieved with **intravenous beta-blockers, calcium channel blockers, or digoxin**, which slow conduction through the AV node. Once the ventricular rate has been controlled, consideration can be given to reversing the underlying causes (e.g., thyrotoxicosis, use of adrenergic stimulants, or worsening heart failure) so that patients may undergo **cardioversion** to sinus rhythm. This may occur spontaneously, or after correction of underlying abnormalities, or it may require pharmacologic or electrical cardioversion. If the duration of **AF exceeds 48 hours, the risk of intraatrial thrombus formation increases.** Cardioverting the patient back to sinus rhythm, the return of coordinated atrial contraction in the presence of an atrial thrombus may lead to clot embolization, leading to a cerebral infarction or other distant ischemic event. Therefore, after 48 hours of AF, patients should receive 3–4 weeks of warfarin prior to and after cardioversion to reduce the risk of thromboembolic phenomena. Alternatively, low-risk patients can undergo transesophageal echocardiography to exclude the presence of an atrial appendage thrombus prior to cardioversion. Postcardioversion anticoagulation is still required for 4 weeks, because even though the rhythm returns to sinus, the atria do not contract normally for some time.

Table 3–1

CAUSES OF ATRIAL FIBRILLATION

Inflammatory Disease (pericarditis, myocarditis)
Surgery (post-bypass surgery, post-valvular surgery)
Medications (theophylline, caffeine, digitalis)
Atherosclerotic coronary artery disease
Rheumatic heart disease (especially with mitral stenosis)
Thyrotoxicosis
Congenital heart disease (atrial septal defect, Ebstein's anomaly)
Hypertensive heart disease
Alcohol consumption (holiday heart syndrome, alcoholic cardiomyopathy)
Pulmonary disease especially pulmonary embolus

Many patients with atrial fibrillation cannot be cardioverted and expect to remain in sinus rhythm. **Two important prognostic factors** are **left atrial dilatation** (an atrial diameter greater than 4.5 cm predicts failure of cardioversion) and **duration of AF**. The longer the patient is in fibrillation, the more likely the patient is to stay there ("atrial fibrillation begets atrial fibrillation") as a consequence of electrical remodeling of the heart. In patients with chronic AF, the management goals are rate control, using drugs to reduce AV nodal conduction as described above, and anticoagulation. Patients with chronic AF who are not anticoagulated have a 5% per year incidence of clinically evident embolization such as stroke. For chronic AF caused by valvular disease such as mitral stenosis, the annual risk of stroke is substantially higher. **Warfarin anticoagulation reduces the risk of stroke in patients with chronic AF by two-thirds**. Warfarin does not produce a predictable dose-related response; therefore, the level of anticoagulation needs to be monitored by regular laboratory testing using the International Normalized Ratio (INR). In AF not caused by valvular disease, the goal INR is 2–3. AF that develops in patients younger than age 60 years without evidence of structural heart disease, hypertension, or other factors for stroke is termed **lone atrial fibrillation,** and the **risk of stroke is very low**, so anticoagulation with warfarin is not used. Instead, low-dosed aspirin may be used.

The major complication of warfarin therapy is bleeding as a consequence of excessive anticoagulation. The risk of bleeding increases as the INR increases. If the INR is markedly elevated, for example, greater than 6, but there is no apparent bleeding, the values will return to normal over several days if the warfarin is held. For higher levels of INR but without bleeding, vitamin K can be administered, orally or intravenously. If clinically significant bleeding is present, warfarin toxicity can be rapidly reversed with administration of vitamin K, and fresh-frozen plasma to replace clotting factors and provide intravascular volume replacement.

Rheumatic Heart Disease In the case presented in the scenario, the cause of this patient's atrial fibrillation appears to be mitral stenosis. Because she has a history of acute rheumatic fever, her mitral stenosis is almost certainly a result of rheumatic heart disease. **Rheumatic heart disease** is a late sequela of acute rheumatic fever, arising many years after the original attack. Valvular thickening, fibrosis, and calcifications lead to valvular stenosis. The **mitral valve is most frequently involved**. The aortic valve may also develop stenosis, but usually in combination with the mitral valve. The right side of the heart is rarely involved.

Almost all cases of **mitral stenosis** in adults are secondary to **rheumatic heart disease**, usually involving women. The physical signs of mitral stenosis are a **loud S1**, and an **opening snap following S2.** The S2-OS interval narrows as the severity of the stenosis increases. There is a **low-pitched diastolic rumble** after the opening snap, heard best at the apex with the bell of the stethoscope. Because of the stenotic valve, pressure in the left atrium is increased, leading to left atrial dilatation and, ultimately, to pulmonary hypertension. Pulmonary hypertension can cause hemoptysis and signs of right-sided heart failure such as peripheral edema. When atrial fibrillation develops, the rapid ventricular response produces pulmonary congestion as a consequence of shortened diastolic filling time. Rate control with intravenous digoxin, beta-blockers, or calcium channel blockers is essential to relief of pulmonary symptoms.

Wolff Parkinson-White Syndrome Another cause of atrial fibrillation is the **Wolff-Parkinson-White (WPW) syndrome**. In these patients, the atrial fibrillation may be life-threatening. In addition to the AV node, patients with WPW have an **accessory pathway** providing an alternate route for electrical communication between the atria and ventricles, leading to **preexcitation**, that is, early ventricular depolarization that begins prior to normal AV nodal conduction. A portion of ventricular activation occurs over the accessory pathway, with the remaining occurring normally through the His-Purkinje system. This preexcitation is recognized on the EKG as a **delta wave**, or early up-slurring of the R wave, which both **widens the QRS complex** and **shortens the PR interval**, which represents the normal AV nodal conduction time (see Figure 3–2). Some patients with the EKG abnormalities of WPW are asymptomatic; others have recurrent tachyarrhythmias. Most of the tachycardia will be caused by paroxysmal supraventricular tachycardia; one-third of patients will have atrial fibrillation. Atrial fibrillation with conduction to the ventricles over an accessory pathway is a special case for two reasons. First, when conducted through the accessory pathway, the **widened QRS** may look like ventricular tachycardia,

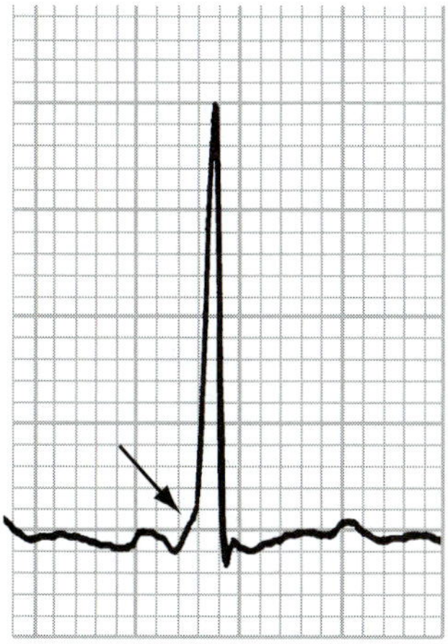

Figure 3–2. EKG revealing the delta wave of Wolff-Parkinson-White. **(Reproduced with permission from Stead LG et al. First aid for the medicine clerkship. New York: McGraw-Hill, 2002:49.)**

except it will have the **irregular RR interval of atrial fibrillation**. Second, because the atrioventricular conduction is occurring through the accessory pathway rather than the AV node, the ventricular rate may be very rapid, and the usual AV nodal blocking drugs given for ventricular rate control will not affect the accessory pathway. In fact, **digoxin and verapamil** can, **paradoxically, increase the ventricular rate** and **should be avoided in WPW patients with AF**. If hemodynamically unstable, **DC cardioversion** should be performed. If hemodynamically stable, the first agent of choice is **procainamide,** to slow conduction and convert the rhythm to sinus.

Comprehension Questions

[3.1] A 28-year-old woman has been told she has rheumatic heart disease, specifically mitral stenosis. Which of following murmurs is most likely present?

A. Diastolic rumble at apex of the heart
B. Early diastolic decrescendo at right upper sternal border
C. Holosystolic murmur at apex
D. Late-peaking systolic murmur at right upper sternal border

[3.2] A 48-year-old woman is noted to have atrial fibrillation with a ventricular heart rate of 140 bpm. She is slightly dizzy with a systolic blood pressure of 75/48 mmHg. Which of the following is the most appropriate next step?

A. Intravenous digoxin
B. DC cardioversion
C. Initiate vagal maneuvers
D. Intravenous Cardizem (diltiazem)

[3.3] Which of the following patients **with atrial fibrillation** is most likely **not** to need anticoagulation?

A. A 45-year-old male who has normal echocardiographic findings and no history of heart disease or hypertension, but a family history of hyperlipidemia
B. A 62-year-old male with mild chronic hypertension and dilated left atrium, but normal ejection fraction
C. A 75-year-old woman who is in good health except for a prior stroke, from which she has recovered nearly all function
D. A 52-year-old man with orthopnea and paroxysmal nocturnal dyspnea

[3.4] A 59-year-old female has been placed on Coumadin after being found to have had chronic atrial fibrillation. She is noted to have an INR of 5.8, is asymptomatic, and has no overt bleeding. Which of the following is the best management for this patient?

A. Transfuse with erythrocytes

B. Give vitamin K
C. Give fresh-frozen plasma
D. Hold Coumadin

Answers

[3.1] **A.** A diastolic rumble at the cardiac apex suggests mitral stenosis. The early diastolic decrescendo murmur is typical of aortic regurgitation, holosystolic murmur at the apex that of mitral regurgitation, and late-peaking systolic murmur at the upper sternal border that of aortic stenosis.

[3.2] **B.** This individual has significant symptoms and hypotension caused by the atrial fibrillation and rapid ventricular rate; consequently, DC cardioversion is the treatment of choice.

[3.3] **A.** Conditions associated with a high risk for embolic stroke include a dilated left atrium, congestive heart failure, prior stroke, and the presence of a thrombus by echocardiogram. The man in answer "A" has "lone atrial fibrillation" and has a low risk for stroke, and thus would not benefit from anticoagulation.

[3.4] **D.** The target INR with Coumadin is 2 to 3; thus, 5.8 is markedly elevated. However, because she has no overt bleeding and is asymptomatic, holding the Coumadin until the INR reaches the acceptable range is a reasonable approach.

CLINICAL PEARLS

❖ The two most common causes of atrial fibrillation are hypertension and atherosclerotic heart disease. The other causes can be remembered with the mnemonic "I SMART CHAP."

❖ Acute atrial fibrillation is treated with DC cardioversion if the patient is unstable. If stable, initial management is ventricular rate control with AV nodal blocking agents such as digoxin, beta-blockers, diltiazem, or verapamil.

❖ Patients with chronic atrial fibrillation generally require long-term anticoagulation to prevent embolic strokes. An exception is "lone atrial fibrillation," where the risk of stroke is low.

❖ WPW is a ventricular preexcitation syndrome defined as symptomatic tachycardia, with a delta wave, a short PR interval (<0.12 seconds), a prolonged QRS interval (>0.12 seconds).

❖ Atrial fibrillation in WPW is treated with DC cardioversion or procainamide; digoxin or verapamil can, paradoxically, increase the ventricular rate.

REFERENCES

Josephson ME, Zimetbaum P. The Tachyarrhythmias. In: Braunwald E, Fauci AS, Kasper KL, et al., eds. Harrison's principles of internal medicine, 15th ed. New York: McGraw-Hill, 2001:1292-1309.

Braunwald E. Valvular Heart Disease. In: Braunwald E, Fauci AS, Kasper KL, et al., eds. Harrison's Principles of internal medicine, 15th ed. New York: McGraw-Hill, 2001:1343-1355.

CASE 4

A 37-year-old executive returns to your office for follow up of recurrent upper abdominal pain. He initially presented 6 weeks ago, complaining of an increase in frequency and severity of burning epigastric pain, which he's had occasionally for more than 2 years. He now has the pain three or four times a week, usually on an empty stomach, and it often awakens him at night. The pain is usually relieved within minutes by food or over-the-counter antacids, but recurs within 2–3 hours. He admitted that stress at work had recently increased and that because of long working hours, he was drinking more caffeine and eating a lot of "take-out" foods. His past medical history and review of systems were otherwise unremarkable, and other than the antacids, he takes no medications. His physical exam was normal, including stool guaiac that was negative for occult blood. You advised a change in diet and started him on an H_2-blocker. His symptoms resolved completely with the diet changes and daily use of the medication. Lab tests done at his first visit shows no anemia, but his serum *Helicobacter pylori* antibody test was positive.

What is your diagnosis?

What is your next step?

ANSWERS TO CASE 4: Peptic Ulcer Disease

Summary: A 37-year-old man presents complaining of chronic and recurrent upper abdominal pain with characteristics suggestive of duodenal ulcer: the pain is burning in quality, occurs when the stomach is empty, and is relieved within minutes by food or antacids. He does not have evidence of gastrointestinal bleeding or anemia. He does not take nonsteroidal antiinflammatory drugs, which might cause ulcer formation, but he does have serological evidence of *H. pylori* infection.

- **Most likely diagnosis:** Peptic ulcer disease.
- **Next step:** Antibiotic therapy for *H. pylori* infection.

Analysis

Objectives

1. Know how to differentiate common causes of abdominal pain by historical clues.
2. Recognize clinical features of duodenal ulcer, gastric ulcer, and features that increase concern for gastric cancer.
3. Understand the role of *Helicobacter pylori* infection and use of NSAIDs in the etiology of peptic ulcer disease.
4. Understand the use and interpretation of tests for *H. pylori.*

Considerations

In this patient, the symptoms are suggestive of duodenal ulcer. He does not have "alarm symptoms" such as weight loss, bleeding or anemia, and his young age and chronicity of symptoms makes gastric malignancy an unlikely cause for his symptoms. *H. pylori* commonly is associated with peptic ulcer disease and requires treatment for cure of the ulcer and prevention of recurrence. This patient's symptoms are also consistent with that of nonulcer dyspepsia.

APPROACH TO PEPTIC ULCER DISEASE

Definitions

Dyspepsia: Pain or discomfort centered in the upper abdomen (mainly in or around the midline), which can be associated with fullness, early satiety, bloating, or nausea. Dyspepsia can be intermittent or continuous, and may or may not be related to meals.

Functional (nonulcer dyspepsia): Symptoms as described above, persisting at least 12 weeks, but without evidence of ulcer on endoscopy.

Helicobacter pylori: A Gram-negative microaerophilic bacillus that resides within the mucus layer of the gastric mucosa, and causes persistent gastric infection and chronic inflammation. It produces a urease enzyme, which splits urea, raising local pH and allowing it to survive in the acidic environment.

Peptic ulcer disease (PUD): The presence of gastric or duodenal ulcers as demonstrated by endoscopy or by upper gastrointestinal barium study.

Clinical Approach

Upper abdominal pain is one of the most common complaints encountered in primary care practice. Many patients have benign functional disorders (i.e., no specific pathology can be identified after diagnostic testing), but others have potentially more serious conditions such as peptic ulcer disease or gastric cancer. Historical clues, knowledge of the epidemiology of diseases, and some simple laboratory assessments can help to separate benign from serious causes of pain. However, endoscopy is often necessary to confirm the diagnosis.

Dyspepsia refers to upper abdominal pain or discomfort that can be caused by peptic ulcer disease, but can also be produced by a number of other gastrointestinal disorders. **Gastroesophageal reflux** typically produces "heartburn," or burning epigastric or mid-chest pain, usually after meals and worse with recumbency. **Biliary colic** caused by gallstones typically has an acute onset of severe pain located in the right upper quadrant or epigastrium, is usually precipitated by meals, especially fatty foods, lasts 30-60 minutes with spontaneous resolution, and is more common in women. **Irritable bowel syndrome** is a diagnosis of exclusion, but is suggested by chronic dysmotility symptoms, that is, bloating, cramping that is often relieved with defecation, without weight loss or bleeding. If one excludes these causes by history or other investigations, it is still difficult to clinically distinguish by symptoms those patients with peptic ulcer disease and those without ulcers, termed nonulcer dyspepsia.

The classic symptoms of **duodenal ulcers** are caused by the presence of acid without food or other buffers. Symptoms are typically produced after the stomach is emptied but food-stimulated acid production still persists, typically 2–5 hours after a meal. They may also wake patients at night, when circadian rhythms increase acid production. The pain is typically relieved within minutes by neutralization of acid by food or antacids (e.g., calcium carbonate, aluminum-magnesium hydroxide). **Gastric ulcers**, by contrast, are more variable in their presentation. Food may actually worsen symptoms in patients with gastric ulcer; or pain might not be relieved by antacids. In fact, many patients with peptic ulcer disease have no symptoms at all. **Gastric cancers** may present with dysphagia if they are located in the cardiac region of the stomach, persistent vomiting if they block the pyloric channel, or early satiety by their mass effect or infiltration of the stomach wall. They may also present with pain symptoms as a result of ulcer formation.

Because the incidence of gastric cancer increases with age, patients **older than 45 years of age** presenting with **new-onset dyspepsia** should generally undergo endoscopy. In addition, those patients with **alarm symptoms** (e.g., weight loss, recurrent vomiting, dysphagia, evidence of bleeding, or anemia) should be referred for prompt endoscopy. Finally, endoscopy should be recommended for patients whose symptoms have **failed to respond** to empiric therapy. When endoscopy is undertaken, besides visualization of the ulcer, biopsies can be taken, to exclude the possibility of malignancy as the cause of a gastric ulcer, and biopsy specimens can be obtained for urease testing or microscopic examination to prove current *H. pylori* infection.

In **younger patients with no alarm features**, an acceptable strategy is to perform a noninvasive ***H. pylori* test** to determine if the patient is infected. *Helicobacter pylori* is more common in older patients, in lower socioeconomic groups, in institutionalized patients, and in developing countries. It has been established as the causative agent in the majority of duodenal and gastric ulcers, as well as being associated with the development of gastric carcinoma and gastric mucosa-associated lymphoid tissue (MALT) lymphoma. The two most common tests are the **urea breath test**, which provides evidence of current active infection, and ***H. pylori* antibody** tests, which provide evidence of prior infection, but will remain positive for life, even after successful treatment. Because chronic infection with *H. pylori* is found in 90–95% of duodenal ulcers and in 80% of patients with gastric ulcers not related to NSAID use, a suggested strategy is to test for infection, and if present, to treat it with an antibiotic regimen such as clarithromycin and amoxicillin, as well as acid suppression with a proton-pump inhibitor. The reason for treating infection with antibiotics is that eradication of the infection will largely prevent recurrence. Whether treatment of *H. pylori* infection reduces or eliminates dyspeptic symptoms in the absence of ulcers (nonulcer dyspepsia) is uncertain. Similarly, it is unclear whether treatment of asymptomatic patients found to be *H. pylori* positive is beneficial. In *H. pylori*-positive patients with dyspepsia, antibiotic treatment may be considered, but a followup visit is recommended within 4–8 weeks. If symptoms persist, or alarm features develop, then prompt upper endoscopy is indicated.

In addition to *H. pylori,* the other major cause of duodenal and gastric ulcers is the use of **nonsteroidal antiinflammatory drugs (NSAIDs)**. They promote ulcer formation by inhibiting gastroduodenal prostaglandin synthesis, resulting in reduced secretion of mucus and bicarbonate and decreased mucosal blood flow. In other words, they impair local defenses against acid damage. The risk of ulcer formation caused by NSAID use is dose-dependent, and can occur within days after treatment is initiated. Misoprostol, a synthetic prostaglandin, has been used to reduce the incidence of NSAID-associated gastric ulcers, but it often induces diarrhea, limiting its usefulness.

A rare cause of ulcer is the **Zollinger-Ellison syndrome**, a condition in which a gastrin-producing tumor (usually pancreatic) causes acid hypersecretion, peptic ulceration, and oftentimes diarrhea. This condition should be suspected if ulcer disease occurs and the patient is *H. pylori* negative and does not use NSAIDs. To diagnose this condition, one should measure serum gastrin levels, which are markedly elevated (>1000 pg/mL), and then try to localize the tumor with an imaging study.

Hemorrhage is the most common severe complication of peptic ulcer disease, and can present with hematemesis or melena. Sometimes in association with hemorrhage, **free perforation** into the abdominal cavity may occur, with a sudden onset of pain and development of peritonitis. If the perforation occurs adjacent to the pancreas, it may induce pancreatitis. Some patients with chronic ulcers later develop **gastric outlet obstruction,** with persistent vomiting and weight loss, but no abdominal distension. Perforation and obstruction are indications for surgical intervention.

Comprehension Questions

[4.1] A 42-year-old overweight, though otherwise healthy, woman presents with the sudden onset of right upper abdominal colicky pain 45 minutes after a meal of fried chicken. The pain is associated with nausea and vomiting, and any attempt to eat since has caused increased pain. The most likely cause is:

A. Gastric ulcer
B. Cholelithiasis
C. Duodenal ulcer
D. Acute hepatitis

[4.2] Which of the following is *not* true of *H. pylori* infection:

A. It is more common in developing countries.
B. It is associated with the development of gastric lymphoma.
C. It is believed to be the cause of nonulcer dyspepsia.
D. The route of transmission is believed to be fecal–oral.
E. It is believed to be a cause of most duodenal and gastric ulcers.

[4.3] A 45-year-old male was brought to the emergency room after vomiting bright red blood. He has a blood pressure of 88/46 mmHg and heart rate of 120 bpm. Which of the following is the best next step?

A. IV fluid resuscitation and preparation for a transfusion
B. Administration of a proton pump inhibitor
C. Guaiac test the stool
D. Treatment for *H. pylori*

[4.4] Which one of the following patients should be promptly referred for endoscopy?

A. A 65-year-old man with a new onset of epigastric pain and weight loss
B. A 32-year-old whose symptoms are not relieved with ranitidine
C. A 29-year-old *H. pylori*-positive patient with dyspeptic symptoms
D. A 49-year-old woman with intermittent right upper quadrant pain following meals

Answers

[4.1] **B.** Right upper abdominal pain that has an acute onset after the ingestion of a fatty meal and that is associated with nausea and vomiting is most suggestive of biliary colic as a result of gallstones. Duodenal ulcer pain is likely to be diminished with food, and gastric ulcer pain is not likely to have the acute severe onset. Acute hepatitis is more likely to produce dull ache and tenderness.

[4.2] **C.** While *H. pylori* is clearly linked to gastric and duodenal ulcers, and probably to gastric carcinoma and lymphoma, it is unclear whether it is more common in patients with nonulcer dyspepsia, or whether treatment in those patients reduces symptoms.

[4.3] **A.** This patient is hemodynamically unstable with hypotension and tachycardia as a consequence of the acute blood loss. Volume resuscitation, immediately with crystalloid or colloid solution, followed by blood transfusion, if necessary, is the initial step to prevent irreversible shock and death. Later, after stabilization, acid suppression and *H. pylori* treatment might be useful to heal an ulcer, if one is present.

[4.4] **A.** Patient "A" has a red flag: he is older than 45 years of age with new onset symptoms. Patient "B" may benefit from the reassurance of a negative endoscopic exam. Patient "C," however, may benefit from treatment of her *H. pylori* first. Some studies indicate this approach may be cost-saving overall. This patient could be sent for an endoscopic examination if she doesn't improve following therapy.

CLINICAL PEARLS

- ❖ The most common cause of duodenal and gastric ulcers are *H. pylori* infection and use of NSAIDs.
- ❖ *H. pylori* is associated with duodenal and gastric ulcers, chronic active gastritis, gastric adenocarcinoma, and gastric MALT (mucosa-associated lymphoid tissue) lymphoma. It is not definitively associated with nonulcer dyspepsia.
- ❖ Treatment of peptic ulcers requires acid suppression with an H_2-blocker or proton pump inhibitor to heal the ulcer, as well as antibiotic therapy of *H. pylori,* if present, to prevent recurrence.
- ❖ Patients with dyspepsia who have "red-flag" symptoms (new dyspepsia after age 45 years, weight loss, dysphagia, evidence of bleeding or anemia) should be referred for an early endoscopic examination.
- ❖ Other patients may be tested for *H. pylori* and treated first. Antibody tests show evidence of infection, but remain positive for life, even after successful treatment. Urea breath tests are evidence of current infection.

❖ Common treatment regimens for *H. pylori* include a 14 day course of bismuth subsalicylate plus metronidazole plus tetracycline; or omeprazole, clarithromycin, and amoxicillin.

REFERENCES

Del Valle J. Peptic Ulcer Disease and Related Disorders. In: Braunwald E, Fauci AS, Kasper KL, et al., eds. Harrison's principles of internal medicine, 15th ed. New York: McGraw-Hill, 2001:1649-1665.

Suerbaum S, Michetti P. Medical Progress: *Helicobacter pylori* infection. *N Engl J Med* 2002;347:1175-1186.

CASE 5

A 65-year-old white woman is brought into the emergency room by her family for increasing confusion and lethargy over the past week. She was recently diagnosed with small-cell cancer of the lung. She has not been febrile or had any other recent illnesses. She is not on any medications. Her blood pressure is 136/82 mmHg, a heart rate of 84 bpm, a respiratory rate of 14 breaths per minute, unlabored, and she is afebrile. On examination, she is an elderly appearing woman who is difficult to arouse and reacts only to painful stimuli. She is able to move her extremities without apparent motor deficits, and her deep tendon reflexes are decreased symmetrically. The remainder of her examination is normal, with a normal jugular venous pressure, and no extremity edema. You order some laboratory tests and the serum sodium is 108 mmol/L; potassium is 3.8 mmol/L; bicarbonate is 24 milliequivalents per liter (mEq/L), blood urea nitrogen is 5 mg/dL; and creatinine is 0.5 mg/dL. The serum osmolality is 220 mOsm/kg and urine osmolality is 400 mOsm/kg. A CT scan of the brain shows no masses or hydrocephalus.

- **What is the most likely diagnosis?**
- **What is your next step in therapy?**
- **What are the complications of therapy?**

ANSWERS TO CASE 5: Hyponatremia, SIADH

Summary: A 65-year-old white woman with small-cell lung cancer has increasing confusion and lethargy over the past week. She is afebrile and normotensive, and has no edema or jugular venous distension. She is lethargic but is able to move her extremities without apparent motor deficits, and her deep tendon reflexes are decreased symmetrically. Her serum sodium is 108 mmol/L; potassium is 3.8 mmol/L; bicarbonate is 24 milliequivalents per liter (mEq/L); blood urea nitrogen is 5 mg/dL; creatinine 0.5 is mg/dL; and serum osmolality is 220 mOsm/kg with a urine osmolality of 400 mOsm/kg. A CT scan of the brain shows no masses or hydrocephalus.

- **Most likely diagnosis:** Coma/lethargy secondary to severe hyponatremia, which is most likely caused by a tumor-related syndrome of inappropriate antidiuretic hormone secretion (SIADH).
- **Next therapeutic step:** Treat the hyponatremia with hypertonic saline.
- **Most serious complication of this therapy:** Osmotic cerebral demyelination, also referred to as central pontine myelinolysis.

Analysis

Objectives

1. Learn the causes of hyponatremia.
2. Understand the use of laboratory testing in the diagnosis of hyponatremia.
3. Know how to treat hyponatremia, and some of the potential complications of therapy.

Considerations

This elderly woman with small-cell lung cancer presents in a stuporous state with hypotonic hyponatremia. She appears euvolemic because she neither has findings suggestive of volume overload (jugular venous distension or peripheral edema) or of volume depletion. She has no focal neurologic deficits or apparent masses on CT scanning of the brain to suggest cerebral metastases. The most likely cause for her mental status alteration is the hyponatremia. The patient does not take medications; thus, with a hypotronic hyponatremia in a euvolemic state, and with an inappropriately concentrated urine, the most likely etiology is inappropriate antidiuretic hormone produced by the lung cancer. Therapy is guided by the severity of the hyponatremia and the symptoms. Because this individual is stuporous and the sodium level is severely decreased, hypertonic saline is required with fairly rapid partial correction. This therapy is not benign and requires an ICU monitoring. Also, the target is not correction of the sodium level to normal, but rather to a level of safety, such as 120-125 mmol/L.

APPROACH TO HYPONATREMIA

Definitions

ADH (antidiuretic hormone): Also referred to as arginine vasopressin (AVP), ADH is the posterior pituitary hormone that controls excretion of free water, and, thus, indirectly, sodium concentration and serum tonicity.

Osmolality: The concentration of osmotically active particles, which draw water into a compartment; normal range is 280–300 mOsm/kg.

SIADH (Syndrome of Inappropriate Antidiuretic Hormone): Nonphysiologic elevation of ADH levels as a consequence of ectopic production, as in malignancy, or stimulation of excess pituitary production by various pulmonary or central nervous system (CNS) diseases.

Clinical Approach

Hyponatremia is defined as a serum sodium level less than 135 mmol/L and is, by far, the **most common electrolyte disturbance among hospitalized patients**. Patients are often asymptomatic, especially if the hyponatremia develops slowly. Depending on the rapidity with which the hyponatremia develops, most patients do not have symptoms until the serum sodium is in the low 120 mmol/L range. The clinical manifestations are related to osmotic water shifts leading to cerebral edema, thus, the symptoms are mainly neurologic: lethargy, confusion, seizures, or coma.

Serum sodium concentrations are important, because they almost always reflect tonicity, the effect of extracellular fluid on cells that will cause the cells (such as brain cells) to swell (hypotonicity) or to shrink (hypertonicity). For purposes of this discussion, we will use serum osmolality as a valid indicator of tonicity, which is almost always true, so we will use the terms interchangeably. Whereas hypernatremia always reflects hyperosmolality, hyponatremia may occur in the setting of hyperosmolality, normal osmolality, or hyposmolality (see Table 5–1).

Hyponatremia associated with a hyposmolar state is more common and more dangerous. Some hyponatremic conditions are associated with hyperosmolarity or with normal osmolarity. **Hyperosmolar hyponatremia** is most often caused by an increase in the serum level of an osmotically active molecule that is confined to the extracellular space and that cannot readily cross cell membranes, such as glucose or mannitol. These solutes draw water out from the intracellular space, leading to relative hyponatremia. Hyperglycemia occurs in the setting of insulin-deficient states such as uncontrolled diabetes mellitus. For glucose, each 100 mg/dL increase in serum glucose leads to roughly a 1.6 mmol/L decrease in the serum sodium. Transurethral resection of the prostate is a common cause of hyponatremia because of the large volume of mannitol-containing bladder irrigation fluid used intraoperatively. For either of these states, correction of the glucose level (or excretion of the mannitol) corrects the hyponatremia.

Table 5–1
CAUSES OF HYPONATREMIA

I. Pseudohyponatremia
   - A. Normal plasma osmolarity
     1. Hyperlipidemia
     2. Hyperproteinemia
     3. Posttransurethral resection of prostate/bladder tumor
   - B. Increased plasma osmolarity
     1. Hyperglycemia
     2. Mannitol

II. Hyposmolar hyponatremia
   - Primary Na+ loss (secondary water gain)
     1. Integumentary loss: sweating, burns
     2. Gastrointestinal loss: vomiting, tube drainage, fistula, obstruction, diarrhea
     3. Renal loss: diuretics, osmotic diuresis, hypoaldosteronism, salt-wasting nephropathy, postobstructive diuresis, nonoliguric acute tubular necrosis
   - A. Primary water gain (secondary Na+ loss)
     1. Primary polydipsia
     2. Decreased solute intake (e.g., beer potomania)
     3. AVP release as a result of pain, nausea, drugs
     4. Syndrome of inappropriate AVP secretion
     5. Glucocorticoid deficiency
     6. Hypothyroidism
     7. Chronic renal insufficiency
   - B. Primary Na+ gain (exceeded by secondary water gain)
     1. Heart failure
     2. Hepatic cirrhosis
     3. Nephrotic syndrome

Reproduced with permission from Braunwald E, Fauci AS, Kasper KL, et al., eds. Harrison's principles of internal medicine, 15th ed. New York: McGraw-Hill, 2001:274

Pseudohyponatremia refers to an artifact of measurement in states where the serum sodium and, thus, the tonicity are in fact normal. This used to occur when high levels of serum proteins (as in a paraproteinemia such as multiple myeloma) or very high lipid levels interfered with the measurement of the serum sodium. With current laboratory technology, the sodium is directly measured, so pseudohyponatremia is not common. One can suspect pseudohyponatremia if the measured and calculated serum osmolarities are different.

Hypotonic hyponatremia *always* occurs because there is water gain, that is, restriction or impairment of free water excretion. If one considers that the normal kidney capacity to excrete free water is about 18-20 L/d, it becomes apparent that it is very difficult to overwhelm this capacity solely through excessive water intake. Therefore, when hyponatremia develops, the kidney is usually holding on to free water, either pathologically, as in SIADH, or physiologically, as an attempt to maintain effective circulating volume when patients are significantly volume depleted. Hyponatremia can also occur when there are sodium losses, for example, as a consequence of diuretic use, or because of aldosterone deficiency, but in those cases, there is then a secondary gain of free water.

To determine the cause of the hypotonic hyponatremia, the physician must clinically assess the volume status of the patient by history and by physical examination. A history of vomiting, diarrhea, or other losses, such as profuse sweating, suggests hypovolemia, as do flat neck veins, dry oral mucous membranes, and diminished urine output. In cases of significant hypovolemia, there is a physiologic increase in ADH in an attempt to retain free water to maintain circulating volume, even at the expense of hypotonicity. In these cases, the excess ADH is not "inappropriate" as in SIADH, but extremely appropriate. At this point, one can check the urinary sodium levels. In hypovolemia, the kidney should be avidly retaining sodium, so the urine sodium level should be <20 mmol/L. If it is >20 mmol/L, the kidneys do not have the ability to retain sodium normally: either it is impaired by the use of diuretics, or it is lacking necessary hormonal stimulation as in adrenal insufficiency, or there is a primary renal problem, such as tubular damage due to acute tubular necrosis. When patients are **hypovolemic**, the treatment of the hyponatremia requires **correction of the volume status, usually replacement with isotonic (0.9%) or "normal" saline.**

Hypervolemia is usually apparent as edema or elevated jugular venous pressure, and commonly occurs as a result **of congestive heart failure, cirrhosis of the liver, or the nephrotic syndrome.** In these edematous disorders, there is usually a total body excess of both sodium and water, yet arterial baroreceptors perceive hypoperfusion or a decrease in intravascular volume, which leads to an increase in the level of ADH, and therefore retention of free water by the kidneys. Renal failure itself can also lead to hypotonic hyponatremia because of an inability to excrete dilute urine. In any of these cases, the usual initial treatment of hyponatremia is to administer diuretics to reduce both salt and water excess. Thus, hypovolemic or hypervolemic hyponatremia is often apparent clinically, and often does not present a diagnostic challenge. Euvolemic hyponatremia, however, is a frequent problem that is not so easily diagnosed. Once the clinician has diagnosed the patient with euvolemic hypotonic hyponatremia, the next step is to measure the urine osmolarity. This is an effort to try to see if the kidney is actually capable of excreting the free water normally (osmolality should be maximally dilute, <100 mOsm/kg), or whether the free water excretion is impaired (urine not maximally concentrated, >150–200 mOsm/kg). If the urine is maximally dilute, it is handling free water normally, but its capacity for excretion has been overwhelmed, as in central polydipsia. More commonly, free water excretion is impaired and the urine is not maximally dilute as it should be. Two important diagnoses must be considered at this point: **hypothyroidism** and **adrenal insufficiency**. **Thyroid hormone and cortisol are both permissive**

for free water excretion, so their deficiency causes water retention. Isolated cortisal deficiency can mimic SIADH. In contrast, patient's with Addison disease also lack aldosterone, so they have impaired ability to retain sodium. Patients with adrenal insufficiency are usually hypovolemic, and often present in shock.

Euvolemic hyponatremia is most commonly caused by **SIADH.** Nonphysiologic nonosmotically mediated (therefore "inappropriate") secretion can occur in the setting of pulmonary disease, central nervous system disease, pain, in the postoperative period, or as part of a paraneoplastic syndrome. Because of the retention of free water, patients actually have mild (although clinically inapparent) volume expansion. Additionally, if they have a normal dietary sodium intake, the kidneys do not retain sodium avidly. Therefore, there is a modest natriuresis that occurs, so urine sodium is elevated to >20 mmol/L. SIADH is a diagnosis of exclusion: the patient must be hyposmolar but euvolemic, with urine that is not maximally dilute (osm >150–200), with urine sodium >20, and have normal adrenal and thyroid function. Some laboratory clues to SIADH are low blood urea nitrogen (BUN) and low uric acid levels. Unless the patient has severe neurologic symptoms, the treatment of SIADH is water restriction.

Patients with **severe neurologic symptoms** such as seizures or coma need partial correction of the sodium level **rapidly**. The treatment of choice is hypertonic (e.g., 3%) saline. When there is concern that the saline infusion might cause volume overload, it can be administered with a loop diuretic such as furosemide. The diuretic will cause the excretion of hypotonic urine that is essentially "half-normal saline," so a greater portion of sodium than water will be retained, helping to correct the serum sodium level.

When hyponatremia occurs for any reason, especially when it occurs slowly, the brain adapts to prevent cerebral edema. Solutes leave the intracellular compartment of the brain over hours to days, so that patients may have few neurological symptoms despite very low serum sodium. If serum sodium is corrected rapidly, the brain does not have time to readjust, and may shrink rapidly as it loses fluid to the extracellular space. It is believed that this rapid shrinkage may trigger demyelination of the cerebellar and pontine neurons. This **osmotic cerebral demyelination**, or **central pontine myelinolysis**, may cause **quadriplegia, pseudobulbar palsies, a "locked-in" syndrome, coma, or death.** Demyelination can occur even when fluid restriction is the treatment used to correct the serum sodium. Therefore, several expert authors have published formulas and guidelines for the slow and judicious correction of hyponatremia, but the general rule is not to correct the serum sodium concentration faster than 0.5–1 mEq per hour.

Comprehension Questions

[5.1] A young man develops seizures following an emergent splenectomy after a car accident. His serum sodium is initially 116 mmol/dL, and is corrected to 120 mmol/dL over the next 3 hours with hypertonic saline. Which of the following factors most likely led to his hyponatremia?

A. Elevation of serum vasopressin
B. Administration of hypertonic solutions
C. Volume depletion
D. Seizure-induced hyponatremia

[5.2] A 56-year-old man presents to the doctor for the first time complaining of fatigue and weight loss. He has never had any health problems, but he has smoked a pack of cigarettes a day for about 35 years. He is a day laborer and is currently homeless and living in a shelter. His exam is notable for a low-normal blood pressure, skin hyperpigmentation, and digital clubbing. He appears euvolemic. You tell him you are not sure of the problem as yet, but you will draw some blood tests and schedule him for follow up in 1 week. The lab calls that night saying his sodium is 126 mmol/dL, potassium is 6.7 mmol/dL, with a normal creatinine and low bicarbonate and chloride levels. What is the likely cause of his hyponatremia given his presentation?

A. SIADH
B. Hypothyroidism
C. Gastrointestinal Losses
D. Adrenal Insufficiency
E. Renal Insufficiency

[5.3] An 83-year-old woman comes to your office complaining of a headache and mild confusion. Her only medical history is of hypertension, which is well controlled with hydrochlorothiazide. Her exam and lab tests show no signs of infection, but her serum sodium is 119 mmol/dL, and plasma osmolarity is 245 mOsm/kg. She appears to be clinically hypovolemic. What is the best initial therapy?

A. Fluid restriction
B. Infusion of 0.9% saline
C. Infusion of 3% saline
D. Infusion of 3% saline with furosemide.

Answers

[5.1] **A.** In the postoperative state, or in situations where the patient is in pain, serum vasopressin may rise, leading to the inappropriate retention of free water, which leads to dilution of the serum. Concomitant administration of hypotonic fluids may exacerbate the situation.

[5.2] **D.** Hyponatremia in the setting of hyperkalemia and acidosis is suspicious for adrenal insufficiency. This patient's exam is also suggestive of the diagnosis, given his complaints of fatigue, weight loss, low blood pressure, and hyperpigmentation. The diagnosis is made by a

24-hour urine cortisol or in measuring the response to adrenocorticotropic hormone (ACTH) stimulation. The underlying cause of the adrenal gland destruction in this patient is probably either tuberculosis or malignancy.

[5.3] **B.** Because the patient is hypovolemic, probably as a result of the use of diuretics, volume replacement with isotonic saline is the best initial therapy. Hyponatremia caused by thiazide diuretics can occur by several mechanisms, including volume depletion. It is most common in elderly women.

CLINICAL PEARLS

❖ Hyponatremia almost always occurs by impairment of free water excretion.

❖ SIADH is a diagnosis of exclusion. Criteria include euvolemic patient, serum hyposmolarity, urine that is not maximally dilute (osM >150–200), urine sodium >20 mmol/L, and normal adrenal and thyroid function.

❖ Hypovolemic patients with hyponatremia should be treated with volume replacement, typically with isotonic (0.9%) saline.

❖ Euvolemic patients with asymptomatic hyponatremia can be treated with fluid restriction. Those with severe symptoms such as coma or seizures should be treated with hypertonic (3%) saline.

❖ The rate of sodium correction generally should not exceed 0.5–1 mEq/h, or central pontine myelinolysis (osmotic demyelination) can occur.

REFERENCES

Androgue H, Madias N. Hyponatremia. *N Engl J Med* 2000;342(21):1581–89.

Singer G, Brenner B. Fluid and Electrolyte Disturbances. In: Braunwald E, Fauci AS, Kasper KL, et al., eds. Harrison's Principles of Internal Medicine, 15th Edition. New York: McGraw-Hill 2001:271-283.

Robertson G. Disorders of the Neurohypophysis. In: Braunwald E, Fauci AS, Kasper KL, et al., eds. Harrison's Principles of Internal Medicine, 15th ed. New York: McGraw-Hill, 2001:2052-2060.

CASE 6

A 42-year-old man is brought to the emergency room by ambulance after a sudden onset of severe retrosternal chest pain that began an hour ago while he was at home mowing the lawn. He describes the pain as sharp, constant, and unrelated to movement. It was not relieved by three doses of sublingual nitroglycerin administered by the paramedics while en route to the hospital. He has never had symptoms like this before. His only medical history is hypertension, for which he takes enalapril. There is no cardiac disease in his family. He does not smoke, drink alcohol, or use illicit drugs. He is a basketball coach at a local high school, and is usually very physically active.

On physical examination, he is a tall man with long arms and legs who appears uncomfortable and diaphoretic; he is lying on the stretcher with his eyes closed. He is afebrile, with a heart rate of 118 bpm, and blood pressure of 156/100 mmHg in the right arm and 188/94 mmHg in the left arm. His head and neck exam is unremarkable. His chest is clear to auscultation bilaterally, and incidental note is made of pectus excavatum. His heart rate is tachycardic and regular, with a soft, early diastolic murmur at the right sternal border. His abdominal exam is benign, and neurologic exam is nonfocal. His chest x-ray shows a widened mediastinum.

- **What is the most likely diagnosis?**

- **What is your next step?**

ANSWERS TO CASE 6: Aortic Dissection, Marfan Syndrome

Summary: A 42-year-old man is brought in with severe chest pain, which was unrelieved by nitroglycerin. His blood pressure is elevated, but asymmetric in his arms, and he has a new murmur of aortic insufficiency. The chest x-ray shows a widened mediastinum. All of these features strongly suggest aortic dissection as the cause of his pain. He is tall with pectus excavatum and other features of Marfan syndrome, which may be the underlying cause of his dissection.

◆ **Most likely diagnosis:** Aortic dissection.

◆ **Next step:** Administer an intravenous beta-blocker and obtain a noninvasive imaging procedure such as transesophageal echocardiography (TEE) or CT angiography or MRI.

Analysis

Objectives

1. Learn the clinical and radiographic features of aortic dissection, as well as complications of dissection.
2. Know the risk factors for aortic dissection.
3. Understand the management of dissection and the indications for surgical versus medical treatment.
4. Learn about other aortic diseases such as abdominal aortic aneurysm, the role for surveillance, and indications for surgical repair.

Considerations

Most patients with chest pain seek medical attention because they are concerned about a myocardial infarction (MI). It is important to differentiate other conditions of chest pain, because some underlying conditions, such as aortic dissection, could be worsened by the treatment of MI by, for example, anticoagulation with heparin or the use of thrombolytics. In hypertensive patients with dissection, urgent blood pressure lowering is indicated to limit propagation of the dissection.

APPROACH TO AORTIC ANEURYSM AND DISSECTION

Definitions

Abdominal aortic aneurysm: Defined as a pathologic dilation to more than 1.5 times the normal diameter of the aorta. Aneurysms can occur anywhere in the thoracic or abdominal aorta, but the large majority occur in the abdomen, below the renal arteries.

Aortic dissection (dissecting hematoma): A tear or ulceration of the aortic intima that allows pulsatile aortic flow to dissect longitudinally along elastic planes of the media, creating a false lumen or channel for blood flow. Sometimes referred to as a "dissecting aneurysm," although the term is misleading, because the dissection typically produces the aneurysmal dilatation, rather than the reverse.

Clinical Approach

The aorta is the largest conductance vessel in the body. It receives most of the shear forces generated by the heart with every heartbeat throughout the lifetime of an individual. The wall of the aorta is composed of three layers: the intima, the media, and the adventitia. These specialized layers allow the aortic wall to distend under the great pressure created by every heartbeat. Some of this kinetic energy is stored as potential energy, thus allowing forward flow to be maintained during the cardiac cycle. One must consider the great tensile stress that the walls of this vessel faces when considering pathological processes that affect it.

Cystic degeneration of the elastic media predisposes patients to aortic dissection. This occurs in various connective tissue disorders that cause cystic medial degeneration, such as Marfan and Ehlers-Danlos syndrome. Other factors predisposing to aortic dissection include hypertension, aortic valvular abnormalities such as aortic stenosis and congenital bicuspid aortic valve, as well as coarctation of the aorta, pregnancy, and atherosclerotic disease. It may also occur iatrogenically after cardiac surgery or catheterization.

A dissection occurs when there is a sudden intimal tear or rupture followed by the formation of a dissecting hematoma within the aortic media, separating the intima from the adventitia and propagating distally. The presence of hypertension and associated shear forces are the most important factors causing propagation of the dissection. Aortic dissection can produce several devastating or fatal complications: it can produce an intraluminal intimal flap, which can occlude branch arteries and cause organ ischemia or infarction; the hematoma may rupture into the pericardial sac causing cardiac tamponade, or into the pleural space causing exsanguination, or it can produce severe acute aortic regurgitation leading to fulminant heart failure.

The clinical features of aortic dissection typically include a **sudden onset of ripping or tearing pain in the chest, which often radiates to the back**, and may radiate to the neck or extremities as the dissection extends (see Table 6-1). It is essential to differentiate from the pain of myocardial ischemia or infarction, **as the use of anticoagulation or thrombolytics in a patient with a dissection may be devastating**. In contrast to anginal pain, which often builds over minutes, the pain of dissection is **often maximal at onset**. In addition, myocardial ischemia pain is usually relieved with nitrates, whereas the pain of dissection is not. Also, because most dissections begin very close to the aortic valve, it may produce the **early diastolic murmur of aortic insufficiency**, and if it occludes branch arteries, it can produce dramatically different pulses and blood pressures in the extremities. Most patients with dissection are hypertensive; if

Table 6–1
CLINICAL MANIFESTATION OF AORTIC DISSECTION

Horner syndrome	Compression of the superior cervical ganglion
Superior vena cava syndrome	Compression of the superior vena cava
Hemopericardium, pericardial tamponade	Thoracic dissection with retrograde flow into the pericardium
Aortic regurgitation	Thoracic dissection involving the aortic root
Bowel ischemia, hematuria	Dissection involving the mesenteric arteries or renal arteries
Hypertension, different blood pressures in arms	Thoracic dissection involving brachiocephalic artery
Hemiplegia	Carotid artery involvement

hypotension is present, one must suspect aortic rupture, cardiac tamponade, or dissection of the subclavian artery supplying the arm where the blood pressure is being measured. Often a widened superior mediastinum is noted on plain chest film because of dissection of the ascending aorta.

When aortic dissection is suspected, it is essential to confirm the diagnosis with an imaging study. Conventional aortography was the traditional diagnostic "gold standard," but in recent years, very sensitive noninvasive studies such as transesophageal echocardiography, dynamic CT scanning, and MRI have gained widespread use. Because of the emergent nature of the condition, the best initial study is the one that can be obtained and interpreted quickly in the given hospital setting.

There are several classification schemes to describe the different types of aortic dissections. Figure 6–1 describes the Stanford classification. Type A dissection always involves the ascending aorta but can involve any other part. Type B dissection does not involve the ascending aorta but can involve any other part.

Two-thirds of aortic dissections originate in the ascending aorta a few centimeters above the aortic valve. The classification system is important because it guides therapy. Virtually all **type A (proximal or ascending) dissections require urgent surgical therapy** with replacement of the involved aorta and sometimes the aortic valve. Without surgery, the mortality rate for type A dissections is 90%. Type B dissections do not involve the ascending aorta and typically originate in the aortic arch distal to the left subclavian artery. Type B dissections are usually first managed medically, and surgery is usually only performed for complications such as rupture or ischemia of a branch artery of the aorta. The aim of medical

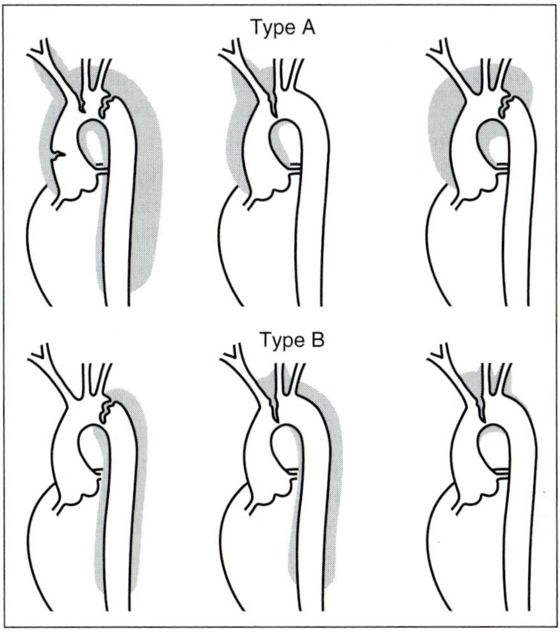

Figure 6–1. Classification of aortic aneurysms. **(Reproduced with permission from Doroghazi RM, Slater EE, eds. Aortic dissection. Harrison's Principles of Internal Medicine. 15th ed. New York: McGraw-Hill, 2001:1432.)**

therapy is to prevent propagation of the dissection by reducing mean arterial pressure and the rate of rise (dP/dT) of arterial pressure, which correlates with arterial shear forces. Intravenous vasodilators, such as sodium nitroprusside to lower blood pressure, can be administered, along with intravenous beta-blockers, such as metoprolol, to reduce shear forces. Alternatively, one may administer intravenous labetalol, which accomplishes both tasks.

In marked contrast to the dramatic presentation of dissection of the thoracic aorta, patients with **aneurysms of the abdominal aorta (AAA) are typically asymptomatic** and are often detected by physical examination, with detection of a midline pulsatile mass, or are noted incidentally on an ultrasound or other imaging procedure. AAA is usually defined as a dilatation of the aorta with a diameter >3 cm, and is found in 1.5–3% of older adults, but in 5–10% of higher risk patients such as those with known atherosclerotic disease. It is a degenerative condition typically found in older men (>50 years of age), most commonly in smokers, who often have atherosclerotic disease elsewhere, such as coronary artery disease or peripheral vascular disease.

The feared complication of AAA is spontaneous rupture. If patients rupture anteriorly into the peritoneal cavity, they usually exsanguinate and die within minutes. If they rupture posteriorly and the bleeding is confined to the retroperitoneum, the peritoneum can produce local tamponade, and they present with severe lower back or midabdominal pain. Overall, the mortality rate of ruptured AAA is 80%, with 50% of patients dead before they reach the hospital.

The risk of rupture is related to the size of the aneurysm: the annual rate of rupture is low if <4.5 cm, it is at least 5–10% per year for 6-cm aneurysms. The risk of rupture must be weighed against the surgical risk of elective repair, which traditionally required excision of the diseased aorta and replacement with a Dacron graft. The Society for Vascular Surgery and the International Society for Cardiovascular Surgery (1992) recommend **elective repair of AAA's 5.0 cm or greater** in diameter, or those expanding more than 0.5 cm per year. As for surveillance of AAA's, the current recommendations are that patients have some sort of imaging of the aneurysm (MRI, CT scan, or ultrasound study) at 3–12-month intervals, depending on the risk of rupture. Recently, endovascular grafts with stents have been used as a less-invasive procedure with less risk than the traditional surgical repair, but the exact role of this procedure remains to be defined.

Comprehension Questions

[6.1] A 59-year-old man complains of severe chest pain that radiates to his back. His brachial pulses appear unequal. He appears hemodynamically stable. On chest radiography, he has a widened mediastinum. Which of the following is the best next step?

A. Initiate thrombolytic therapy
B. CT of chest with contrast
C. Initiate aspirin and heparin
D. Serial cardiac enzymes

[6.2] A 45-year-old woman with new-onset aortic regurgitation is found to have aortic dissection of the ascending aorta and aortic arch by echocardiography. She is relatively asymptomatic. Which of the following is the best management?

A. Oral atenolol therapy and monitor the dissection
B. Angioplasty
C. Surgical correction
D. Oral Coumadin therapy

[6.3] A healthy 75-year-old man undergoing an ultrasound examination for suspected gallbladder disease is found incidentally to have a 6.0-cm abdominal aneurysm of the aorta. Which of the following is the best management for this patient?

A. Surgical repair of the aneurysm
B. Serial ultrasound examinations every 6 months
C. Urgent MRI
D. Beta-agonist therapy

Answers

[6.1] **B.** A CT scan of the chest is a quick imaging test to confirm the aortic dissection. Thrombolytic therapy or anticoagulation can worsen the process.

[6.2] **C.** Surgery is urgently required in the event of aortic root dissection.

[6.3] **A.** When an AAA reaches 5 cm or greater, surgery is usually indicated, because the risk of rupture is increased.

CLINICAL PEARLS

- Hypertension is an underlying factor that predisposes to aortic dissection in the majority of cases. Other patients at risk include those with Marfan syndrome, congenital aortic anomalies, or otherwise normal women in the third trimester of pregnancy.
- Urgent surgical repair is indicated for type A (ascending) aortic dissections. Uncomplicated, stable, type B (transverse or descending) aortic dissections can be managed medically.
- Medical therapy for aortic dissection includes intravenous beta-blockers such as metoprolol or labetalol to lower cardiac contractility, arterial pressure, and shear stress, and thus limit the propagation of the dissection.
- Anticoagulation or thrombolytic therapy is usually contraindicated in aortic dissection.

  Aortic dissection may be complicated by rupture, occlusion of any branch artery of the aorta, or retrograde dissection with hemopericardium and cardiac tamponade.
- The risk of rupture of abdominal aortic aneurysms increases with size. Those larger than 5 cm should undergo elective surgical repair; those smaller than 4.5 cm may be monitored with serial ultrasonography or other imaging procedure.
- Chest pain in the face of a widened mediastinum or chest x-ray should suggest aortic dissection.

REFERENCE

Isselbacher EM, Eagle KA, Zipes DP, et al. Diseases of the aorta. In: Braunwald E, ed. Heart disease: a textbook of cardiovascular medicine, 5th ed. Philadelphia: WB Saunders, 1997:1546–1581.

❖ CASE 7

A 32-year-old man infected with HIV, whose last CD4 count is unknown, presents to the emergency room with a fever of 102.5°F, progressively worsening shortness of breath, and nonproductive cough. He was diagnosed with HIV infection about 3 years ago when he presented to his doctor with oral thrush. He was offered highly active antiretroviral therapy (HAART) and stayed on this regimen until about 10 months ago, when he lost his job and insurance and could no longer pay for the drugs and discontinued all treatment. He has felt more "run down" recently. For the last 2–3 weeks he has had fever, a nonproductive cough, and felt short of breath with mild exertion, such as cleaning his house. He now feels short of breath at rest. On exam his blood pressure is 134/82 mmHg, his pulse is 110 bpm, his respiratory rate is 28 breaths per minute, and his oxygen saturation on room air at rest is 89% which drops to 80% when he walks 100 feet. He is in mild distress. His lungs are clear and there are white patches that don't scrape off covering his buccal mucosa. Otherwise, his exam is unremarkable. Laboratory testing shows a leukocyte count of 2800 cells/mm^3 with 78% polymorphonuclear cells, 15% lymphocytes, and 7% eosinophils. The serum LDH (lactic [acid] dehydrogenase) is 540 IU/L. His chest radiograph is shown in Figure 7–1.

- **What is the most likely diagnosis?**
- **What is your next step?**
- **What other diagnoses should be considered?**

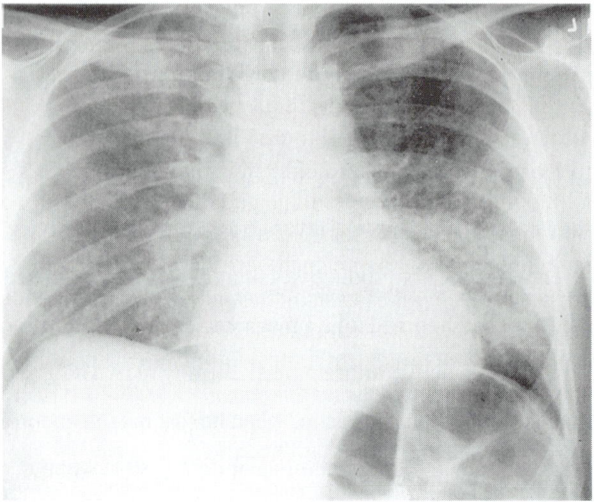

Figure 7–1. Chest radiograph. **(Reproduced with permission from Walzer P. Pneumocystis carinii infecion. In: Braunwald E, Fauci AS, Kasper KL, et al., eds. Harrison's Principles of Internal Medicine, 15th ed. New York: McGraw-Hill, 2001:1183.)**

ANSWERS TO CASE 7: HIV and Pneumocystis Pneumonia

Summary: A 32-year-old man with known HIV infection but unknown CD4 count presents with a subacute onset of fever, dry cough, and gradually worsening dyspnea. He is not taking any antiretroviral therapy or prophylactic medications. Diffuse bilateral pulmonary infiltrate is seen on chest x-ray, and he is tachypneic and hypoxemic. The presence of oral thrush suggests that he is immunosuppressed. His leukocyte count is 2800 cells/mm^3 and his LDH level is 540 IU/L.

- **Most likely diagnosis:** AIDS and probable PCP (*Pneumocystis carinii* pneumonia).*
- **Next step:** The next step is to stabilize the patient, who is tachypneic and hypoxic, but only in mild distress and hemodynamically stable. Therefore, there is time to further evaluate him. An arterial blood gas measurement can be done to quantify his degree of hypoxemia, as it will impact the treatment.
- **What other diagnoses must be considered?** In patients with AIDS, other opportunistic infections must be considered. Other respiratory

* As of 2002, the organism has been renamed *Pneumocystis jiroveci*. The abbreviation PCP remains for *Pneumocystis pneumonia*.

infections such as tuberculosis, atypical mycobacteria, cryptococcosis, disseminated histoplasmosis must be considered. In addition, HIV-infected patients are also susceptible to the usual causes of community-acquired pneumonias: streptococcus pneumonia, mycoplasma, and viruses such as influenza.

Analysis

Objectives

1. Understand the natural history of HIV infection.
2. Know the types of opportunistic infections that typically affect HIV-infected patients at various levels of immunocompromise.
3. Be familiar with respiratory infections in patients with AIDS.
4. Be familiar with indications for antiretroviral therapy and for prophylactic medications against opportunistic infections.

Considerations

This individual with HIV, currently not on antiviral medication, presents with subacute dyspnea and cough. His lack of sputum production and **elevated LDH** is suggestive of *Pneumocystis carinii* pneumonia (PCP). The presence of oral thrush suggests a CD4 count of less than 250. If it is less than 200, then PCP seems the most likely explanation of his symptoms and chest x-ray findings. The PO_2 (partial pressure of oxygen) level by arterial blood gas gives information about prognosis and therapy. Arterial oxygen concentration <70 torr or A-a (alveolar-arterial) gradient >35 mmHg suggests a worse prognosis and preantibiotic steroids may be helpful. In our patient, the oxygen saturations by pulse oximetry are 89%, and oxygen desaturation with minimal exertion are hallmarks of PCP. He is quite tachypneic. He therefore is likely to have a respiratory alkalosis, and the low pCO_2 (partial pressure of carbon dioxide) will result in an increased A-a gradient. He may benefit from steroid therapy followed by trimethoprim-sulfamethoxazole treatment.

Clinical Approach

In evaluating a patient with HIV and suspected opportunistic infection, it is essential to know or estimate the patient's level of immunodeficiency. This is reflected by the CD4 (T4) cell count. Normal CD4 levels in adults range from 600 to 1500 cells/mm^3. As levels decline below 500/mm^3, immune function is compromised, and patients become increasingly susceptible to unusual infections or malignancies.

Approximately 30% of patients first infected with HIV will develop an **acute HIV syndrome** characterized by a sudden-onset of a mononucleosis-like illness with fever, headaches, lymphadenopathy, pharyngitis, and sometimes a macular rash. The rest remain asymptomatic and have a clinically **latent period** of 8–10 years, on average, before the clinical manifestations of immunocompromise appear. As CD4 levels decline, various opportunistic infections appear. At levels below **500**, patients are susceptible to infections such as recurrent pneumonias, tuberculosis, vaginal candidiasis, or herpes zoster. At levels below **200**, patients are significantly immunocompromised and develop infections with organisms that rarely cause significant illness in immunocompetent hosts, such as *Pneumocystis carinii*, toxoplasmosis, cryptococcosis, histoplasmosis or cryptosporidiosis. At levels below **50**, patients are severely immunocompromised and are susceptible to disseminated infection with histoplasmosis, *Mycobacterium avium-intracellulare* complex (MAC), as well as development of cytomegalovirus (CMV) retinitis colitis, or esophagitis, or primary CNS lymphoma.

PCP is the **most common opportunistic infection affecting AIDS patients**, but is often very difficult to diagnose. The clinical presentation ranges from fever without respiratory symptoms, to mild, persistent, **dry cough**, to significant hypoxemia and respiratory compromise. In addition, the radiographic presentation can be highly variable, ranging from a near-normal chest film to a diffuse bilateral infiltrate, to large cysts or blebs (but almost never causes pleural effusion). The blebs can rupture causing spontaneous pneumothorax. PCP is often diagnosed presumptively when patients present with a subacute onset of fever and respiratory symptoms. **Definitive diagnosis can be established by use of Giemsa or silver stain** to visualize the cysts, but usually requires induction of sputum using aerolized hypertonic saline to induce cough, or bronchoalveolar lavage to obtain a diagnostic specimen. **Elevated LDH** is often used as an indirect marker for PCP, although it is nonspecific, and may also be elevated in disseminated histoplasmosis or lymphoma. It is useful as a negative predictor, because **patients with an LDH <220 IU/L are very unlikely to have PCP**. Similarly, if patients have a CD4 count greater than 250/mm^3, or if they were taking PCP prophylaxis with trimethoprim-sulfamethoxasole, the diagnosis of PCP should be considered highly unlikely.

The level of oxygenation of PCP patients by arterial blood gas is useful because it may affect prognosis and therapy. **Patients with an arterial PO_2 <70 mmHg, or an alveolar-arterial gradient >35 mmHg,** have significant disease and have an **improved prognosis** if **prednisone is given during antimicrobial therapy**. After prednisone is given to patients with hypoxia, the usual treatment for PCP is trimethoprim-sulfamethoxazole (TMP-SMX). Patients who are allergic to sulfa may be treated with alternative regimens, including pentamidine or clindamycin with primaquine.

Many other respiratory infectious are possible and should be considered in patients with AIDS. Diagnosis can be suggested by chest radiography. Diffuse interstitial infiltrates are seen with PCP, disseminated histoplasmosis, *M. tuberculosis,* and *M. kansasii.* Patchy infiltrates and pleural-based infiltrates can be seen with tuberculosis and cryptococcal lung disease. Cavitary lesions can be seen with TB, PCP, and coccidiomycosis. Clinical history should also be considered. Because the **most common cause of pneumonia in AIDS**

patients are the same organisms that cause pneumonia in immunocompetent hosts, an acute onset of fever and productive cough, with a pulmonary infiltrate, is most consistent with **community-acquired pneumonia.** A more indolent or chronic history of cough, weight loss, especially in a patient who has a high-risk background (prison, homeless, immigrant) should raise the question of **tuberculosis.** In patients with CD4 >200, the radiographic appearance of TB is likely to be similar to that of other hosts, for example, bilateral apical infiltrate with cavitation; in those with CD4 <200, the radiographic appearance is extremely variable. Because tuberculosis involves both the alveoli and the pulmonary circulation, it is rare for patients with TB to be hypoxic with minimal infiltrate on chest x-ray (although this is relatively common in PCP). Patients with suspected pulmonary TB should be placed in respiratory isolation until it is assured they are not spreading airborne tuberculous infection. Diagnosis and treatment of TB is discussed in Chapter 31. In HIV patients, ***M. kansasii*** can cause identical pulmonary disease and radiographic findings as *M. tuberculosis.*

Several other opportunistic infections in AIDS also deserve mention. **Cerebral toxoplasmosis** is the **most common CNS mass lesion in HIV patients**. It typically presents with headache, seizures, or focal neurologic deficits, and is seen on CT or MRI scanning, usually as multiple enhancing lesions, often located in the basal ganglia. Presumptive diagnosis is often made based on the radiologic appearance, supported by serologic evidence of infection. The major alternative diagnosis for CNS mass lesions is **CNS lymphoma.** This diagnosis is considered if there is a single mass lesion, or if it the lesions do not regress after 2 weeks of empiric toxoplasmosis therapy with sulfadiazine with pyrimethamine. If this is the case, historically, the next diagnostic step has been stereotactic brain biopsy. However, recent evidence indicates that examination of the cerebrospinal fluid (CSF) for **Epstein-Barr virus DNA** is a useful strategy, because it is present in >90% of cases of patients with **CNS lymphoma**.

Another CNS complication that requires a high index of suspicion is **cryptococcal meningitis.** It is a chronic indolent infection, which often presents with vague symptoms of mood or personality changes, headaches, or visual disturbance. If the diagnosis is considered, one can screen for evidence of cryptococcal infection by a serum cryptococcal antigen, or perform a lumbar puncture. CSF frequently shows a lack of inflammatory response (i.e., normal white blood cell [WBC] count), but often presents with elevated intracranial pressures. Diagnosis can be confirmed by seeing the yeast by India ink stain, by fungal culture, or by measuring the level of cryptococcal antigen from CSF. Treatment of cryptococcal meningitis requires induction with intravenous amphotericin B plus flucytosine, then chronic suppression with oral fluconazole. At times, frequent lumbar punctures with removal of large volumes of CSF are required to treat the intracranial hypertension, and CSF shunts may be required.

At very low CD4 counts ($<50/mm^3$), patients with AIDS are also susceptible to **CMV** infections. This can be manifested as viremia with persistent fever and constitutional symptoms, retinitis that can lead to blindness, esophagitis that can cause severe odynophagia, colitis, and necrotizing adrenalitis, which occasionally destroys sufficient adrenal tissue to produce clinical adrenal insufficiency. Therapy for severe CMV infections includes intravenous ganciclovir, foscarnet or cidofovir.

Mycobacterium avium-intracellulare complex (MAC) is one of the most frequent opportunistic infections in patients with very low CD4 counts. The most frequent presentations are disseminated infection with persistent fevers, weight loss, and constitutional symptoms, as well as GI symptoms such as abdominal pain or chronic watery diarrhea. It is often diagnosed by obtaining a mycobacterial blood culture. Treatment with clarithromycin and ethambutol and rifabutin is required for weeks to try to clear the bacteremia.

Because of the frequency and severity of common opportunistic infections, **antimicrobial prophylaxis** is routinely given as a patient's immune status declines. With CD4 counts $<200/mm^3$, PCP prophylaxis should be given as one double-strength tablet of TMP-SMX three times a week. When counts fall below $100/mm^3$ and patients have a positive toxoplasma serology, toxoplasmosis can be prevented by increasing the dosing of the TMP-SMX to daily. If CD4 levels are below $50/mm^3$, MAC prophylaxis consists of clarithromycin 500 mg daily or azithromycin 1200 mg weekly. Prophylaxis can be discontinued if highly active antiretroviral therapy (HAART) is started and the patient's CD 4 levels recover.

HAART therapy includes a combination at least 3 drugs consisting of nucleoside analog or nonnucleoside analog reverse transcriptase inhibitors, or protease inhibitors. Recently, a new medication to inhibit fusion of the HIV virus with target CD4 cells has gained FDA approval. HAART therapy is very potent and has dramatically revolutionized treatment of HIV patients, producing suppression of viral replication and allowing a patient's CD4 count to recover. However, initiation of HAART is not likely practical in acutely ill patients, because the medications are not easy to take and often cause side effects that can be confused with the underlying disease process. Additionally, within 1–2 weeks of starting HAART, improvement in the immune system can actually cause worsening symptoms as a result of host responses, termed the "immune reconstitution syndrome." It is, therefore, better to wait until the acute illness has resolved, and initiate antiretroviral therapy after the patient has recovered, in consultation with an infectious diseases expert, when reliable followup has been assured.

Comprehension Questions

[7.1] A 32-year-old woman with a 5-year history of HIV infection is noted to have a CD4 count of 100 cells/mm^3. She is admitted to the hospital with a 2-week history of fever, shortness of breath, and a dry cough. Which of the following diagnostic tests would most likely confirm the diagnosis?

A. Silver stain of the sputum
B. Gram stain of the sputum showing Gram-positive diplococci

C. Acid-fast smear of the sputum
D. Nitrogen diffusion test

[7.2] Which of the following is the most likely organism to cause pneumonia in a patient with AIDS?

A. *Pneumocystis carinii*
B. Mycobacterium tuberculosis
C. Histoplasmosis capsulatum
D. Streptococcus pneumoniae

[7.3] A 44-year-old woman infected with HIV is noted to have a CD4 count of 180 cells/mm^3. Which of the following is recommended as a useful prophylactic agent in this patient at this point?

A. Fluconazole
B. Azithromycin
C. Trimethoprim-sulfamethoxazole
D. Ganciclovir

[7.4] A 36-year-old woman with HIV is admitted with new-onset seizures. A CT of the head reveals multiple enhancing lesions of the brain. Which of the following is the best therapy for the likely condition?

A. Rifampin, isoniazid, ethambutol
B. Ganciclovir
C. Penicillin
D. Sulfadiazine with pyrimethamine

Answers

[7.1] **A.** This clinical history is consistent with PCP, which is diagnosed by silver stain of the sputum.

[7.2] **D.** The same organisms that cause community-acquired pneumonia in immunocompetent individuals are causative in HIV patients. Additionally, HIV patients are susceptible to other opportunistic infections such as *Pneumocystis*.

[7.3] **C.** When the CD4 count falls below 200 cells/mm^3, trimethoprim-sulfamethoxazole (Bactrim) prophylaxis is generally initiated to prevent PCP. Prophylaxis against *Mycobacterium avium-intracellulare* complex is usually started when the CD4 count is <50 cells/mm^3, and toxoplasmosis prophylaxis is usually started when the CD4 count is <100 cells/mm^3.

[7.4] **D.** The most common cause of a mass lesion of the brain in an HIV patient is toxoplasmosis, which is treated with sulfadiazine with pyrimethamine.

CLINICAL PEARLS

- *Pneumocystis carinii* pneumonia typically has a subacute presentation with fever and a dry cough, almost always in patients with a CD4 count of less than 200. It often has a diffuse bilateral infiltrate on chest x-ray and an elevated serum LDH.
- Pulmonary tuberculosis should always be considered in AIDS patients with respiratory symptoms and suggestive history; its radiographic presentation may be atypical.
- The most common causes of pneumonia in AIDS patients are the same as in immunocompetent patients, that is, community-acquired organisms such as Streptococcus pneumoniae.
- In patients with CD4 counts less than 200, TMP-SMX (Bactrim) prophylaxis is effective in preventing PCP, and in preventing toxoplasmosis when the CD4 count is <100. With a CD4 count of <50, clarithromycin or azithromycin can prevent MAC.
- HAART is effective in reducing viral replication and increasing CD4 counts, and restoring immunocompetence, but generally should not be initiated during an acute illness.

REFERENCES

Fauci AS, Lane HC. HIV Disease: AIDS and Related Disorders. In: Braunwald E, Fauci AS, Kasper KL, et al., eds. Harrison's principles of internal medicine, 15th ed. New York: McGraw-Hill, 2001:1852–913.

Walzer P. Pneumocystis carinii infection. In: Braunwald E, Fauci AS, Kasper KL, et al., eds. Harrison's Principles of Internal Medicine. 15th ed. New York: McGraw-Hill, 2001:1182-1185.

Huan L, Stansell JP. Pneumocystis carinii pneumonia. In: Sande MA, Volberding PA, eds. The Medical management of AIDS, 6th ed. Philadelphia: WB Saunders, 1999:305-330.

CASE 8

A 58-year-old man presents to the emergency room complaining of severe pain in his left foot that woke him from sleep. He has a prior history of chronic stable angina, hypercholesterolemia, and hypertension, for which he takes aspirin and atenolol. He has had pain in both calves and feet with walking for several years, which has gradually progressed so that he can now only walk 100 feet before he has to stop because of pain. He occasionally has had mild pain in his feet at night, but it usually gets better when he sits up and hangs his feet off the bed. This time, the pain was more severe, did not improve, and he now feels like the foot is numb and he cannot move his toes.

On physical examination, he is afebrile, his heart rate is 72 bpm, and his blood pressure is 125/74 mmHg. His head and neck examination is significant for a right carotid bruit. His chest is clear to auscultation; his heart is regular with a nondisplaced apical impulse, an S4 gallop, and no murmurs. His abdomen is benign, with no tenderness or masses. He has bilateral femoral bruits, and palpable femoral and popliteal pulses bilaterally, with the left popliteal more pronounced than the right. His pedal pulses are diminished but present on the right, but absent on the left, and the left distal leg and foot are pale and cold to touch, with very slow capillary refill.

- **What is the most likely diagnosis?**

- **What is your next step?**

ANSWER TO CASE 8: Limb Ischemia (Peripheral Vascular Disease)

Summary: A 58-year-old man presents to the emergency room with severe pain and numbness of his left foot. He has angina, hypertension, hypercholesterolemia, and a carotid bruit. He has had symptoms previously of left calf pain with exertion, but now has a sudden onset of pain, pallor, and pulselessness. His pulses are absent distal to the left popliteal artery, but that popliteal artery pulse is bounding.

- **Most likely diagnosis:** Acute limb ischemia, possibly thrombotic arterial occlusive vascular disease.
- **Next step:** Angiogram of the lower extremity.

Analysis

Objectives

1. Understand the clinical presentation of a patient with atherosclerotic peripheral vascular disease, including acute limb ischemia.
2. Know the evaluation and the medical management of peripheral vascular disease.
3. Understand the indications for extremity revascularization.

Considerations

This patient has diffuse atherosclerotic vascular disease including coronary artery disease, carotid disease, and peripheral vascular disease. His **history of calf pain with walking, but resolution with rest, is classic for claudication**. Recently, the perfusion of his left leg was likely worsening, requiring his waking up and dangling his leg to enable blood flow and to help the pain. **Rest pain is a warning sign of possible critical limb vascular insufficiency.** The patient complains of a sudden onset of **pain, pallor, and pulselessness**, indicative of acute arterial occlusion. His limb ischemia may result from acute arterial occlusion caused by emboli, usually arising from a dislodged thrombus from the heart, or a previously diseased vessel. Depending on the level of occlusion, the patient may require urgent arterial thromboembolectomy, or possibly arteriography, to first determine the arterial anatomy and define the best mode of revascularization.

APPROACH TO PERIPHERAL VASCULAR DISEASE

Definitions

Ankle-Brachial Index (ABI): Ratio of ankle to brachial systolic blood pressure using Doppler ultrasound flow.

Claudication syndrome: Calf pain that increases with walking or leg exertion in a predictable manner, and resolves with rest.

Clinical Approach

While atherosclerosis is a systemic disease, clinicians often focus on the coronary circulation, and are less attentive to the extremities. Yet atherosclerotic peripheral arterial disease (PAD) is estimated to affect up to 16% of Americans aged 55 years or older, and may exist without clinically recognized coronary or cerebrovascular disease. Furthermore, PAD confers the same risk of cardiovascular death as persons with a prior myocardial infarction or stroke. **The most important risk factors** for peripheral arterial disease are **cigarette smoking and diabetes** mellitus. Hypertension, dyslipidemia, and elevated levels of homocysteine are also play significant roles.

Diagnosis The most common symptom associated with chronic arterial insufficiency caused by PAD is **intermittent claudication,** characterized by pain, ache, a sense of fatigue, or other discomfort that occurs in one or both leg during exercise, such as walking, and is relieved with rest. It is ischemic pain, and occurs distal to the site of the arterial stenosis, most commonly in the calves. The symptoms are often progressive, and may severely limit a patient's activities and reduce the patient's functional status. An individual with proximal stenosis, such as aortoiliac disease, may complain of exertional pain in the buttocks and thighs. Severe occlusion may produce **rest pain**, which often occurs at night, and may be relieved by sitting up and dangling the legs, using gravity to assist blood flow to the feet.

On physical examination, palpation of the **peripheral pulses may be diminished** or absent below the level of occlusion; **bruits** may indicate accelerated blood flow velocity and turbulence at the sites of stenosis. Bruits may be heard in the abdomen with aortoiliac stenosis, and in the groin with femoral artery stenosis. **Elevation of the feet** above the level of the heart in the supine patient often induces **pallor in the soles**. If the legs are then placed in the dependent position, they frequently develop rubor as a result of reactive hyperemia. Chronic arterial insufficiency may cause **hair loss on the legs and feet**, thickened and brittle toenails, and shiny atrophic skin, and severe ischemia may produce ulcers or gangrene.

When PAD is suspected, the most commonly used test to evaluate for arterial insufficiency is the **ankle-brachial index (ABI).** Systolic blood pressures are measured by Doppler ultrasonography in each arm, and in the dorsalis pedis and posterior tibial arteries in each ankle. Normally, blood pressures in the large arteries of the legs and arms are similar. In fact, blood pressures in the legs are often higher than the arms because of an artifact of measurement, so the normal ratio of ankle to brachial pressures is >1.0. Patients with claudication typically have ankle–brachial index values ranging from 0.41 to 0.90, and those with critical leg ischemia have values of 0.40 or less. Further evaluation with exercise treadmill testing can clarify the diagnosis when symptoms are equivocal, can allow for assessment of functional limitations (e.g., maximal walking distance), and can also evaluate for concomitant coronary artery disease.

Management The goals of therapy include a reduction in cardiovascular morbidity and mortality, improvement in quality of life by decreasing symptoms of claudication and eliminating rest pain, and preserving limb viability.

The first step in managing patients with PAD is risk factor modification. Because of the likelihood of coexisting atherosclerotic vascular disease, patients with **symptomatic PVD** have an estimated **mortality** rate of **50% in 10 years**, most often as a consequence of cardiovascular events. **Smoking cessation** is, by far, the **single most important risk factor** impacting both claudication symptoms and overall cardiovascular mortality. Besides slowing the progression to critical leg ischemia, **tobacco cessation reduces the risk of fatal or nonfatal myocardial infarction by as much as 50%,** more than any other medical or surgical intervention. In addition, treatment of hypercholesterolemia, control of hypertension and diabetes, and use of antiplatelet agents such as aspirin or clopidogrel have all been shown to improve cardiovascular health, and may have an effect on peripheral arterial circulation. Carefully supervised exercise programs can improve muscle strength and prolong walking distance.

Specific medications to improve claudication symptoms have been used, with some benefit. Pentoxyphylline, a substituted xanthine derivative that increases erythrocyte elasticity, has been reported to decrease blood viscosity to allow improved blood flow to the microcirculation; however, results from clinical trials are conflicting and its benefit, if present, appears small. A newer agent, cilostazol, a phosphodiesterase inhibitor with vasodilatory and antiplatelet properties, has been approved by the FDA for treatment of claudication. It is a has been shown in randomized controlled trials to improve maximal walking distance. See Figure 8–1 for a management algorithm.

Patients with **critical leg ischemia**, defined as having an **ABI <0.40, severe or disabling claudication**, **rest pain**, or **nonhealing ulcers**, should be **evaluated for a revascularization procedure**. This may be accomplished by percutaneous angioplasty, with or without placement of intraarterial stents, or surgical bypass grafting. Angiography (either conventional or magnetic resonance arteriography) should be performed to define the flow-limiting lesions prior to any vascular procedure. Ideal candidates for arterial revascularization are those with discrete stenosis of large vessels, while diffuse atherosclerotic and small vessel disease respond poorly.

Less-common causes of chronic peripheral arterial insufficiency include thromboangiitis obliterans, or **Buerger disease,** which is an inflammatory condition of small and medium-size arteries, which may affect upper or lower extremities, and is found almost exclusively in smokers, especially males younger than age 40 years. **Fibromuscular dysplasia** is a hyperplastic disorder **affecting medium and small arteries that usually affects women;** generally, the renal or carotid arteries are involved, but when the arteries to the limbs are affected, the clinical symptoms identical to atherosclerotic peripheral arterial disease (PAD). **Takayasu arteritis** is an inflammatory condition seen primarily in younger women that usually affects branches of the aorta, most commonly the subclavian arteries, and causes **arm claudication and**

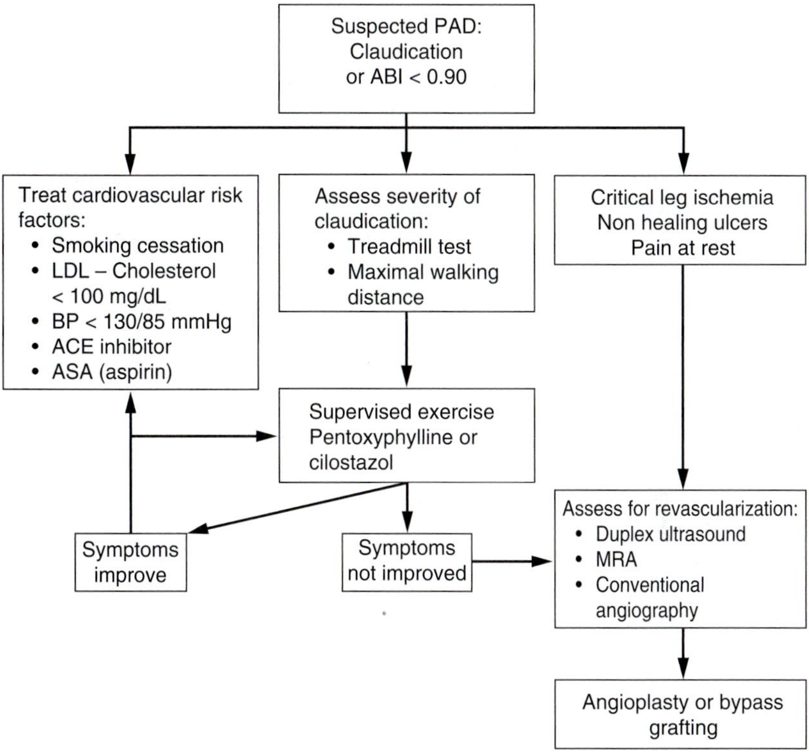

Figure 8–1. Management algorithm of peripheral arterial disease. **(Adapted from Hiatt W. Medical treatment of peripheral arterial disease and claudication. N Engl J Med 2001;344(21):1608–21.)**

Raynaud phenomenon, along with constitutional symptoms such as **fever** and **weight loss**.

Patients with chronic peripheral arterial insufficiency who present with sudden unremitting pain may have an **acute arterial occlusion,** most commonly a result of **embolism** or **in situ thrombosis**. **The heart is the most common source of emboli**; conditions that may cause cardiogenic emboli include atrial fibrillation, dilated cardiomyopathy, or endocarditis. Artery-to-artery embolization of atherosclerotic debris from the aorta or large vessels may occur spontaneously, or, more often, after an intravascular procedure, such as arterial catheterization. Emboli tend to lodge at the bifurcation of two vessels, most often in the femoral, iliac, popliteal, or tibioperoneal arteries. Arterial thrombosis may occur in atherosclerotic vessels at the site of stenosis, or in an area of aneurysmal dilatation, which may also complicate atherosclerotic disease.

When patients have acute arterial occlusion, they may present with a number of signs, which can be remembered as **"six P's:" pain, pallor, pulselessness, paresthesias, poikilothermia (coolness), and paralysis.** The first five signs occur fairly quickly with acute ischemia; paralysis will develop if the arterial occlusion is severe and persistent.

Rapid restoration of arterial supply is mandatory in patients with an **acute arterial occlusion that threatens limb viability**. Initial management includes anticoagulation with heparin to prevent propagation of the thrombus. The affected limb should be placed below the horizontal plane without any pressure applied to it. Conventional arteriography is usually indicated to identify the location of the occlusion and to evaluate potential methods of revascularization. Surgical removal of an embolus or arterial bypass may be performed, particularly if a large proximal artery is occluded. A balloon catheter may also be attempted to try removing the clot Alternatively, a catheter can be used to deliver intraarterial thrombolytic therapy directly into the thrombus. In comparison with systemic fibrinolytic therapy, localized infusion is associated with fewer bleeding complications.

Comprehension Questions

[8.1] A 49-year-old smoker with hypertension, diabetes, and hypercholesterolemia comes to the office complaining of pain in his calves when he walks 2–3 blocks. What therapy might offer him the greatest benefit in symptom reduction and in overall mortality?

A. Aspirin
B. Revascularization procedure
C. Ramipril
D. Smoking cessation
E. Pravastatin

Match the most likely cause (A-E) of arterial insufficiency to the patient described [8.2–8.4]:

A. Cholesterol embolism
B. Fibromuscular dysplasia
C. Thromboangiitis obliterans (Buerger disease)
D. Takayasu aortitis
E. Psychogenic pain

[8.2] A 31-year-old male smoker with resting pain in his legs and a nonhealing foot ulcer.

[8.3] A 21-year-old woman with fever, fatigue, and unequal pulses and blood pressures in her arms.

[8.4] A 62-year-old man with livido reticularis, three blue toes, including one with gangrene following cardiac catheterization.

Answers

[8.1] **D.** Tobacco cessation is the most important intervention to improve cardiovascular morbidity and mortality in high-risk patients such as those with PAD, and to improve claudication symptoms. Bupropion is an antidepressant medication that reduces nicotine craving and is a useful adjunct to smoking cessation efforts. Cilostazol may help with claudication symptoms, but will not affect cardiovascular mortality. The use of aspirin, ACE inhibitors, and HMG-CoA (beta-hydroxy-beta-methylglutaryl-coenzyme A) reductase inhibitors are important adjuncts for risk factor modification, and for symptoms relief, but their benefits pale in comparison to smoking cessation.

[8.2] **C.** Thromboangiitis obliterans, or Buerger disease, is a disease of young male smokers, and may cause symptoms of chronic arterial insufficiency in either legs or arms.

[8.3] **D.** Takayasu aortitis is associated with symptoms of inflammation such as fever, and most often affects the subclavian arteries, producing stenotic lesions that may cause unequal blood pressures, diminished pulses, and ischemic pain in the affected limbs.

[8.4] **A.** Embolism of cholesterol and other atherosclerotic debris from the aorta or other large vessels to small vessels of skin or digits may complicate any intraarterial procedure.

CLINICAL PEARLS

❖ Smoking cessation is the single most important intervention for atherosclerotic peripheral vascular disease. Other treatments include pentoxifylline or cilostazol, regular exercise, and cardiovascular risk factor modification.

❖ Revascularization by angioplasty or bypass grafting may be indicated for patients with debilitating claudication, ischemic rest pain, or tissue necrosis.

❖ Acute arterial occlusion that threatens limb viability is a medical emergency.

❖ Acute severe ischemia of an extremity causes the "six Ps": *pain, pallor, pulselessness, paresthesias, poikilothermia,* and *paralysis.* Chronic incomplete arterial occlusion may result only in exertional pain or fatigue, pallor on elevation of the extremity, and rubor on dependency.

REFERENCES

Creager M, Dzau VJ. Vascular disease of the extremities. In: Braunwald E, Fauci AS, Kasper DL, et al. Harrison's principles of internal medicine, 15th ed. New York: McGraw-Hill, 2001:1434–1438.

Hiatt W. Medical treatment of peripheral arterial disease and claudication. N Engl J Med 2001:344(21):1608–1621.

CASE 9

A 56-year-old man comes into your office as a new patient. Seven years ago at a work-related health screening, he was diagnosed with hypertension and hypercholesterolemia. At that time, he saw a physician who prescribed a diuretic and encouraged him to lose some weight with diet and exercise. Since that time, the patient has not sought medical attention. During the past 2 months, he has been experiencing occasional headaches, which he attributes to increased stress at work. He denies chest pain, shortness of breath, dyspnea on exertion, or paroxysmal nocturnal dyspnea. He smokes one pack of cigarettes per day and has done so since he was 15 years old. He typically drinks two glasses of wine with dinner. His father was diagnosed with heart disease in his early fifties and underwent coronary artery bypass surgery at age 76 years. On examination, the patient is obese, you calculate his body mass index (BMI) as 30 kg/m^2. His blood pressure is 190/100 mmHg (right arm) and 192/100 mmHg (left arm). His blood pressure did not change with changes in position. His heart rate is 84 bpm. There is a right carotid bruit present. He has no thyromegaly or lymphadenopathy. The funduscopic examination reveals narrowing of the arteries, arteriovenous *nicking,* and flame-shaped hemorrhages with cotton wool exudates. The cardiac examination reveals that his point of maximal impulse (PMI) is displaced 2 cm left of the midclavicular line. There is an S4 gallop. No murmurs are auscultated. The lung and abdomen examinations are normal. The extremities show diminished dorsalis pedis and posterior tibialis pulses. There is no clubbing, cyanosis, or edema.

What are your next steps?

ANSWER TO CASE 9: Hypertension, Outpatient

Summary: A 56-year-old hypertensive male is being evaluated as a new patient. Seven years ago he was diagnosed with hypertension and hypercholesterolemia, with no followup since. He has had occasional headaches for 2 months, but denies chest pain or symptoms of heart failure. He smokes one pack of cigarettes per day and drinks two glasses of wine a day. His father was diagnosed with heart disease. He is obese. His blood pressures are in the range of 190/100 mmHg. The funduscopic examination reveals hypertensive retinopathy. His PMI is displaced laterally, suggesting cardiomegaly, and there is a fourth heart sound, consistent with a thickened, noncompliant ventricle. In addition, he has multiple cardiovascular risk factors, including his age, obesity, smoking, a family history of heart disease, and his carotid bruit and diminished pedal pulses suggest he may already have diffuse arterial atherosclerosis.

◆ **Next steps:** (a) Measurement of serum glucose, creatinine (or an estimate of the glomerular filtration rate), calcium, fasting lipid profile that includes high-density lipoprotein (HDL), low-density lipoprotein (LDL), and triglycerides, urinalysis, and electrocardiogram. (b) Start the patient on a two-drug antihypertensive regimen that includes a thiazide diuretic. (c) Recommend life-style changes, most importantly tobacco cessation.

Analysis

Objectives

1. Know the risk factors for cardiovascular disease.
2. Understand how treatment decisions are made in the management of hypertension.
3. Be familiar with the various causes of secondary hypertension and when to pursue these diagnoses.

Considerations

This is a 56-year-old male with severe hypertension, who has evidence, on physical examination, of hypertensive end-organ damage, that is, hypertensive retinopathy and left ventricular hypertrophy. In addition, he has multiple risk factors for atherosclerotic disease, and may already have developed carotid and peripheral arterial disease. The most likely diagnosis is essential hypertension, but secondary causes still need to be considered. Although many of the end-organ effects are apparent, a thorough evaluation for other modifiable risk factors for coronary artery disease is fundamental. Lifestyle modification, including smoking cessation, diet, weight loss, and aerobic exercise, cannot be overemphasized in conjunction with pharmacological therapy. If we specifically look at our patient, we realize that he already has risk factors for cardiovascular disease: he is a smoker; he is known to have both hypertension and high cholesterol; and he has a positive family history of heart disease. As previously stated, he also has indications of end-organ damage, and although you have only measured his BP once in your office, he has been told before that he is hypertensive. His blood pressure is above 160/100 mmHg, which places him in **stage 2 hypertension, which warrants starting him on two-drug therapy without further delay**. One of the drugs should be a thiazide diuretic.

APPROACH TO HYPERTENSION

Definitions

Essential hypertension: Also known as idiopathic or primary hypertension. It has no known cause, yet comprises approximately 95% of all cases of hypertension.

Lifestyle modification: A cornerstone in the treatment of hypertension, consisting of regular aerobic activity, weight loss, decreased salt intake, and an increase in the amount of fruit and vegetables, while decreasing the amount of total fat, especially saturated fat, in the diet. Alcohol consumption should also be moderated, no more than two glasses of wine a day for men and one glass a day for women.

Secondary hypertension: Elevated arterial blood pressure with a known underlying cause, such as renal artery stenosis or primary aldosteronism. Prevalence is approximately 5–6% of all cases of hypertension.

Clinical Approach

The Initial Evaluation and Management. Stage I hypertension is generally diagnosed by two or more blood pressures exceeding or equal to 140 mmHg systolic and/or 90 mmHg diastolic at two separate visits after the initial screening. Prehypertension is defined as blood pressures between 120 and 139 mmHg systolic or 80 and 89 mmHg diastolic (see Table 9–1). Essential or idiopathic hypertension is the most common form of hypertension, comprising 92–95% of cases, but approximately 5–7% of cases of hypertension are caused by secondary causes (see Table 9–2). To identify the secondary (and potentially reversible) causes of hypertension, the clinician must be aware of the clinical and laboratory manifestations of the processes. A secondary cause of hypertension, and thus, more extensive testing is indicated when patients have any of the following clinical features: age of onset before 25 years or after 55 years, presenting with malignant hypertension, requiring 3 or more anti-hypertensive medications, hypertension that has suddenly become uncontrolled, a rising creatinine level with the use of ACE inhibitors, or overt clinical signs of a secondary cause. (see Table 9–3)

Other Cardiac Risk Factors and Evaluation for Target Organ Damage Cardiac risk evaluation and treatment is extremely important to establish prognosis, identify organ dysfunction, and dictate therapy. Cardiovascular risk fac-

Table 9–1

CLASSIFICATION AND MANAGEMENT OF HYPERTENSION*

BP CLASSIFICATION	SYSTOLIC BP mmHg	DIASTOLIC BP mmHg	LIFESTYLE MODIFICATIONS	INITIAL DRUG THERAPY
Normal	<120	<80	Advised	None
Prehypertensive	120–139	80–89	Yes	No antihypertensive indicated; give drugs for any compelling indication.
Stage I hypertension	140–159	90–99	Yes	Thiazide diuretic for most; may need other drugs; choice depends upon other medical diagnoses.
Stage II hypertension	≥ 160	≥ 100	Yes	Two-drug combination will be needed by most patients; at least one drug should be a thiazide diuretic.

*For all stages of hypertension, prehypertension to stage II, either the systolic or the diastolic blood pressure elevation may be diagnostic.

(Reproduced with permission from Chobanian AV, Bakris GL, Black HR et al. The Seventh Report of the Joint National Committee on Prevention, Detection, Evaluation and Treatment of High Blood Pressure; 289(19): 2561)

Table 9–2
SECONDARY CAUSES OF HYPERTENSION

Renal diseases
- Parenchymal (Glomerulonephritis, polycystic renal disease, diabetic nephropathy)
- **Renovascular**

Endocrine
- Primary aldosteronism
- Cushing syndrome
- Pheochromocytoma
- Hyperthyroidism
- Growth hormone excess (acromegaly)
- Oral contraceptives

Miscellaneous
- Coarctation of the aorta
- Increased intravascular volume (posttransfusion)
- Hypercalcemia
- Medications (sympathomimetics, glucocorticoids)

Table 9-3
CLUES TO RENOVASCULAR HYPERTENSION*

Epigastric or flank bruits

Accelerated or malignant hypertension

Severe hypertension in individuals younger than age 25 years or older than age 55 years

Sudden development or worsening of hypertension at any age

Hypertension with unexplained impairment of kidney function

Hypertension refractory to appropriate (three) drug regimen

Extensive occlusive disease in the peripheral circulation

Coronary and cerebral vascular disease

*Renovascular hypertension is the most common cause of secondary hypertension

tors and hypertensive target organ damage should be identified (listed in Table 9–4). The major risk factors of cardiovascular disease are age, cigarette smoking, dyslipidemia, diabetes mellitus, obesity, kidney disease, and a family history of premature cardiovascular disease. Target organ damage includes the heart, brain, kidneys, peripheral arteries, and eyes. Although treatment decisions in the management of hypertension depend more upon the level of the blood pressure (modified perhaps in the presence of diabetes mellitus), the presence of other cardiovascular risk factors and/or evidence of target organ

Table 9–4
CARDIOVASCULAR RISK FACTORS AND TARGET ORGANS

Cardiovascular risk factors (compelling indications)
Smoking
Dyslipidemia (elevated LDL, low HDL)
Diabetes mellitus
Age older than 60 years
Gender (men and postmenopausal women)
Family history of cardiovascular disease
Target organ damage
Heart disease
Left ventricular hypertrophy
Prior myocardial infarction
Angina
Heart failure
Transient ischemic attack or stroke
Nephropathy
Peripheral arterial disease
Retinopathy

damage may further guide therapy and give some prognostic information (see Table 9–4). A complete history and physical exam, including funduscopic examination, auscultation of the major arteries for bruits, palpation of the abdomen for enlarged kidneys, masses, or an enlarged abdominal aorta, evaluation of the lower extremities for edema and perfusion, and a neurological exam should be standard. Some initial laboratory testing is also indicated (see Table 9–5). Counseling patients on lifestyle changes is important at any level of blood pressure and includes weight loss, limitation of alcohol intake, increased aerobic physical activity, reduced sodium intake, cessation of smoking, and reduced intake of dietary saturated fat and cholesterol.

Therapy For most patients, a low dose of the initial drug of choice should be used slowly, titrating upward at a schedule dependent on the patient's age, needs, and responses. The **target blood pressure is typically 135/85 mmHg, unless the patient has diabetes or renal disease, in which the target would be lower than 130/80**. A long-acting formulation that provides 24-hour efficacy is preferred over short-acting agents for better compliance and more consistent blood pressure control. The list of oral and hypertensive drugs is extensive (Table 9–6). Because they are associated **with a decrease in mortality in all types of patients, thiazide diuretics** should be considered in all patients with hypertension (including diabetics) who do not have compelling contraindications to this class of drugs. Both thiazide diuretics and beta-block-

Table9-5

BASIC TESTS FOR INITIAL EVALUATION OF HYPERTENSION

Urine for protein, blood, glucose, and microscopic examination
Hemoglobin or hematocrit; leukocyte count
Serum potassium
Serum calcium and phosphate
Serum creatinine or blood urea nitrogen
Fasting glucose
Total, HDL, and LDL cholesterol; triglycerides
Electrocardiogram
Consider thyroid-stimulating hormone

ers should be used first in uncomplicated hypertension, unless there are specific compelling indications to use other drugs, for example **ACE inhibitors in patients with diabetes or heart failure**. Most patients ultimately need more than one drug to control their blood pressure. It is critical to tailor the treatment to the patient's personal, financial, lifestyle, and medical factors, and to periodically review compliance and adverse effects.

Selected Causes of Secondary Hypertension **The most common cause of secondary hypertension is renal disease (renal parenchymal or renal vascular).** Renal artery stenosis is caused by atherosclerotic disease with hemodynamically significant blockage of the renal artery in older patients (less than 40 years) or by fibromuscular dysplasia in younger adults. Table 9–3 summarizes the clues to renal vascular hypertension. The clinician must have a high index of suspicion, and further testing may be indicated, for instance, in an individual with diffuse atherosclerotic disease. Potassium level may be low or borderline-low in patients with renal artery stenosis caused by secondary hyperaldosteronism. A captopril-enhanced radionuclide renal scan is often helpful in establishing the diagnosis; other diagnostic tools include MR angiography and spiral computed tomography. Surgical or angioplastic correction of the vascular occlusion may be considered.

Pheochromocytoma is a catecholamine-releasing tumor that typically produces hypertension. Approximately 90% of pheochromocytomas arise from the adrenal medulla and 10% from the extra-adrenal sympathetic ganglia. The vast majority of pheochromocytomas release norepinephrine. The clinical manifestations include headaches, palpitations, diaphoresis, and chest pain. Other symptoms include anxiety, nervousness, tremor, pallor, malaise, and, occasionally, nausea and/or vomiting. Symptoms are typically paroxysmal and associated with hypertension. Also, patients with pheochromocytoma may

Table 9-6
PARTIAL LISTING OF ANTIHYPERTENSIVE AGENTS

CATEGORY	AGENT	MECHANISM OF ACTION	SIDE EFFECTS	CONTRAINDICATIONS
Diuretic	Thiazide diuretic	Sodium diuresis, volume depletion, possible lower peripheral vascular resistance	Hypokalemia, carbohydrate intolerance, hyperuricemia, hyperlipidemia	Diabetes mellitus, gout, primary aldosteronism
	Loop diuretic **(furesomide)**		**Hypokalemia**, hyperglycemia, hypocalcemia, rash, hyperuricemia	Gout, primary aldosteronism
	Potassium sparing (spironolactone)	Competitive inhibitor of aldosterone, causing renal sodium loss	**Hyperkalemia**, gynecomastia, diarrhea	Renal failure
Antiadrenergic	Clonidine	Stimulation of alpha-2 vasomotor center of brain	Postural hypotension, drowsiness, dry mouth, **rebound hypertension** with abrupt withdrawal	
	Methyldopa	Similar to clonidine	Postural hypotension, sedation, fatigue, hemolysis, lupuslike syndrome	Active hepatic disease
	Beta-blocker (cardio-selective agents may have less bronchospasm)	Block sympathetic effect of heart and kidneys (renin)	**Bronchospasm**, heart failure, hyperlipidemia, gastrointestinal symptoms, depression	Congestive heart failure, asthma, heart block

	Alpha-beta blocker	Same as beta-blockers and also direct vasodilation	Similar to beta-blockers	Similar to beta-blockers
Vasodilator	Hydralazine	Arterial vasodilation, produces reflex tachcardia	Headache, tachycardia, angina, lupuslike syndrome	Lupus erythematosus, severe coronary artery disease
	Nitroprusside	Direct arterial and venous dilator	Weakness, fatigue, nausea, muscle twitching, **cyanide toxicity**	
ACE inhibitor	Catopril, enalapril, etc.	Inhibit conversion of angiotensin I to angiotensin II (powerful vasoconstrictor)	Leukopenia, pancytopenia, hypotension, **cough**, angioedema, urticarial rash, **hyperkalemia**, acute renal failure	Renal failure, bilateral renal artery stenosis, pregnancy
Angiotension-receptor antagonist	Losartan	Competitive inhibition of the angiotensin II receptor	Similar to ACE inhibitors but no cough or angioedema	Pregnancy, bilateral renal artery stenosis
Calcium-channel antagonist	Dihydropyridines (nifedipine, nicardipine)	Modify calcium transport into cells by interacting with alpha subunit of L-type voltage-dependent calcium channel, causing vasodilation	Tachycardia, flushing, gastro-intestinal side effects, hyperkalemia, **edema**	Heart failure, significant heart block
	Benzothiazpines (diltiazem)	Similar to dihydropyridines	**Heart block**, constipation, liver dysfunction	Heart failure, significant heart block
	Phenylalkylamine (verapamil)	Similar to dihydropyridines	Hypotension, **heart block**, constipation, GI side effects	Heart failure, significant heart block

(Source: Braunwald E, Fuaci AS, Kasper KL, et al. eds., Harrison's 15th ed. Pp1420-24)

have orthostatic hypotension. Thus, in the evaluation of newly diagnosed hypertension, orthostatic blood pressure measurements may be helpful.

Hyperthyroidism presents with symptoms of nervousness, tremor, weight loss usually with increased appetite, palpitations, heat intolerance, excessive perspiration, emotional lability, muscle weakness, and diarrhea. The patient will have a widened pulse pressure with increased systolic blood pressure and decreased diastolic blood pressure, as well as a hyperdynamic precordium. The patient may have warm skin, tremor, and thyroid gland enlargement or other thyroid abnormalities. A low serum thyroid-stimulating hormone (TSH) and elevated thyroid hormones (such as free T4) are diagnostic.

Obstructive sleep apnea is another fairly common cause of hypertension. The definitive event in obstructive sleep apnea is the critical narrowing of the upper airway that occurs when the resistance of the upper airway musculature fails against the negative pressure generated by inspiration. In most patients this is a result of a reduced airway size that is congenital, or perhaps complicated by obesity. Some patients have obvious anatomical defects contributing to the occlusion of the airway. Alcohol, because it decreases arousal, is a common confounding factor. These patients frequently become hypoxic and hypercarbic multiple times during sleep, which, among other things, can eventually lead to systemic vasoconstriction and systolic hypertension, as well as pulmonary hypertension. Usually, the patient will present complaining of excessive daytime sleepiness and perhaps difficulties functioning at work or school. Often, the patient's bed-partner will force him/her to see the doctor, as the patient's noisy attempts to breathe while sleeping can be alarming to observe.

Glucocorticoid excess states, including Cushing syndrome, and iatrogenic (treatment with glucocorticoids) states usually present with weakness, fatigue, thinning of the skin with easy bruising, thinning of the extremities with truncal obesity, round moon face, supraclavicular fat pad, buffalo hump, purple striae, acne, and possible psychiatric symptoms, such as depression, emotional lability, irritability, and headache. An excess of glucocorticoid can cause secondary hypertension because glucocorticoid hormones have mineralocorticoid activity. Dexamethasone suppression testing of the serum cortisol level aids in the diagnosis of Cushing syndrome.

Carcinoid syndrome is caused by the overproduction of serotonin. Carcinoid tumors arise from the enterochromaffin cells located in the gastrointestinal tract and in the lungs. The clinical manifestations include cutaneous flushing, headache, diarrhea, and bronchial construction with wheezing. Carcinoid syndrome is also accompanied by hypertension.

Coarctation of the aorta is a congenital narrowing of the aortic lumen, more commonly seen in males and may be associated with cardiac malformations such as aortic stenosis, ventricular septal defect, and bicuspid aortic valve. It is usually diagnosed in younger patients and most commonly in the pediatric age group by discordant upper and lower extremity blood pressures. Coarctation of the aorta can cause leg claudication, cold extremities, and diminished or absence of femoral pulses as a result of decreased blood pressure in the lower extremities. Other symptoms include throbbing headaches and possible epistaxis as a result of increased blood pressure above the area of coarctation. In more severe cases, collateral arterial vessels may be visible on inspection of the trunk.

Polycystic kidney disease is inherited as an autosomal dominant trait. The classical clinical findings are positive family history of polycystic kidney disease, bilateral flank masses, flank pain, elevated blood pressure, and hematuria. Other causes of chronic renal disease can also lead to hypertension. Other causes of secondary hypertension include **primary hyperaldosteronism,** which will typically cause hypertension and hypokalemia. Anabolic steroids, sympathomimetic drugs, tricyclic antidepressants, nonsteroidal antiinflammatory agents, and illicit drugs such as cocaine, as well as licit ones such as caffeine and tobacco, are also included in possible secondary causes of hypertension.

Comprehension Questions

[9.1] A 30-year-old woman is noted to have blood pressures in the 160/100 mmHg range. She also has increased obesity, especially around her abdomen, with striae. She has been bruising very easily and has hirsutism. Which of the following is the most likely diagnosis?

A. Hyperthyroidism
B. Coarctation of the aorta
C. Cushing syndrome
D. Pheochromocytoma

[9.2] Which of the following would most likely provide prognostic information regarding a hypertensive patient?

A. Vascular biopsy
B. End-organ effects from hypertension such as left ventricular hypertrophy
C. Patient's enrollment in a clinical trial
D. Measurement of serum homocysteine levels

[9.3] Which of the following antihypertensive agents are generally considered first-line agents in uncomplicated hypertension?

A. Thiazide diuretics
B. ACE inhibitors
C. Alpha-blocking agents
D. Nitrates
E. Calcium channel blockers

Answers

[9.1] **C.** The central obesity, abdominal striae, hirsutism, and easy bruisability are consistent with Cushing syndrome, a disease of adrenal steroid overproduction.

[9.2] **B.** Prognosis in hypertension depends on the patient's other cardiovascular risks and observed end-organ effects from the hypertension.

[9.3] **A.** Thiazide diuretics and beta-blockers are generally considered first-line agents for uncomplicated hypertension because of their effect in reducing cardiovascular mortality and their cost-effectiveness.

CLINICAL PEARLS

- ❖ In general, the diagnosis of hypertension requires two or more blood pressure measurements on at least two visits.
- ❖ Cardiovascular disease risk evaluation consists of identifying target organ dysfunction and cardiovascular risk factors, such as diabetes.
- ❖ Most patients with hypertension have essential hypertension, but secondary causes of hypertension should be evaluated when clinically indicated.
- ❖ Renovascular hypertension is the most common cause of secondary hypertension.
- ❖ Atherosclerotic renal artery stenosis may develop in individuals with essential hypertension.
- ❖ Lifestyle modification consisting of dietary, exercise, and stress relief measures are the cornerstone of hypertension control, and lower cardiovascular risk.
- ❖ Consider diuretics and beta-blockers as first-line agents in uncomplicated hypertension, unless there are compelling indications for using other drugs.

REFERENCES

Chobanian AV, Aram GL, Bakris GL, Black HR. The seventh report of the Joint National Committee on Prevention, Detection, Evaluation, and Treatment of High Blood Pressure. The JNC 7 Report. JAMA 2003;289(19):2560–2572.

Williams GH. Hypertensive Vascular Disease. In: Braunwald E, Fauci AS, Kasper KL, et al., eds. Harrison's principles of internal medicine, 15th ed. New York: McGraw-Hill, 2001:1413–1430.

Williams GH. Approach to the Patient with Hypertension. In: Braunwald E, Fauci AS, Kasper KL, et al., eds. Harrison's principles of internal medicine, 15th ed. New York: McGraw-Hill, 2001:211–214.

CASE 10

A 39-year-old man is brought to the emergency room by ambulance after he was found wandering in the street in a disoriented state. He is confused and agitated, and further history is obtained from his wife. She reports that for the last several months he has been complaining of intermittent headaches, palpitations, and had experienced feelings of light-headedness and flushed skin when playing basketball. Three weeks ago, he was diagnosed with hypertension, and was started on clonidine twice a day. He took it for 2 weeks, but because it made him feel sedated, he was instructed by his physician 5 days ago to stop the clonidine and to begin metoprolol twice daily. On examination, he is afebrile, with a heart rate of 110 bpm, a respiratory rate of 26 breaths per minute, an oxygen saturation of 98%, and blood pressure of 215/132 mmHg, equal in both arms. He is agitated, diaphoretic, and is looking around the room, but does not appear to recognize his wife. His pupils are dilated but reactive, and he has papilledema and scattered retinal hemorrhages. He has no thyromegaly. His heart, lung, and abdominal examinations are normal. His pulses are bounding and are equal in his arms and legs. He moves all of his extremities well, his reflexes are brisk and symmetric, and he is slightly tremulous. A noncontrast CT of the head is read as negative for hemorrhage. Laboratory studies include a normal leukocyte count and a hemoglobin level of 16.5 g/dL. Serum Na is 139 mEq/L, K is 4.7mEq/L, Cl is 105mEq/L, HCO_3 is 29 mEq/L, blood urea nitrogen (BUN) is 32 mg/dL, and creatinine is 1.3 mg/dL. A urinalysis is normal and a urine drug screen is negative. A lumbar puncture is performed, with an opening pressure of 18 mm H_2O, and the cerebrospinal fluid (CSF) has no cells and a normal protein and glucose.

- **What is the most likely diagnosis?**
- **What is the underlying etiology?**
- **What is the next step?**

ANSWERS TO CASE 10: Hypertensive Encephalopathy/Pheochromocytoma

Summary: A 39-year-old man recently diagnosed with hypertension is now in the emergency room with an acute confusional state and blood pressures of 215/132 mmHg. He has been having episodes of palpitations, headaches, and lightheadedness. His medication was recently changed from clonidine to metoprolol. His examination is significant for dilated pupils, papilledema, and bounding peripheral pulses. The urine drug screen is negative. A CT scan of the head is normal, and a lumbar puncture reveals no erythrocytes or leukocytes, but an opening pressure of 18 mmH_20.

- **Most likely diagnosis:** Hypertensive encephalopathy.
- **Possible etiology:** Pheochromocytoma.
- **Next step:** Admit to the intensive care unit, begin immediate lowering of blood pressure with a parenteral agent, and closely monitor arterial pressure.

Analysis

Objectives

1. Learn the definition and management of hypertensive emergencies and urgencies.
2. Understand the relationship between systemic blood pressure and cerebral blood flow.
3. Know how to diagnose and medically treat a patient with a pheochromocytoma.

Considerations

This is a relatively young male with severely elevated blood pressures and presents with **altered mental status**. Illicit drug use, such as with cocaine, must be considered. This patient's drug screen was negative. **Hypertensive encephalopathy**, a symptom complex of **severely elevated blood pressures, confusion, increased intracranial pressure, and/or seizures**, is a diagnosis of exclusion, meaning other causes for the patient's acute mental decline, such as stroke, subarachnoid hemorrhage, meningitis, or mass lesions, must be ruled out. It is not necessary to know the specific etiology of the patient's hypertension to treat his encephalopathy; urgent blood pressure lowering is indicated. However, it is not necessary, and **may be harmful, to normalize the blood pressure too quickly**, because it may cause cerebral hypoperfusion. **Parenteral medications should be used to lower the diastolic blood pressure to 100–110 mmHg**. The patient has tachycardia, hypertension, diaphoresis, dilated pupils, and a slight tremor, all signs of a hyperadrenergic state. Pheochromocytoma must be considered as a possible underlying etiology of his hypertension. His antihypertensive medication changes may also be contributory—perhaps clonidine rebound.

APPROACH TO HYPERTENSIVE EMERGENCIES

Hypertensive crises are critical elevations in blood pressure, which are usually classified as either hypertensive emergencies or urgencies. The presence of acute end-organ damage constitutes a **hypertensive emergency**, whereas the absence of such complications is thought of as **hypertensive urgency**. Examples of acute end-organ damage include hypertensive encephalopathy, myocardial ischemia or infarction associated with markedly elevated blood pressure, aortic dissection, pulmonary edema secondary to acute left ventricular failure and eclampsia.

Hypertensive emergencies require reduction in blood pressure over a few hours, typically with intravenous medications and close monitoring in an intensive care unit. Hypertensive urgencies also require prompt medical attention, but the blood pressure can be lowered over 1–2 days, and can be monitored in the outpatient setting for patients with reliable followup.

Hypertensive crises are uncommon, but most often occur in patients with an established history of so-called essential hypertension; that is, hypertension without an apparent underlying cause. A crisis may be precipitated by use of sympathomimetic agents such as cocaine, or by conditions that produce excess sympathetic discharge, such as clonidine withdrawal. Hypertensive crises may also be caused by underlying diseases that cause hypertension, such renovascular disease (e.g., renal artery stenosis), renal parenchymal disease (e.g., glomerulonephritis), and pheochromocytoma.

Although the pathophysiology is not completely understood, abrupt rises in vascular resistance are met with endothelial compensation by the release of vasodilator molecules such as nitric oxide. If the increase in arterial pressure persists, the endothelial response is overwhelmed and decompensates, leading to a further rise in pressure and endothelial damage and dysfunction.

Cerebral blood flow is a good example of vascular compensation by vasodilation or vasoconstriction in response to changes in arterial pressure (see Figure 10–1). In normotensive adults, cerebral blood flow remains relatively constant over a range of mean arterial pressures between 60 and 120 mmHg, because of cerebral vasoconstriction limiting excessive cerebral perfusion. As the mean arterial pressure increases beyond the normal range of cerebral autoregulation, there is cerebrovascular endothelial dysfunction, increased permeability of the blood–brain barrier, leading to vasogenic edema and the formation of microhemorrhages. Patients then manifest symptoms of hypertensive encephalopathy such as lethargy, confusion, headaches, or vision changes. Typical imaging findings on MRI include posterior leukoencephalopathy, usually in the parietooccipital regions, which may or may not be seen on CT scanning. Without therapy, this can lead to seizures, coma, and death.

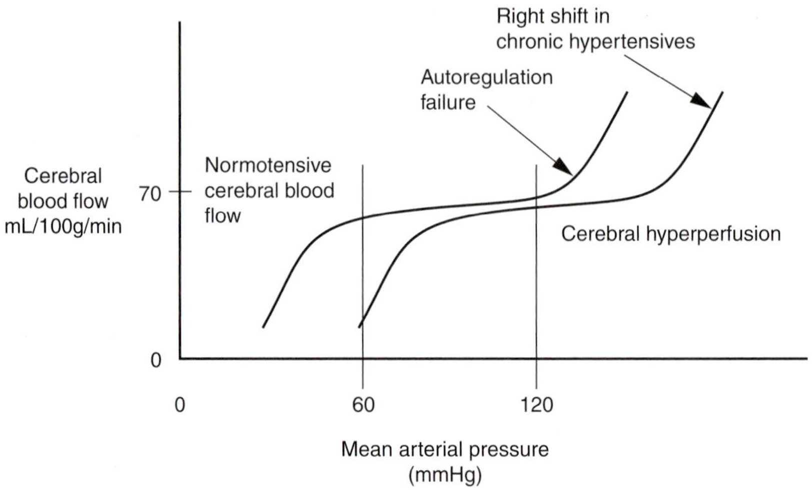

Figure 10–1. Cerebral blood flow autoregulation. Cerebral blood flow is fairly constant over a range of blood pressures. Chronic hypertensive patients have an adaptive mechanism that shifts the curve to the right.

The **definition of hypertensive emergency does not require numerical thresholds** of arterial pressure, but **is based on end-organ effect**s. Autoregulation failure can occur in previously normotensive individuals at blood pressures as low as 160/100 mmHg; however, individuals with longstanding hypertension frequently develop adaptive mechanisms (such as cerebral arterial autoregulation), and may not show clinical manifestations until the blood pressure rises to above 220/110 mmHg. Thus, the **emergent treatment of hypertensive encephalopathy** (and indeed, all hypertensive emergencies) should be **focused on the symptoms** rather than the numbers. In fact, it may be dangerous to "normalize" the blood pressure of patients with chronic hypertension. As a consequence of the right shift in the autoregulation curve, these "normal" blood pressures may lead to decreased perfusion to the brain leading to infarction, or similar renal or coronary hypoperfusion, and resultant ischemic injury. Usually, a reasonable goal is reduction of mean arterial pressures by **no more than 25%**, or to a diastolic blood pressure of 100–110 mmHg over a period of minutes to hours.

The treatment of **hypertensive emergencies usually necessitates parenteral medication and without delay;** direct blood pressure monitoring with an arterial catheter is often necessary. One of the most commonly used medications to treat hypertensive emergencies is **sodium nitroprusside**. It has the advantage of nearly instantaneous onset of action, and its dose can be easily titrated for a smooth reduction in blood pressure. However, its metabolite may accumulate, resulting in cyanide or thiocyanate toxicity when it is given for more than 2–3 days. **Fenoldopam**, a new **dopamine receptor agonist**, has gained FDA approval for the treatment of hypertensive emergencies. It causes peripheral vasodilatation by stimulating dopamine-1 receptors, increasing renal blood flow, and perhaps **improving renal function** in individuals with renal insufficiency.

Certain clinical situations may favor the use of other medications. Intravenous loop diuretics and vasodilators such as nitroglycerin decrease the preload (central venous pressure) in acute pulmonary edema. Myocardial ischemia or infarction is treated with intravenous nitroglycerin to improving coronary perfusion, and beta-blockers to reduce the blood pressure, heart rate, and myocardial oxygen demand. Patients with aortic dissection benefit from medications that reduce the shear forces affecting the aorta, which will help limit the propagation of the dissection. A useful technique in treating these individuals is to use intravenous nitroprusside to lower the arterial blood pressure and a beta-blocker to blunt reflex tachycardia; alternatively, intravenous labetalol, a combined alpha- and beta-blocker, alone may be used. Patients presenting with acute cerebral infarction generally should not have acute blood pressure lowering because of the possibility of worsening cerebral ischemia.

The vast majority of hypertension has no discernible cause, so-called essential hypertension. Some patients have secondary causes, such as renal artery stenosis, hyperaldosteronism, aortic stenosis, or pheochromocytoma. A history of headaches, palpitations, and hyperadrenergic state (flushing, dilated pupils, diaphoresis) suggests the diagnosis of **pheochromocytoma;** pheochromocytomas are catecholamine-producing tumors that arise from chromaffin cells of the adrenal medulla. Other symptoms may include episodic anxiety, tremor, and orthostatic hypotension caused by volume contraction from pressure-induced natriuresis. Although uncommon, accounting for only 0.01–0.1% of hypertensive individuals, these tumors have important therapeutic considerations.

The diagnosis is established by measuring increased concentrations of catecholamines or their metabolites in either urine or plasma. Usually, **a 24-hour urine collection** is assayed for **metanephrines, vanillylmandelic acid (VMA), and unconjugated, or "free," catecholamines**. After the biochemical tests document the excess catecholamines, the next step is to locate the tumor for surgical removal. Approximately 90% of pheochromocytomas are in the adrenal gland, usually identified by computed tomography or magnetic resonance imaging. If the initial imaging is unrevealing, scintigraphic localization with ^{123}I-metaiodobenzylguanidine (^{123}I-MIBG) scan is indicated, because this radioisotope is preferentially taken up in catecholamine-producing tumors.

The treatment of choice for these tumors is surgical resection, but it is critical to reverse the acute and chronic effects of the excess catecholamines prior to excision. Alpha-adrenergic blocking agents, such as phenoxybenzamine, an irreversible, long-acting agent, begun 1 week prior to surgery helps to prevent hypertensive exacerbations, especially worrisome during surgery. To expand the commonly seen contracted blood volume, a liberal salt diet is initiated. **Sometimes, a beta-blocking agent is started, but only after alpha-blockade is established**. The products of pheochromocytomas stimulate both the alpha- and beta-adrenergic receptors; thus, using a beta-blocker alone may worsen the hypertension because of unopposed alpha-adrenergic stimulation. Also, beta-blockade may result in acute pulmonary edema, especially if there is a cardiomyopathy secondary to chronic catecholamine exposure.

Surgery for these tumors is associated with a morbidity rate as high as 40%. An experienced anesthesia team is vital in anticipating the drastic hemodynamic changes that occur intraoperatively. Parasympathetic nervous system blockade should be avoided (to limit tachycardia), and often, intravenous nitroprusside is needed to treat an acute hypertensive crises. If an adrenal gland is involved, it should be removed entirely, with care given to provide glucocorticoid stress coverage if a bilateral adrenalectomy is planned (10% are bilateral). Approximately 2 weeks after surgery, urine and plasma catecholamines should be measured for metanephrines, which would indicate metastatic disease. Metastasis are usually resected, but may be treated with chemotherapy and/or external radiation therapy.

Less than 10% of pheochromocytomas are familial, and these tend to be bilateral. One should consider screening for the presence of the *RET* protooncogene seen in multiple endocrine neoplasia type II (MEN II), the *VHL* gene for von Hippel-Lindau syndrome, or screening family members for these diseases as well as familial pheochromocytoma and neurofibromatosis.

Comprehension Questions

[10.1] A 30-year-old man with chronic hypertension is seen in the clinic having run out of his medication, hydrochlorothiazide. He has no complaints and has a blood pressure of 200/120 mmHg. Which of the following is the best management?

A. Admit in the hospital and initiate intravenous nitroprusside
B. Restart the hydrochlorothiazide and recheck the blood pressure in 48 hours
C. Change to an ACE inhibitor
D. Refer to a social worker and don't prescribe an antihypertensive agent

[10.2] An 80-year-old woman without a history of hypertension undergoes surgery for a hip fracture. Her blood pressure on postoperative day 1 is 178/110 mmHg. She is asymptomatic. What is the best next step?

A. Transfer the patient to the intensive care unit, obtain cardiac enzymes, and lower the blood pressures to the 140/90 mmHg range.
B. Pain control and monitor the blood pressure.
C. Start the patient on a beta-blocker and monitor the blood pressure.
D. Restrict visitors and turn down television, alarms, and other noise.

[10.3] A 61-year-old man with coronary artery disease complains of progressive orthopnea and pedal edema. He is hospitalized with a blood pressure of 190/105 mmHg. The cardiac enzymes and EKG are normal. Intravenous furosemide has been administered. What is the best next step?

A. Prescribe a beta-blocker to decrease myocardial oxygen demands
B. Start intravenous dopamine
C. Observe
D. Start an ACE inhibitor

[10.4] A 58-year-old woman is seen in the emergency room with aphasia and right-arm weakness of 8 hours duration. Her blood pressure is 169/108 mmHg. Which of the following is the best next step?

A. Normalize the blood pressure with beta-blockade
B. Start an anticoagulating medication
C. Normalize the blood pressure with an ACE inhibitor
D. Observation of the blood pressure

Answers

[10.1] **B.** This man has a hypertensive urgency—elevated blood pressures without end-organ symptoms. The appropriate treatment is initiation of blood pressure medication and reassessment in 24–48 hours.

[10.2] **B.** Elevated blood pressures without symptoms may occur acutely after surgery, particularly as a consequence of postoperative pain. Generally, this hypertension, unless markedly elevated, does not need to be treated, and can lead to orthostatic hypotension when the patient gets out of bed.

[10.3] **D.** Elevated blood pressures may exacerbate congestive heart failure and need to be treated. Generally, beta-blockers are avoided when patients are volume-overloaded because they decrease myocardial contractility, exacerbating the decreased ejection fraction.

[10.4] **D.** In general, hypertension should not be acutely decreased in an individual suspected of having a stroke because of the concern of cerebral hypoperfusion and worsening brain ischemia.

CLINICAL PEARLS

❖ A hypertensive emergency is defined as an episode of elevated blood pressure associated with acute end-organ damage or dysfunction, and requires immediate lowering of the blood pressure.

❖ Asymptomatic patients with elevated blood pressure can usually be started back on an oral regimen and reassessed as outpatients in 24–48 hours.

- The cerebral autoregulation curve of individuals with chronic hypertension is shifted to the right. Nevertheless, marked elevations in mean arterial pressure can exceed the ability the of cerebral vessels to constrict, causing hyperperfusion, cerebral edema, and hypertensive encephalopathy.
- Pheochromocytomas may cause paroxysmal blood pressure elevations, but the majority of patients have sustained hypertension, in association with episodic headaches, palpitations, and diaphoresis.
- Preoperative blood pressure control in pheochromocytoma can be achieved by using alpha-blockers such as phenoxybenzamine. Beta-blockers used alone can, paradoxically, increase blood pressure because of unopposed alpha-adrenergic effects.

REFERENCES

Dluhy RG, Lawrence JE, Williams GH. Endocrine hypertension. In: Larsen PR, Kronenberg HM, Melmed S, Polonsky KS, eds. Williams' textbook of endocrinology, 10th ed. Philadelphia, WB Saunders, 2003:555–562.

O'Connor DT. The adrenal medulla, catecholamines, and pheochromocytoma. In: Goldman L, Bennett JC, eds. Cecil's textbook of medicine, 21st ed. Philadelphia, WB Saunders, 2000:1259–1262.

Vaughan CJ, Delanty N. Hypertensive emergencies. Lancet 2000;356:411–417.

CASE 11

A 28-year-old man comes to your office complaining of a 5-day history of nausea, vomiting, diffuse abdominal pain, fever to 101°F, and muscle aches. He has lost his appetite, but is able to tolerate liquids, and has no diarrhea. He has no significant past medical history or family history, and has not traveled outside the United States. He admits to having 12 different lifetime sexual partners, denies illicit drug use, and he drinks alcohol occasionally, but not since this illness began. He takes no routine medications, but has been taking acetaminophen, approximately 30 tablets per day for 2 days for fever and body aches since this illness began. On examination, his temperature is 100.8°F, his heart rate is 98 bpm, and his blood pressure is 120/74 mmHg. He appears jaundiced, his chest is clear to auscultation, and his heart is regular without murmurs. His liver percusses 12 cm, and is smooth and slightly tender to palpation. He has no abdominal distension or peripheral edema. Laboratory values are significant for a normal complete blood count, a creatinine of 1.1 mg/dL, alanine aminotransferase (ALT) 3440 IU/L, aspartate aminotransferase (AST) 2705 IU/L, total bilirubin 24.5 mg/dL, direct bilirubin 18.2 mg/dL, alkaline phosphatase 349 IU/L, serum albumin 3.0 g/dL, and a prothrombin time of 14 seconds.

- **What is the most likely diagnosis?**

- **What is the most important immediate diagnostic test?**

ANSWERS TO CASE 11: Acute Viral Hepatitis, Acetaminophen Exacerbation

Summary: A 28-year-old man complains of nausea, vomiting, diffuse abdominal pain, fever, and myalgias. He has had 12 different lifetime sexual partners and is currently taking acetaminophen. He appears icteric and has a low-grade fever and tender hepatomegaly. His laboratory studies are consistent with severe hepatocellular injury and somewhat impaired hepatic function.

- **Most likely diagnosis:** Acute hepatitis, either viral infection or toxic injury, possibly exacerbated by acetaminophen use.

- **Most important immediate diagnostic test:** Acetaminophen level, because acetaminophen toxicity may greatly exacerbate liver injury, but is treatable.

Analysis

Objectives

1. Understand the use of viral serologic studies to diagnose hepatitis A, B, and C infections.
2. Know the prognosis for acute viral hepatitis and recognize fulminant hepatic failure.
3. Know measures to prevent hepatitis A and B infection.
4. Understand the use of the acetaminophen nomogram and the treatment of acetaminophen hepatotoxicity.

Considerations

This patient has an acute onset of hepatic injury and systemic symptoms that predate his acetaminophen use. The markedly elevated hepatic transaminase and bilirubin levels are consistent with viral hepatitis, or possibly toxic injury. This patient denied intravenous drug use, which would be a risk factor for hepatitis B and C infection. His sexual history is a possible clue. The degree and pattern of transaminase (ALT and AST) elevation can provide some clues to help differentiate possible etiologies. Transaminase levels greater than 1000 IU/L are seen in conditions that produce extensive hepatic necrosis such as toxic injury, viral hepatitis, or ischemia ("shock liver"). Alcoholic hepatitis almost always has levels less than 500 IU/L, and often with an AST:ALT ratio of 2:1. In this case, it is important to consider the possibility of acetaminophen toxicity, both because it can produce fatal liver failure and because there is an effective antidote available. By obtaining a serum acetaminophen level, and knowing the time of his last ingestion, this data can be plotted on a nomogram (Figure 11–1) to help predict acetaminophen-related liver damage and the possible need for *N*-acetylcysteine.

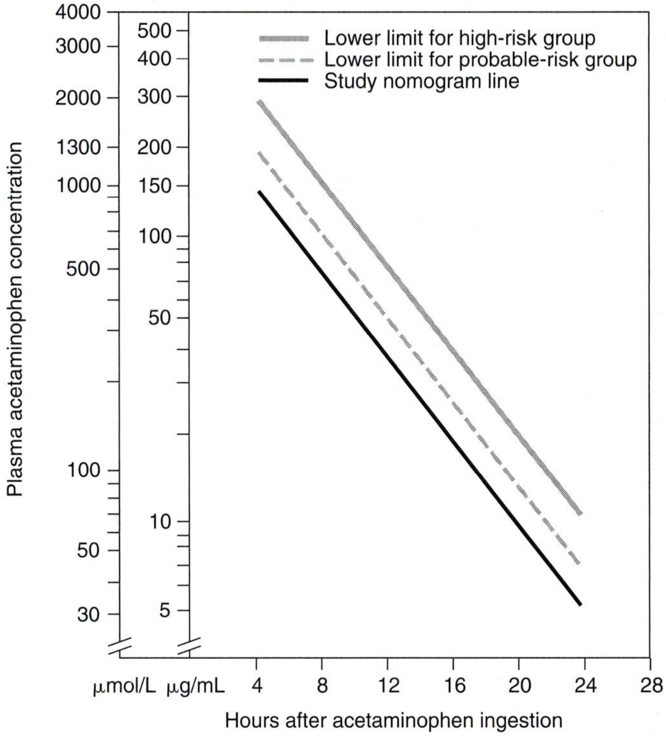

Figure 11–1. Acetaminophen nomogram. **(Reproduced with permission from Poisoning and Drug Overdose. In: Braunwald E, Fauci AS, Kasper KL, et al., eds. Harrison's Principles of Internal Medicine, 15th ed. New York: McGraw-Hill, 2001:2602.)**

APPROACH TO SUSPECTED HEPATITIS

Viral Hepatitis

Most cases of acute hepatitis are caused by infection with one of five viruses: hepatitis A, B, C, D, or E. They can produce virtually indistinguishable clinical syndromes although it is unusual to observe acute hepatitis C. Affected individuals often complain of a prodrome of nonspecific constitutional symptoms, including fever, nausea, fatigue, arthralgias, myalgias, and headache, and sometimes pharyngitis and coryza. This is followed by the onset of visible jaundice caused by hyperbilirubinemia, with tenderness and enlargement of the liver, and dark urine caused by bilirubinuria. The clinical course, and prognosis then vary based on the type of virus causing the hepatitis.

Hepatitis A and E are both very contagious and transmitted by fecal–oral route, usually by contaminated food or water where sanitation is poor, and in daycare by children. **Hepatitis A** is found worldwide and is the **most common**

cause of acute viral hepatitis in the United States. Hepatitis E is much less common and is found in Asia, Africa, Central America and the Caribbean. Both hepatitis A and E infections usually lead to self-limited illnesses, and generally resolve within weeks. Almost all patients with hepatitis A recover completely and have no long-term complications. A few may have fulminant disease resulting in liver failure. Most patients with hepatitis E also have uncomplicated courses, but some patients, particularly pregnant women, have been reported to develop severe hepatic necrosis and fatal liver failure.

Hepatitis B is the second most common type of viral hepatitis in the United States, and it is **usually sexually transmitted**. It may also be acquired parenterally, such as by intravenous drug use, and during birth from chronically infected mothers. The outcome depends on the age at which the infection was acquired. Up to 90% of infected newborns develop chronic hepatitis B infection, which places the affected infant at significant risk of hepatocellular carcinoma later in adulthood. For those individuals infected later in life, approximately 95% of patients will recover completely without sequelae. Between 5 and 10% of patients will develop chronic hepatitis, which may progress to cirrhosis. Also, a chronic carrier state may be seen in which the virus continues to replicate, but does not cause irreversible hepatic damage in the host.

Hepatitis C is transmitted **parenterally by blood transfusions or intravenous drug use**, and rarely by sexual contact. The mode of transmission is unknown in about 40% of cases. It is uncommonly diagnosed as a cause of acute hepatitis, often producing subclinical infection, but is frequently diagnosed later as a cause of chronic hepatitis.

Hepatitis D is a defective RNA virus that requires the presence of the hepatitis B virus to replicate. It can be acquired as a coinfection simultaneously with acute hepatitis B, or as a later superinfection in a person with a chronic hepatitis B infection. Patients afflicted with chronic hepatitis B virus who then become infected with hepatitis D may suffer clinical deterioration; in 10–20% of these cases, individuals develop severe fatal hepatic failure.

Fortunately, in most cases of acute viral hepatitis, patients recover completely, so that the treatment is generally supportive. However, **fulminant hepatic failure** as a result of massive hepatic necrosis may progress over a period of weeks. This is usually caused by infection by the hepatitis B and D viruses, or is drug-induced. This syndrome is characterized by rapid progression of encephalopathy from confusion or somnolence to coma. Patients also have worsening coagulopathy as measured by increasing prothrombin times, rising bilirubin levels, ascites and peripheral edema, hypoglycemia, hyperammonemia, and lactic acidosis. Fulminant hepatitis carries a poor prognosis (the mortality for comatose patients is 80%) and is often fatal without an emergency liver transplant.

Diagnosis

Clinical presentation does not reliably establish the viral etiology, so serologic studies are used to establish a diagnosis. Anti-Hepatitis A IgM establishes an

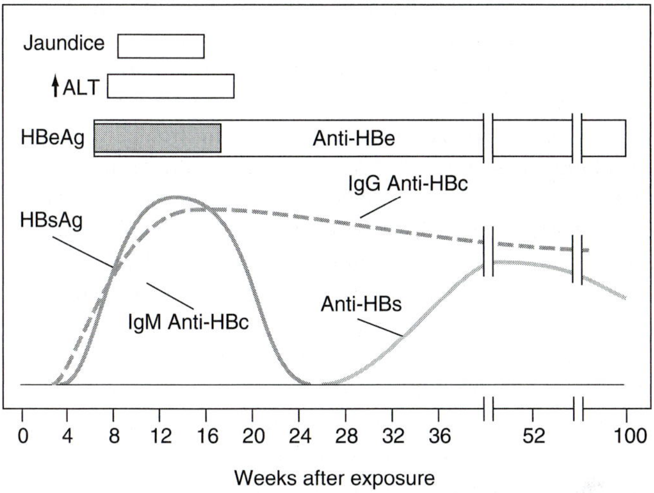

Figure 11–2. Serologic markers in acute hepatitis B infection. **(Reproduced with permission from Dienstag JL, Isselbacher KJ. Acute Viral Hepatitis. In: Braunwald E, Fauci AS, Kasper KL, et al., eds. Harrison's Principles of Internal Medicine, 15th ed. NewYork: McGraw-Hill, 2001:1724.)**

acute hepatitis A infection. Anti-Hepatitis C antibody is present, in acute hepatitis C, but it may be negative for several weeks. The hepatitis C polymerase chain reaction (PCR) assay, which becomes positive earlier in the disease course, often aids in the diagnosis. Acute hepatitis B infection is diagnosed by the presence of hepatitis B surface antigen (HBsAg) in the clinical context of elevated serum transaminase levels and jaundice. HBsAg later disappears when the antibody (anti-HBs) is produced (see Figure 11–2). There is often an interval of a few weeks between the disappearance of HBsAg and the appearance of anti-HBsAb, which is referred to as the "window period." During this interval, the presence of anti-Hepatitis B core antigen IgM (anti-HBc IgM) is indicative of an acute hepatitis B infection. Hepatitis B precore antigen (HBeAg) represents a high level of viral replication. It is almost always present during acute infection, but its persistence after 6 weeks of illness is a sign of chronic infection and high infectivity. Persistence of HBsAg or HBeAg is a marker for chronic hepatitis or a chronic carrier state; elevated versus normal serum transaminase levels distinguish between these two entities, respectively.

Prevention

The efficacy of the hepatitis A vaccine for hepatitis A (available in two doses given 6 months apart) exceeds 90%. It is indicated for individuals planning to travel to endemic areas. Postexposure prophylaxis with hepatitis A immune globulin, along with the first injection of the vaccine should be given to household and intimate contacts within 2 weeks of exposure. The Hepatitis B vaccine (given in three doses over 6 months) provides effective immunity in more than 90% of patients. It is recommended for health care workers, as well as for universal vaccination of infants in the United States. Hepatitis B immune globulin (HBIg) is given after exposure such as a needle-stick injury from an infected patient or to a newborn of infected mothers; the first inoculation of the vaccine is usually given concurrently. There is no immunization and no proven postexposure prophylaxis for persons exposed to hepatitis C. **Interferon treatment** may be used in individuals with hepatic injury.

Acetaminophen Hepatitis

Acetaminophen-induced hepatocellular injury may result after a single, large ingestion, as in a suicide attempt, or by chronic usage of multiple over-the-counter acetaminophen-containing preparations to treat pain or fever. **Hepatic toxicity** most often occurs after an acute ingestion of **10g or more**, but lower doses may cause injury in patients with preexisting liver disease, or particularly in those who abuse alcohol. Acetaminophen is metabolized in the liver by the cytochrome P450 enzyme system, which produces a toxic metabolite; this metabolite is detoxified by binding to glutathione. Potential hepatic injury is greater when P450 activity is augmented by drugs such as ethanol or phenobarbital, or when less glutathione is available, as in alcoholism, malnutrition, or AIDS. Acetaminophen levels are measured between 4 and 24 hours after an acute ingestion and plotted on a **nomogram** to predict possible hepatotoxicity and determine if treatment is necessary (see Figure 11–1). Sometimes, emperic therapy is started even before labe results return.

If acetaminophen levels are above the level that predisposes to hepatic injury, treatment is started with gastric decontamination with charcoal, and administration of ***N*-acetylcysteine**, which provides cysteine to replenish glutathione stores. *N*-acetylcysteine should be started within the first 10 hours to prevent liver damage; it is continued for 72 hours. Meanwhile, the patient should not receive any medications that are known to be hepatotoxic.

Comprehension Questions

[11.1] A 25-year-old medical student is stuck with a hollow needle during a procedure on a patient known to have hepatitis B and C viral infection, but who is HIV-negative. The student's baseline laboratory studies include serology: HBsAg negative, anti-HBsAb positive, anti-HBc IgG negative. Which of the following is true regarding this medical student's hepatitis status?

A. Prior vaccination with hepatitis B vaccine.
B. Acute infection with hepatitis B virus.

C. Prior infection with hepatitis B virus.
D. The student was vaccinated for hepatitis B, but is not immune.

[11.2] What postexposure prophylaxis should the student described in question [11.1] receive?

A. Hepatitis B immune globulin (HBIg)
B. Oral lamivudine
C. Intravenous immune globulin (IVIg)
D. Reassurance

[11.3] In a suicide attempt, an 18-year-old woman takes 4 g of acetaminophen, approximately 8 hours previously. Her acetaminophen level is 30 mcg/mL. What should be done for this patient?

A. Immediately start *N*-acetylcysteine
B. Observation
C. Alkalinize the urine
D. Intravenous activated charcoal

Answers

[11.1] **A.** This student's serology is most consistent with vaccination and not prior infection. Like all health care workers, the student should have been vaccinated against the hepatitis B virus, which induces anti-HBs IgG antibody, which is thought to be protective. Not all people receiving the vaccine develop an adequate antibody titer; if none were detected, it would indicate the need for revaccination. Patients with prior hepatitis B infection will also likely have anti-HBsAb, but will also have anti-HBc IgG. Acute infection would be signified by the presence of either HBsAg or anti-HBc IgM.

[11.2] **D.** No postexposure prophylaxis is definitively indicated. The student has detectable protective antibody levels against the hepatitis B virus, and if the levels are judged to be adequate, the student is protected against infection. Oral lamivudine is a treatment for chronic hepatitis B infection, and is part of an antiretroviral prophylaxis if the patient was HIV-positive. There is no effective prophylaxis for hepatitis C exposure.

[11.3] **B.** The serum acetaminophen level of 30 mcg/mL, with last ingestion 8 hours previously, is plotted on the nomogram and falls below the "danger zone" of possible hepatic injury. Thus, this patient should be observed. Sometimes, patients will take more than one medication, so that serum and/or urine drug testing may be worthwhile. Gastrointestinal activated charcoal, not intravenous charcoal, is used for other ingestions.

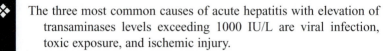

CLINICAL PEARLS

- ❖ The three most common causes of acute hepatitis with elevation of transaminases levels exceeding 1000 IU/L are viral infection, toxic exposure, and ischemic injury.
- ❖ The large majority of adults with acute hepatitis B viral infection recover completely, but 5–10% develop chronic hepatitis.
- ❖ Fulminant hepatic failure, characterized by the rapid development of hepatic encephalopathy, coagulopathy, peripheral edema, and ascites, is usually fatal unless a liver transplant is performed.
- ❖ Prevention of hepatitis B viral infection hinges on long-term immunity with a highly effective recombinant vaccine, and short-term postexposure prophylaxis with hepatitis B immune globulin (HBIg).
- ❖ The likelihood of toxic acetaminophen injury and need for treatment can be predicted from a nomogram based on serum level and the time since last ingestion.

REFERENCES

Bass NM. Toxic and drug-induced liver disease. In: Cecil RL, Bennett JC, Goldman L, eds. Cecil's textbook of medicine, 21st ed. Philadelphia, WB Saunders, 2000:781–82.

Deinstag JL, Isselbacher KJ. Acute viral hepatitis. In: Braunwald E, Fauci AS, Kasper KL, et al., eds. Harrison's principles of internal medicine, 15th ed. New York: McGraw-Hill, 2001:1721-1737.

Dienstag JL, Isselbacher KJ. Toxic and Drug-Induced Hepatitis. In: Braunwald E, Fauci AS, Kasper KL, et al., eds. Harrison's Principles of Internal Medicine, 15th ed. New York: McGraw-Hill, 2001:1737-1742.

Hoofnagle JH, Lindsay KL. Acute viral hepatitis. In: Cecil RL, Bennett JC, Goldman, L eds. Cecil's textbook of medicine, 21st ed. Philadelphia, WB Saunders, 2000:783–90.

Luis S, Marsano MD. Hepatitis. Prim Care Clin Office Pract 2003;30(1):81-107.

CASE 12

A 38-year-old woman who is in her third pregnancy, presents to your office for evaluation of menstrual irregularity. She states that her periods started when she was 12 years old, and have been fairly regular ever since, coming once every 28–30 days. However, about 9 months ago, her cycles seemed to lengthen, and the last 3 months she has not had a period at all. She stopped breastfeeding 3 years ago, but over the last 3 months she noticed that she could express a small amount of milky fluid from her breasts. She had a bilateral tubal ligation after her last pregnancy, and has no other past medical or surgical history. She takes no medications except multivitamins. Over the last year or so, she thinks she's gained about 10 pounds, and she feels as if she has no energy despite adequate sleep. She has noticed some mild thinning of her hair, and slightly more coarse skin texture. She denies headaches or visual changes. Her physical exam, including a pelvic exam and breast exam, are normal; she is not obese or hirsute. You elicit slight whitish nipple discharge. Her pregnancy test is negative

- **What is the most likely diagnosis?**

- **What is the most likely etiology for the condition?**

ANSWERS TO CASE 12: Oligomenorrhea Caused by Hypothyroidism

Summary: A 38-year-old Gravida 3, Para 3 woman complains of amenorrhea. Her menarche began at age 12 years and occurred every 28–30 days. However, about 9 months ago, her cycles seemed to lengthen, and for the last 3 months she has not had a period at all. She has milky breast leakage. She had a bilateral tubal ligation after her last pregnancy, has no other past medical or surgical history, and takes no medications except multivitamins. Over the last year, she thinks she's gained about 10 pounds, has fatigue, mild thinning of her hair, and slightly more coarse skin. She denies headaches or visual changes. Her physical exam, including a pelvic exam and breast exam, is normal, she is not obese or hirsute. You can elicit slight whitish nipple discharge.

- **Most likely diagnosis:** Oligomenorrhea, galactorrhea, and hypothyroidism.
- **Most likely etiology:** In this patient, with her symptoms of weight gain, fatigue, thinning hair, and galactorrhea in the setting of previously normal menses, hypothyroidism is the most likely diagnosis.

Analysis

Objectives

1. Understand the differential diagnosis of secondary amenorrhea and the approach to the investigation of possible hormonal causes.
2. Understand the interactions of the hormones involved in the hypothalamic–pituitary–gonadal axis.
3. Recognize the clinical features and diagnostic evaluation of hypothyroidism.
4. Be familiar with the treatment of hypothyroidism.

Considerations

This 38-year-old woman presents with oligomenorrhea, weight gain, fatigue, and galactorrhea despite having previously normal menses and discontinuing breast-feeding 3 years ago. Her history of fatigue, weight gain, and hair loss suggest a systemic cause of her symptoms, specifically hypothyroidism. However, her normal physical exam with lack of myxedema or bradycardia, normal reflexes, normal cognition, and nondisplaced point of maximal impulse (PMI) suggests mild hypothyroidism. Lack of virilization or obesity does not exclude polycystic ovarian syndrome, but their absence make this diagnosis less likely. Hypothyroidism alone could attribute to galactorrhea, because hypothyroidism can be associated with hyperprolactinemia. Although prolactinomas can also cause galactorrhea, as well as secondary amenorrhea, the lack of visual disturbance in this patient is reassuring.

A variety of other disorders could lead to the symptoms exhibited by this woman (e.g., hypopituitarism, adrenal insufficiency); the definitive workup, aside from a thorough history and physical exam, will invariably include laboratory studies. To make informed and cost-effective choices, a carefully formulated stepwise approach should be undertaken by the physician.

APPROACH TO OLIGOMENORRHEA

Definitions

Amenorrhea: *Primary*–Absence of menarche by the age of 16 years regardless of the presence or absence of secondary sex characteristics. *Secondary*–Absence of menstruation for 3 or more months in women with normal past menses.

Galactorrhea: Any white discharge from the nipple that is persistent and looks like milk.

Oligomenorrhea: Menses occurring at infrequent intervals of more than 40 days or having fewer than 9 menses per year.

Polycystic ovarian syndrome: A syndrome characterized by infertility, hirsutism, obesity, and amenorrhea or oligomenorrhea.

Clinical Approach

The assessment of oligomenorrhea is similar to the workup for secondary amenorrhea with the understanding that secondary amenorrhea is present when a normally menstruating woman stops having periods for 3 consecutive months or more. **The most common cause of both symptoms, and the easiest to exclude in the office, is pregnancy**. A negative in-office pregnancy test should be confirmed with a serum beta-hCG (human chorionic gonadotropin). Primary amenorrhea is present when the first menses has not appeared in a girl by the age of 16 years and is generally caused by a variety of genetic or congenital defects and is commonly associated with disorders of puberty. Given this patient's age and history, primary amenorrhea is not a consideration, thus a diagnostic pathway for secondary amenorrhea/oligomenorrhea should be undertaken.

Problems of the Hypothalamic–Pituitary–Ovarian Axis Excluding pregnancy and problems in the genital outflow tract, disorders of the hypothalamic–pituitary–ovarian axis account for the largest number of cases of oligomenorrhea and amenorrhea. Disorders of the hypothalamus account for the largest percentage of abnormality (>45%); these include problems of nutrition (rapid weight loss/anorexia), excessive exercise, stress, and infiltrative diseases (i.e., craniopharyngioma, sarcoidosis, histiocytosis). The largest single cause of oligomenorrhea is polycystic ovarian syndrome (PCOS), accounting for 30% of all cases. PCOS was once thought to be a disease originating in the ovary; however, it is now known that **PCOS is a much more complicated neuroendocrine disorder** with evidence of **estrogenization,** as well as early or **insulin**

resistance. Other important causes of amenorrhea include diseases of the pituitary, specifically neoplasms (i.e., prolactinomas, functioning or nonfunctioning adenomas), accounting for 18% of cases. Empty sella syndrome, caused by cerebrospinal fluid (CSF) herniation into the pituitary fossa, and Sheehan syndrome, caused by severe obstetric hemorrhage and/or maternal hypotension at delivery, are important causes of atrophy and ischemia of the pituitary, and if suspected, should be investigated by MRI. Finally, disorders such as premature ovarian failure (loss of all functional ovarian follicles before age 40 years), diseases of the thyroid, and adult-onset adrenal hyperplasia should be considered and investigated if supported by history and physical exam with the appropriate laboratory studies (see Table 12–1).

The history and physical examination will narrow the range of possible causes. In this patient, the history of fatigue, weight gain, and galactorrhea, along with previously normal menses and a normal physical exam, place hypothyroidism at the top of the list. Because of the lack of headaches or visual field changes, a prolactinoma is less likely; however, a prolactin level that is very high would direct investigation toward this entity, given the history of galactorrhea. In the workup of secondary amenorrhea, these two diagnoses are the easiest to start with because the tests are minimally invasive, relatively inexpensive, and the treatment is straightforward.

Table 12-1

DIFFERENTIAL DIAGNOSIS OF OLIGOMENORRHEA*

	HISTORY	LABORATORY	THERAPY
Polycystic ovarian syndrome	Irregular menses since menarche, obesity, hirsutism	Slightly elevated testosterone, elevated LH/FSH	Oral contraceptive agent
Hypothyroidism	Fatigue, cold intolerance	Elevated TSH	Thyroxine replacement
Hyperprolactinemia	Headache, bitemporal hemianopsia, galactorrhea, medications, hypothyroidism	Elevated prolactin level	Depends on etiology
Ovarian failure	Hot flushes, hypoestrogenemia	Elevated FSH and LH	Replacement of hormones
Sheehan syndrome	Postpartum hemorrhage, unable to breast feed	Low pituitary hormones (FSH, TSH, ACTH)	Replacement of pituitary hormones

* Pregnancy must always be suspected with oligo- or amenorrhea.

Abbreviations: ACTH = adrenocorticotropic hormone; FSH = follicle-stimulating hormone; LH = luteinizing hormone; TSH = thyroid-stimulating hormone.

Hypothyroidism is defined as the insufficient production of thyroid hormone. Secondary hypothyroidism as a result of dysfunction of hypothalamic and pituitary hormone secretion are much less common, but should be suspected in a patient with a history suggestive of Sheehan syndrome or symptoms or signs of a tumor in the region of the sella. **Ninety-five percent of cases of hypothyroidism** are caused by **primary thyroid gland failure**, resulting in insufficient thyroid hormone production. In the United States**, the most common cause of hypothyroidism is lymphocytic (Hashimoto) thyroiditis**, in which cytotoxic antibodies are produced, which leads to thyroid atrophy and fibrosis. The next most common cause is the surgical or radioactive iodine treatment for hyperthyroidism, or Graves disease. **Worldwide, iodine deficiency** is the **most common cause of goitrous (enlarged thyroid) hypothyroidism**, but in the United States, this is rare.

Most hypothyroid patients present with vague and nonspecific symptoms. **Elderly** individuals may be suspected of having **dementia or depression**, when the cause is really hypothyroidism. In general, symptoms of fatigue, weight gain, muscle cramping, cold intolerance, hair thinning, menstrual changes, or carpal tunnel syndrome are common symptoms that should prompt an investigation of thyroid function. In severe, prolonged hypothyroidism, a syndrome termed **myxedema** may develop. These patients present with dull facies, swollen eyes and doughy extremities from the accumulation of hydrophilic polysaccharides in the dermis, sparse hair, and a thickened tongue. They may have an enlarged heart, nonmechanical intestinal obstruction (ileus), and a delayed relaxation phase of their deep tendon reflexes. Without treatment, they may become stuporous and hypothermic, especially if challenged with an intercurrent illness. This is a life-threatening emergency with a high mortality, even when managed aggressively with intravenous levothyroxine.

In testing outpatients for hypothyroidism, the measurement of the **serum thyroid-stimulating hormone (TSH)** is the most sensitive and useful test. Because almost all cases of hypothyroidism are caused by thyroid gland failure, the normal pituitary response is to markedly increase the TSH levels in an attempt to stimulate the failing gland. Falling levels of thyroid hormone produce logarithmic increases in the TSH concentration. Measurements of the thyroid hormone level can also be performed, but one needs to remember that almost all thyroxine (T4) circulates bound to protein, but it is the free fraction that is able to diffuse into cells and become active. So, one can **either measure the free T4** directly in some laboratories, or it can be **estimated by using the triiodothyronine (T3) uptake**, which is a measure of available protein binding, to calculate the free thyroxine index (FTI). When there is **excess thyroid-binding globulin (TBG), as in pregnancy or oral contraceptive use, the T4 levels will be high (as a consequence of the large amount of carrier protein),** but the **T3 uptake will be low** (the value varies inversely with the amount of TBG present.) Conversely, when there is a low level of TBG, as in a hypoproteinemic patient with nephrotic syndrome, the level of T4 will necessarily also be low (not much carrier protein), but the T3 uptake will be high. An easy way to remember this is by like vector analysis: **when the T4 and the T3 uptake are both high, the patient really is hyperthyroid; when they are both low, the patient is hypothyroid**. However, when they vary in opposite directions, for example, high T4 with low T3 uptake, they "cancel each other out," that is, it is a protein-binding abnormality as described above.

In mild cases, or "subclinical hypothyroidism," the TSH is mildly elevated, but the measured free T4 or FTI is within the normal range (although probably lower than what it would be if the patient were really euthyroid.) Patients may be asymptomatic, or report the vague and subtle symptoms of hypothyroidism such as fatigue. About half of such patients will progress to overt hypothyroidism within 5 years. They often have some **derangement of cholesterol metabolism, such as elevated total and low-density lipoprotein (LDL) cholesterol**. Thyroid hormone replacement can be prescribed in an attempt to relieve symptoms, or possibly to reduce cardiovascular risk.

In overt hypothyroidism, the TSH is markedly elevated, and a low free T4 or free thyroxine index (low T4, low T3 uptake) is also seen. T3 levels can be normal, because the elevated TSH levels may induce hypersecretion of T3 from the gland. Elevated cholesterol levels are also common.

The overwhelming majority of patients with hypothyroidism can be treated with once-daily dosing of synthetic levothyroxine, which is biochemically identical to the natural hormone. **Levothyroxine is relatively inexpensive, has a long half-life (6–7 days), allowing once-daily** dosing, and gives a predictable response. Older thyroid preparations such as desiccated thyroid extract are also available, but are not favored because they have a high content of T3, which is rapidly absorbed and can produce tachyarrhythmias, and the T4 content is less predictable. In **older patients and in those with known cardiovascular disease, dosing should start at a low level,** such as 25–50mcg/d, and increased at similar increments once every 4–6 weeks to an average dose of 1.7-2.1 micrograms/kg body weight. Overly rapid replacement with the sudden increase in metabolic rate can overwhelm the coronary or cardiac reserve. Depending on the cause of hypothyroidism, and the amount of residual gland function, individual patient needs will vary widely. The **TSH level will take 6–8 weeks to readjust to a new dosing level**, so follow-up laboratory testing should be scheduled accordingly.

Comprehension Questions

[12.1] A 42-year-old woman presents to your office for her annual physical. On exam, you note neck fullness, and when you palpate her thyroid, it is enlarged, smooth, rubbery, and nontender**.** The patient is asymptomatic. You send her for thyroid function testing: her T4, free T4, and T3 are normal, but her TSH is slightly elevated. What is the most likely diagnosis?

A. Iodine deficiency
B. Thyroid cancer

C. Hashimoto thyroiditis
D. Graves disease
E. Multinodular goiter

[12.2] What laboratory tests could be performed to confirm your diagnosis of the patient in case [12.1]?

A. Repeat thyroid function tests
B. Thyroid ultrasound
C. Nuclear thyroid scan
D. Antithyroid antibody tests
E. Complete blood count with differential

[12.3] A 19-year-old gymnast active in national competition is brought to your office by her mother because her menses have ceased for the last 3 months. Prior to this, she was always regular. She denies excess dieting, although she does work out with her team 3 hours daily. On exam, her body mass index (BMI) is 20 kg/m^2 and is completely normal. Which laboratory test should be ordered first?

A. Thyroid function tests
B. Complete blood count
C. LH/FSH
D. Prolactin
E. Beta-hCG

[12.4] A 35-year-old woman who was diagnosed with hypothyroidism 4 weeks ago presents to your office complaining of persistent feelings of fatigue and sluggishness. After confirming your diagnosis with a measurement of the TSH, you started her on 50 mcg of levothyroxine daily. She has been reading about her diagnosis on the Internet and wants to try desiccated thyroid extract instead of the medicine you gave her. On examination, she weighs 175 lb, her heart rate is 64 bpm at rest, and her blood pressure is normal. What is the best next step?

A. Tell her that this delay in resolution of symptoms is normal and have a followup visit with her in 2 months.
B. Change her medication, as requested, to thyroid extract and titrate.
C. Increase her dose of levothyroxine and have her come back in 4 weeks.
D. Tell her to start a multivitamin with iron to take with her levothyroxine.

Answers

[12.1] **C.** Hashimoto thyroiditis is the most common cause of hypothyroidism with goiter in the United States. It is most commonly found in middle-aged women, although it can be seen in all age groups. Patients can present with a rubbery, nontender goiter that may have "scalloped" borders. Iodine deficiency is exceedingly uncommon in the United States because of iodized salt. Graves disease is a hyperthyroid condition. Patients with multinodular goiter are usually euthyroid. Patients with thyroid cancer are usually euthyroid and have a history of head and neck irradiation.

[12.2] **D.** Hashimoto thyroiditis is an autoimmune disease of the thyroid. Several different autoantibodies directed toward components of the thyroid gland will be present in the patient's serum; however, of these, antithyroperoxidase antibody is almost always detectable (also called antimicrosomal antibody). These antibodies are markers, not the cause, of the destruction of the gland. On thyroid biopsy, lymphocytic infiltration and fibrosis of the gland are pathognomonic. The presence of these autoantibodies predicts progressive gland failure and need for hormone replacement. None of the other tests will be helpful.

[12.3] **E.** In a young woman with oligomenorrhea, pregnancy should always be the first diagnosis considered. Urine pregnancy tests are easily performed in the office, and are highly sensitive. Serum beta-hCG can be measured to confirm a negative test. In this patient, the next most likely diagnosis is hypothalamic hypogonadism, secondary to her strenuous exercise regimen. These young women are at risk of osteoporosis, and should be counseled as to adequate nutrition and offered combined oral contraceptives if the amenorrhea persists.

[12.4] **C.** Levothyroxine is the preferred replacement hormone for hypothyroidism. The amount of hormone batch to batch, as well as the patient dose response, are believed to be more predictable than with other forms of hormone replacement, such as thyroid extract, which is made from desiccated beef or pork thyroid glands. There is no evidence that the natural hormone replacement is superior to the synthetic. The dose of levothyroxine should be titrated to relief of symptoms, as well as to normalization of the TSH. Other medications, especially iron-containing vitamins, should be taken at different times than levothyroxine, because they may interfere with absorption.

CLINICAL PEARLS

- ❖ The most common causes of oligomenorrhea are disorders of the hypothalamic–pituitary–gonadal axis, such as polycystic ovarian syndrome and hypothyroidism.
- ❖ Hypothyroidism is a cause of hyperprolactinemia. Both hypothyroidism and hyperprolactinemia may cause hypothalamic dysfunction, leading to menstrual irregularities.
- ❖ The most common cause of hypothyroidism is primary thyroid gland failure as a result of Hashimoto thyroiditis.

- ❖ A low free T4 or FTI and a high TSH characterize primary hypothyroidism.
- ❖ Synthetic levothyroxine (T4) replacement is the treatment of choice for hypothyroidism; in older patients, you need to "start low and go slow."
- ❖ The goal of therapy is to normalize the TSH in primary hypothyroidism and to relieve symptoms.

REFERENCES

Carr BR, Bradshaw KD. Disturbances of menstruation and other common gynecologic complaints in women. In: Braunwald E, Fauci AS, Kasper KL, et al, eds. Harrison's principles of internal medicine, 15th ed. New York: McGraw-Hill, 2001:295–7.

Jameson JL, Weetman AP. Disorders of the thyroid gland. In: Braunwald E, Fauci AS, Kasper KL, et al, eds. Harrison's principles of internal medicine, 14th ed. New York: McGraw-Hill, 2001:2066–9.

CASE 13

A 49-year-old woman presents to the emergency room complaining of a 4-week history of progressive abdominal swelling and discomfort. She has no other gastrointestinal symptoms, and has a normal appetite and normal bowel habits. Her past medical history is significant only for three pregnancies, one of which was complicated by excessive blood loss, requiring a blood transfusion. She is happily married for 20 years, exercises, doesn't smoke, and only drinks occasionally. On pointed questioning, however, she does admit that she was "wild" in her youth, and did snort cocaine once or twice at parties many years ago. She does not use drugs now. She was HIV-negative at the time of the birth of her last child.

On examination, her temperature is 100.3° F, her heart rate is 88 bpm, and her blood pressure is 94/60 mmHg. She is thin, her complexion is sallow, her sclerae are icteric, her chest is clear, and her heart is regular with no murmur. Her abdomen is distended and with mild diffuse tenderness, hypoactive bowel sounds, shifting dullness to percussion, and a fluid wave. She has no peripheral edema. Laboratory studies are normal except that her Na is 129 mEq/L, her albumin is 2.8 mg/dL, her total bilirubin is 4 mg/dL, her prothrombin time is 15 seconds, her hemoglobin is 12 g/dL with a mean cell volume (MCV) of 102 fL, and her platelet count is $78{,}000/mm^3$.

- **What is the most likely diagnosis?**

- **What is your next step?**

ANSWERS TO CASE 13: Cirrhosis, Probable Hepatitis C Related

Summary: A 49-year-old woman presents with new-onset abdominal swelling. Her past history reveals a blood transfusion with postpartum hemorrhage and use of cocaine. On examination, her temperature is 100.3° F, her heart rate is 88 bpm, and her blood pressure is 94/60 mmHg. Her sclerae are icteric. Her abdomen is distended with mild diffuse tenderness, shifting dullness to percussion, and a fluid wave, consistent with ascites. She has no peripheral edema. Laboratory studies show the following levels: Na 129 mmol/L, albumin 2.8 mg/dL, prothrombin time 15 seconds, hemoglobin 12 g/dL with an MCV 102 fL, and a platelet count of 78,000/mm^3.

- **Most likely diagnosis:** Ascites caused by portal hypertension as a complication of hepatic cirrhosis.
- **Next step:** Perform a paracentesis to evaluate the ascitic fluid to try to determine its likely etiology, as well as evaluate for the complication of spontaneous bacterial peritonitis.

Analysis

Objectives

1. Know the causes of chronic hepatitis, especially hepatitis C virus.
2. Learn the complications of chronic hepatitis, such as cirrhosis and portal hypertension.
3. Understand the utility of the serum-ascites albumin gradient (SAAG) to differentiate causes of ascites.
4. Know how to diagnose spontaneous bacterial peritonitis.

Considerations

This 49-year-old woman had been in good health until recently, when she noted increasing abdominal swelling and discomfort, indicative of ascites. The physical examination is consistent with ascites with the fluid wave and shifting dullness. Her icteric suggests the liver as the etiology of the ascites. Her laboratory studies are significant for hypoalbuminemia and coagulopathy (prolonged prothrombin time), indicating probable impaired hepatic synthetic function and advanced liver disease. She does have prior exposures, most notably a blood transfusion, which put her at risk for hepatitis viruses, especially hepatitis C. Currently, she also has a low-grade fever and mild abdominal tenderness, both signs of infection. Bacterial infection of the ascitic fluid needs to be considered, because untreated cases have a high mortality.

While the large majority of patients with ascites and jaundice have cirrhosis, other etiologies of the ascites must be considered, including malignancy. Thus, a paracentesis using a needle introduced through the skin into the peritoneal cavity can be used to assess for infection, as well as to seek an etiology of the ascites.

APPROACH TO CHRONIC HEPATITIS

Definitions

Ascites: Abnormal accumulation (>25 mL) of fluid within the peritoneal cavity.

Chronic hepatitis: Evidence of hepatic inflammation and necrosis, usually found by elevated transaminases, for at least 6 months.

Cirrhosis: A histologic diagnosis reflecting irreversible chronic hepatic injury, which includes extensive fibrosis and formation of regenerative nodules.

Portal hypertension: Increased pressure gradient (>10 mmHg) in the portal vein, usually resulting from resistance to portal flow, and most commonly caused by cirrhosis.

Spontaneous bacterial peritonitis: Bacterial infection of ascitic fluid without any intraabdominal source of infection. Occurs in 10–20% of cirrhotic patients with ascites.

Clinical Approach

Chronic hepatitis is diagnosed when patients have evidence of hepatic inflammation and necrosis (usually found by elevated transaminases) for at least 6 months. The **most common causes of chronic hepatitis are viral infections**, such as **hepatitis B and C, alcohol use, chronic exposure to other drugs or toxins, and autoimmune hepatitis**. Less-common causes are inherited metabolic disorders, such as hemochromatosis, Wilson disease, or alpha-1-antitrypsin deficiency. Table 13–1 lists the diagnostic markers for these disorders.in

Table 13-1
CAUSES OF CHRONIC HEPATITIS

CAUSE	TEST
Hepatitis C	Anti-HCV Ab, presence of HCV RNA
Hepatitis B	Persistent HBsAg, presence of HBeAg
Autoimmune	ANA, anti-LKM (liver kidney microsome)
Hemochromatosis	High transferrin saturation (>50%), high ferritin
Wilson disease	Low serum ceruloplasmin
Alpha-1-antitrypsin deficiency	Low alpha-1-antitrypsin enzyme activity

Hepatitis C infection is most commonly acquired through percutaneous exposure to blood. It can also be transmitted through exposure to other body fluids, although this method is less effective. Risk factors for acquisition of hepatitis C include intravenous drug use, sharing of straws to snort cocaine, hemodialysis, blood transfusion, tattooing, and piercing. In contrast to hepatitis B, sexual transmission is rare. Vertical transmission from mother to child is also uncommon, but occurs more often when the mother has high viral titers or is HIV-positive.

Most patients with hepatitis C are asymptomatic. The clinician must have a high index of suspicion and offer screening to those individuals with risk factors for infection. To date, the best methods for detecting infection include the ELISA (enzyme-linked immunoabsorbent assay) test, which detects anti-HCV antibody, or hepatitis C virus polymerase chain reaction (PCR). Approximately 70–80% of all patients infected with hepatitis C will develop chronic hepatitis in the 10 years following infection. Within 20 years, 30% of those will develop cirrhosis, and over 30 years, 30% of those with cirrhosis may develop hepatocellular carcinoma. Therapy is directed at reducing the viral load to prevent the sequelae of end-stage cirrhosis, liver failure, and hepatocellular carcinoma. Currently, the **only available treatment for hepatitis C remains combination therapy with alpha-interferon and ribavirin**. However, trials have demonstrated a sustained response (undetectable viral levels) in only 40% of those undergoing 48 months of therapy. Pegylated interferons have increased the observed response rate to approximately 50–60%. The therapy, however, has many side effects, such as influenza-like symptoms and depression. The goal of interferon therapy for hepatitis C is to prevent the complications of chronic hepatitis.

Cirrhosis is the end result of chronic hepatocellular injury that leads to both **fibrosis and nodular regeneration**. With ongoing hepatocyte destruction and collagen deposition, the liver shrinks in size and becomes nodular and hard. Alcoholic cirrhosis is one of the most common forms of cirrhosis encountered in the United States. It is related to chronic alcohol use, but there appears to be some hereditary predisposition to the development of fibrosis, and the process is enhanced by concomitant infection with hepatitis C. Clinical symptoms are produced by the hepatic dysfunction, as well as by portal hypertension, which is produced by increased resistance to portal blood flow, producing portal hypertension, and sometimes to resultant portosystemic shunting (Table 13–2). Loss of functioning hepatic mass leads to jaundice, as well as impaired synthesis of albumin (leading to edema), and of clotting factors (leading to coagulopathy). Fibrosis and increased sinusoidal resistance lead to portal hypertension and its complications, such as esophageal varices, ascites, and hypersplenism. Portosystemic shunting via natural collaterals or iatrogenic shunts causes hepatic encephalopathy.

The most common cause of ascites is portal hypertension as a consequence of cirrhosis. The pathogenesis involves a combination of decreased effective circulatory blood volume because of portal hypertension (underfill theory),

Table 13-2

COMPLICATIONS OF CIRRHOSIS

DISORDER	DIAGNOSIS	CLINICAL PRESENTATION	TREATMENT
Portal hypertension	Diagnosis is made by the appearance of the above features, and evaluation of portal blood flow using Doppler ultrasonography	The clinical features are related to portal hypertension and its sequelae—ascites, splenomegaly, hypersplenism, encephalopathy, and bleeding varices	Nonselective beta-blockers such as propranolol lower portal pressure; during acute variceal hemorrhage, Sandostatin or octreotide cause splanchnic vasoconstriction
Ascites	Made by finding free peritoneal fluid on physical exam, or by an imaging study	Abdominal distension, sometimes with peripheral edema	Sodium restriction, Spironolactone; loop diuretics; large-volume paracentesis
Spontaneous bacterial peritonitis	A diagnosis can be made when the ascitic fluid contains more than 250 polymorphonuclear neutrophils/mL and confirmed with a positive culture; the most common organisms are Escherichia coli, Klebsiella, other enteric flora or enterococci, pneumococci	Abdominal pain, distension,fever, decreased bowel sounds, or sometimes few abdominal symptoms but worsening encephalopathy	IV antibiotics, such as cefotaxime or ampicillin/sulbactam

inappropriate renal sodium retention leading to expansion of plasma volume (overfill theory), and decreased plasma oncotic pressure. When not caused by portal hypertension, ascites may be a result of exudative causes such as infection (e.g., tuberculous peritonitis) or malignancy. The patient usually presents with abdominal swelling and demonstration of free fluid by physical examination or imaging procedures such as ultrasonography.

It is important to try to determine the cause of ascites in order to look for reversible causes and for serious causes, such as malignancy, and to guide therapy. Ascitic fluid is obtained by paracentesis and examined for protein, albumin, cell count with differential, and culture. The first step in trying to determine the cause of ascites (see Table 13–3) is to determine whether it is caused by portal hypertension or to an exudative process by calculating serum ascites albumin gradient (SAAG):

serum ascites albumin gradient = serum albumin – ascitic albumin

The treatment of ascites usually consists of dietary sodium restriction coupled with diuretics. Loop diuretics are often combined with spironolactone to provide effective diuresis and to maintain normal potassium levels. **Spontaneous bacterial peritonitis** is a relatively common complication of ascites, thought to be caused by translocation of gut flora into the peritoneal fluid. Symptoms include fever and abdominal pain, but often there is paucity of signs and symptoms. Diagnosis is established by paracentesis and finding >250 polymorphonuclear neutrophils/mm^3, or a positive culture. Culture of ascitic fluid often fails to yield the organism, but when fluid cultures are positive, it is usually with a single organism, most often gram-negative enteric flora, or occasionally enterococci or pneumococci. This is in contrast to

Table 13-3

DIFFERENTIAL DIAGNOSIS OF ASCITES BASED ON SAAG*

High gradient >1.1 g/dL = Portal hypertension
- Cirrhosis
- Portal vein thrombosis
- Budd-Chiari syndrome
- Congestive heart failure
- Constrictive pericarditis

Low gradient <1.1 g/dl = nonportal hypertension
- Peritoneal carcinomatosis
- Tuberculous peritonitis
- Pancreatic ascites
- Bowel obstruction or infarction
- Serositis, e.g., as in lupus
- Nephrotic syndrome

*SAAG: serum ascites albumin gradient = serum albumin – ascitic albumin

secondary peritonitis, for example, as a consequence of intestinal perforation, which is usually polymicrobial. Empiric therapy includes coverage for Gram-positive cocci and Gram-negative rods, such as intravenous ampicillin and gentamicin, or a third-generation cephalosporin or a quinolone antibiotic.

Comprehension Questions

Match the probable cause of cirrhosis or liver failure (A to G) with the patient and the patient's presentation [13.1 to 13.5]:

A. Wilson disease
B. Hematochromatosis
C. Primary biliary cirrhosis
D. Sclerosing cholangitis
E. Autoimmune hepatitis
F. Alcohol-induced hepatitis
G. Viral hepatitis

[13.1] A 15-year-old girl with elevated liver enzymes and a positive ANA (antinuclear antibody).

[13.2] A 56-year-old man with brittle diabetes, tan skin, and a family history of cirrhosis.

[13.3] A 35-year-old man with ulcerative colitis.

[13.4] A 56-year-old woman who presented complaining of pruritus and fatigue.

[13.5] A 32-year-old man with Kayser-Fleischer rings, dysarthria, and spasticity.

Answers

[13.1] **E.** Idiopathic or autoimmune hepatitis is a less-well-understood cause of hepatitis that seems to be caused by autoimmune cell-mediated damage to hepatocytes. A subgroup of these patients includes young women with positive antinuclear antibodies and hypergammaglobulinemia who may have other symptoms and signs of systemic lupus erythematosus.

[13.2] **B.** Hemochromatosis is a genetic disorder of iron metabolism. Progressive iron overload leads to organ destruction. Diabetes mellitus, cirrhosis of the liver, hypogonadotrophic hypogonadism, arthropathy, and cardiomyopathy are among the more common end-stage developments. Skin deposition of iron leads to "bronzing" of the skin, which could be mistaken for a tan. Diagnosis is made early in the course of disease through demonstrating elevated iron stores, but can be made through liver biopsy with iron stains. Genetic testing is also available. Therapy involves phlebotomy to remove excess iron stores.

[13.3] **D.** Sclerosing cholangitis is an autoimmune destruction of both the intra- and extrahepatic bile ducts and is often associated with inflammatory bowel disease, most commonly ulcerative colitis. Patients present with jaundice or symptoms of biliary obstruction; cholangiography reveals the characteristic beading of the bile ducts.

[13.4] **C.** Primary biliary cirrhosis is also thought to be an autoimmune disease leading to destruction of the small- to medium-size bile ducts. Most patients are women between the ages of 35 and 60 years, who usually present with symptoms of pruritus and fatigue. An alkaline phosphatase level elevated two to five times above the baseline in an otherwise asymptomatic patient should also raise suspicion for the disease. There is no specific therapy available.

[13.5] **A.** Wilson disease is an inherited disorder of copper metabolism. The inability to excrete excess copper leads to deposition of the mineral in the liver, brain, and other organs. Patients can present with fulminant hepatitis, acute nonfulminant hepatitis, or cirrhosis, or with bizarre behavioral changes as a result of neurologic damage. Kayser-Fleischer rings develop when copper is released from the liver and deposits in Descemet membrane of the cornea.

CLINICAL PEARLS

- ❖ The most common causes of cirrhosis are alcohol use, hepatitis B and C, and autoimmune disorders.
- ❖ Hepatitis C is most commonly contracted through blood exposure, rarely through sexual contact, and most patients are asymptomatic until they develop complications of chronic liver disease.
- ❖ A serum ascites albumin gradient (SAAG) >1.1 g/dL suggests that ascites is caused by portal hypertension, as occurs in cirrhosis.
- ❖ Treatment of cirrhotic ascites requires sodium restriction and, usually, diuretics, such as spironolactone and furosemide.
- ❖ Spontaneous bacterial peritonitis is infection of the ascitic fluid characterized by >250 polymorphonuclear cells/mm^3, sometimes with a positive monomicrobial culture.

REFERENCES

Shara A. Hepatitis C. Ann Intern Med 1996;125(8):658–668.

Dienstag JL, Isselbacher KJ. Chronic Hepatitis. In: Braunwald E, Fauci AS, Kasper KL, et al., eds. Harrison's Principles of Internal Medicine, 15th ed. New York: McGraw-Hill, 2001:1742-1752.

Chung RT, Podolsky DK. Cirrhosis and its Complications. In: Braunwald E, Fauci AS, Kasper KL, et al., eds. Harrison's Principles of Internal Medicine, 15th ed. New York: McGraw-Hill, 2001:1754-1767.

CASE 14

A 42-year-old Hispanic woman presents to the emergency department complaining of 24 hours of severe, steady epigastric abdominal pain, radiating to her back, with several episodes of nausea and vomiting. She has had similar painful episodes in the past, usually in the evening following heavy meals, but they always resolved spontaneously within an hour or two. This time the pain did not improve, so she sought medical attention. She has no prior medical history and takes no medications. She is married, has three children, and does not drink alcohol or smoke cigarettes.

On examination, she is afebrile, tachycardic with a heart rate of 104 bpm, blood pressure of 115/74 mmHg, and shallow respirations of 22 breaths per minute. She is moving uncomfortably on the stretcher, her skin is warm and diaphoretic, and she has scleral icterus. Her abdomen is soft, mildly distended with marked right upper quadrant and epigastric tenderness to palpation, hypoactive bowel sounds, and no masses or organomegaly appreciated. Her stool is negative for occult blood. Laboratory studies are significant for a total bilirubin (9.2 g/dL) with a direct fraction of 4.8 g/dL, an alkaline phosphatase of 285 IU/L, aspartate aminotransferase (AST) of 78 IU/L, alanine aminotransferase (ALT) of 92 IU/L, and elevated amylase level of 1249 IU/L. Her leukocyte count is 16,500/mm^3 with 82% polymorphonuclear cells, and 16% lymphocytes. A plain film of the abdomen shows a nonspecific gas pattern and no pneumoperitoneum.

- **What is the most likely diagnosis?**
- **What is the most likely underlying etiology?**
- **What is your next diagnostic step?**

ANSWERS TO CASE 14: Pancreatitis, gallstones

Summary: An older woman with a prior history consistent with symptomatic cholelithiasis now presents with epigastric pain and nausea for 24 hours, much longer than would be expected with uncomplicated biliary colic. Her symptoms are consistent with acute pancreatitis. She also has hyperbilirubinemia and elevated alkaline phosphatase, suggesting obstruction of the common bile duct caused by a gallstone, which is the likely cause of her pancreatitis.

- **Most likely diagnosis:** Acute pancreatitis
- **Most likely etiology:** Choledocholithiasis (common bile duct stone).
- **Next diagnostic step:** Right upper quadrant abdominal ultrasonography.

Analysis

Objectives

1. Know the causes, clinical features, and prognostic factors in acute pancreatitis.
2. Learn the principles of treatment and complications of acute pancreatitis.
3. Know the complications of gallstones.
4. Understand the medical treatment of a patient with biliary sepsis and the indications for endoscopic retrograde cholangiopancreatography (ERCP) or surgical intervention.

Considerations

This 42-year-old woman complained of episodes of mild right upper quadrant abdominal pain with heavy meals in the past. These prior episodes were short-lived. This is very consistent with biliary colic. However, this episode is different in severity and location of pain (now radiating straight to her back and accompanied by nausea and vomiting). The elevated amylase level confirms the clinical impression of acute pancreatitis. She likely has acute pancreatitis caused by a stone in the common bile duct. Biliary obstruction is suggested by the elevated bilirubin level. She is moderately ill, but is hemodynamically stable and has only one prognostic feature to predict mortality—her elevated white blood cell (WBC) count (see Table 14–1). She can likely be managed on a hospital ward without need for intensive care.

APPROACH TO ACUTE PANCREATITIS

Acute pancreatitis is an inflammatory process in which pancreatic enzymes are activated and cause autodigestion of the gland. It can be caused by many processes, but in the United States, **alcohol use is the most common cause**, and episodes are often precipitated by binge drinking. The next most common

Table 14-1
RANSON CRITIERIA FOR SEVERITY OF PANCREATITIS

Initial:
- Age >55 years
- WBC >16,000 /mm^3
- Serum glucose >200
- Serum lactate dehydrogenas (LDH) >350 IU/L
- AST >250 IU/L

Within 48 hours of admission
- Hematocrit drop >10 points
- Blood urea nitrogen (BUN) rise >5 mg/dL after intravenous hydration
- Arterial PO_2 < 60 mmHg
- Serum calcium < 80 mg/dL
- Base deficit >4 mEq/L
- Estimated fluid sequestration of >6 L

Source: Ranson JHC. Am J Gastroenterol 1982; 77:633.

cause is biliary tract disease, usually due to passage of a gallstone into the common bile duct. Hypertriglyceridemia is also a common cause, and occurs when serum triglyceride levels are >1000 mg/dL, as is seen in patients with familial dyslipidemias or diabetes (see Table 14–2 for etiologies). When patients appear to have "idiopathic" pancreatitis, that is, no gallstones are seen on ultrasonography and no other predisposing factor can be found, biliary tract disease is still the most likely cause—either biliary sludge (microlithiasis) or sphincter of Oddi dysfunction.

Abdominal pain is the cardinal symptom of pancreatitis and is often severe, typically in the **upper abdomen with radiation to the back**. The pain is often relieved by sitting up and bending forward, and is exacerbated by food. Patients also **commonly experience nausea and vomiting**, that is precipitated by oral intake. They **may have low-grade fever** (if it is >101°F, one should suspect infection), and are often volume-depleted, because of the vomiting, inability to tolerate oral intake, and also because the inflammatory process may cause third-spacing with sequestration of large volumes of fluid in the peritoneal cavity.

The most common test used to diagnose pancreatitis is an **elevated serum amylase**. It is released from the inflamed pancreas within hours of the attack, and remains elevated for 3–4 days. Amylase undergoes renal clearance, and after serum levels decline, it remains elevated in the urine. **Amylase is not specific to the pancreas**, however, and can be elevated as a consequence of many other abdominal processes such as **gastrointestinal ischemia with infarction or perforation; even just the vomiting** associated with pancreatitis can cause elevated amylase of **salivary origin.** Elevated **serum lipase,** also seen in acute pancreatitis, is **more specific than amylase to pancreatic origin, and**

Table 14-2
CAUSES OF ACUTE PANCREATITIS

Biliary tract disease (e.g., gallstones)
Alcohol use
Drugs (e.g., the antiretroviral didanosine [ddl], pentamidine, thiazides, furosemide, sulfonamides, azathioprine, L-asparaginase)
Surgical manipulation of the gland or ERCP
Hypertriglyceridemia/hypercalcemia
Infections such as mumps or cytomegalovirus
Trauma such as blunt abdominal trauma

remains elevated longer than amylase. When the diagnosis is uncertain, or when complications of pancreatitis are suspected, **CT imaging of the abdomen is highly sensitive** for showing the inflammatory changes in patients with moderate to severe pancreatitis.

Treatment of pancreatitis is mainly supportive, and includes "pancreatic rest," that is, **withholding food or liquids by mouth until symptoms subside**, and adequate **narcotic analgesia, usually with meperidine**. **Intravenous fluids** are necessary for maintenance and to replace any deficits. In patients with severe pancreatitis who sequester large volumes of fluid in their abdomen as pancreatic ascites, sometimes prodigious amounts of parenteral fluid replacement is necessary to maintain intravascular volume. Patients with adynamic ileus and abdominal distension or protracted vomiting may benefit from nasogastric suction. When pain has largely subsided and the patient has bowel sounds, oral clear liquids can be started, and the diet advanced as tolerated.

The large majority of patients with acute pancreatitis will recover spontaneously and have a relatively uncomplicated course. Several criteria have been developed to try to identify the 15–25% of patients who will have a more complicated course. These include the Ranson (US) and Glasgow/Imrie (UK) criteria, as well as the APACHE (Acute Physiology and Chronic Health Evaluation) II scoring system. When three or more of the following are present, a severe course complicated by pancreatic necrosis can be predicted by Ranson's criteria (see Table 14–1). **The most common cause of early death in patients with pancreatitis is hypovolemic shock**, which is multifactorial: third-spacing and sequestration of large fluid volumes in the abdomen, as well as increased capillary permeability. Others develop pulmonary edema, which may be noncardiogenic as a consequence of acute respiratory distress syndrome (ARDS), or cardiogenic as a consequence of myocardial dysfunction.

Pancreatic complications include a **phlegmon**, which is a solid mass of inflamed pancreas, often with patchy areas of necrosis. Sometimes, extensive areas of **pancreatic necrosis** develop within a phlegmon. Either necrosis or a phlegmon can become secondarily infected, resulting in **pancreatic abscess.** Abscesses typically develop 2–3 weeks after the onset of the illness, and should be suspected if there is fever or leukocytosis. If pancreatic abscesses are not drained, the mortality approaches 100%. Pancreatic necrosis and abscess are the leading causes of death in patients after the first week of illness. A **pancreatic pseudocyst** is a collection of inflammatory fluid and pancreatic secretions with a high enzyme content. Most will resolve spontaneously within 6 weeks, especially if they are <6 cm, but if they are causing pain, if they are large or expanding, or if they become infected, they usually require drainage. Any of these local complications of pancreatitis should be suspected if persistent pain, fever, abdominal mass, or persistent hyperamylasemia occurs.

Gallstones

Gallstones are usually formed as a consequence of precipitation of cholesterol microcrystals in bile, and are very common, occurring in 10–20% of patients older than 65 years of age. They are often asymptomatic, and when discovered incidentally, may be followed without intervention, as only 10% of patients will develop any symptoms related to their stones within 10 years. When patients do develop symptoms because of a stone in the cystic duct or Hartmann pouch, the typical attack of **biliary colic** usually has a sudden onset, often precipitated by a large or fatty meal, with severe steady pain in the right upper quadrant or epigastrium, lasting between 1 and 4 hours. They may have mild elevations of the alkaline phosphatase and slight hyperbilirubinemia, but elevations of the bilirubin over 3g/dL suggest a common duct stone. The first diagnostic test in a patient with suspected gallstones is usually an **ultrasonogram**. It is noninvasive and very sensitive for detecting stones in the gallbladder, as well as intrahepatic or extrahepatic biliary duct dilatation.

One of the most common complications of gallstones is **acute cholecystitis**, which occurs when a stone becomes impacted in the cystic duct, and edema and inflammation develop behind the obstruction. This is apparent ultrasonographically as gallbladder wall thickening and pericholecystic fluid, and is characterized clinically as a persistent right upper quadrant abdominal pain, with fever and leukocytosis. Cultures of bile in the gallbladder often yield enteric flora such as *Escherichia coli* and *Klebsiella.* If the diagnosis is in question, nuclear scintigraphy with a **hepatoiminodiacetic acid (HIDA) scan** may be performed. The positive test shows visualization of the liver by the isotope, but nonvisualization of the gallbladder, may indicate an obstructed cystic duct. Treatment of acute cholecystitis usually involves making the patient NPO (nil per os), intravenous fluids and antibiotics, and early cholecystectomy within 48–72 hours.

Another complication of gallstones is **cholangitis**, which occurs when there is intermittent obstruction of the common bile duct, allowing reflux of bacteria up the biliary tree, followed by development of purulent infection behind the obstruction. If the patient is septic, it requires urgent decompression of the biliary tree, either surgically or by endoscopic retrograde cholangiography (ERCP), to remove the stones endoscopically after performing a papillotomy, which allows the other stones to pass.

Comprehension Questions

[14.1] A 43-year-old man who is an alcoholic is admitted to the hospital with acute pancreatitis. He is given intravenous hydration and is placed NPO. Which of the following findings is a poor prognostic sign?

A. His age
B. Initial serum glucose of 60 mg/dL
C. Blood urea nitrogen (BUN) rise of 7 mg/dL over 48 hours
D. Hematocrit drop of 3%
E. Amylase level of 1000 IU/L

[14.2] A 37-year-old woman is noted to have gallstones on ultrasonography. She is given a low-fat diet. After 3 months she is noted to have severe right upper quadrant pain, fever to 102°F, and nausea. Which of the following is the most likely diagnosis?

A. Acute cholangitis
B. Acute cholecystitis
C. Acute pancreatitis
D. Acute perforation of the gallbladder

[14.3] A 45-year-old male was admitted for acute pancreatitis thought to be a result of blunt abdominal trauma. After 3 months he persists with epigastric pain, but is able to eat solid food. His amylase level is elevated at 260 IU/L. Which of the following is the most likely diagnosis?

A. Recurrent pancreatitis
B. Diverticulitis
C. Peptic ulcer disease
D. Pancreatic pseudocyst

Answers

[14.1] **C.** When the BUN rises by 5 mg/dL after 48 hours despite IV hydration, it is a poor prognostic sign. Notably, the amylase level does not correlate to the severity of the disease.

[14.2] **B.** Acute cholecystitis is one of the most common complication of gallstones. This patient with fever, right upper quadrant pain, and a history of gallstones, likely has acute cholecystitis.

[14.3] **D.** A pancreatic pseudocyst has a clinical presentation of abdominal pain and mass, and persistent hyperamylasemia in a patient with prior pancreatitis.

CLINICAL PEARLS

- ❖ The most common causes of acute pancreatitis in the United States are alcohol, gallstones, and hypertriglyceridemia.
- ❖ Acute pancreatitis is usually managed with pancreatic rest, intravenous hydration, and analgesia, often with narcotics.
- ❖ Patients with pancreatitis who have zero to two of Ranson's criteria are expected to have a mild course; those with three or more can have significant mortality.
- ❖ Pancreatic complications (phlegmon, necrosis, abscess, pseudocyst) should be suspected if persistent pain, fever, abdominal mass, or persistent hyperamylasemia occurs.
- ❖ Patients with asymptomatic gallstones do not require treatment; they may be observed and treated if symptoms develop. Cholecystectomy is performed for patients with symptoms of biliary colic, or for those with complications.
- ❖ Acute cholecystitis is best treated with antibiotics, and then cholecystectomy generally within 48–72 hours.

REFERENCES

Greenberger NJ, Toskes PP. Acute and Chronic Pancreatitis. In: Braunwald E, Fauci AS, Kasper KL, et al., eds. Harrison's Principles of Internal Medicine, 15th ed. New York: McGraw-Hill, 2001:1792-1804.

Greenberger NJ, Paumgartner G. Diseases of the Gallbladder and Bile Ducts. In: Braunwald E, Fauci AS, Kasper KL, et al., eds. Harrison's Principles of Internal Medicine, 15th ed. New York: McGraw-Hill, 2001:1776-1788.

CASE 15

A 72-year-old man is brought to the emergency room after fainting while in church. He had stood up to sing a hymn and then fell to the floor. His wife, who witnessed the episode, reports that he was unconscious for approximately 5 minutes. When he awakened, he was groggy for another minute or two, then seemed himself. No abnormal movements were noted. This has never happened to him before, but she does report that for the last several months he has had to curtail activities such as mowing the lawn, because he becomes weak and feels light-headed. His only medical history is osteoarthritis of his knees, for which he takes acetaminophen.

On examination, he is alert, talkative, and smiling. He is afebrile, his heart is regular with a rate of 35 bpm, and his blood pressure is 118/72 mmHg, which remains unchanged on standing. He has a contusion on his face, left arm, and chest wall, but no lacerations. His chest is clear to auscultation, and his heart is regular but bradycardic with a nondisplaced apical impulse. He has no focal deficits. Laboratory exam shows normal blood counts, normal renal function and serum electrolytes, and negative cardiac enzymes. His EKG is shown in Figure 15–1.

- **What is the most likely diagnosis?**

- **What is your next step?**

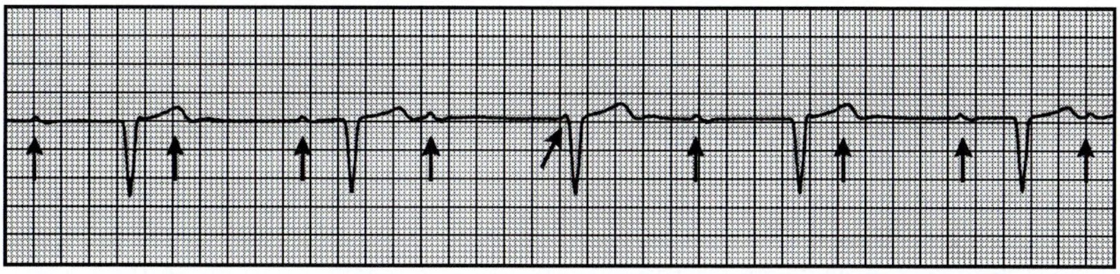

Figure 15–1. EKG. **(Reproduced with permission from Stead LG, Stead SM, Kaufman MS. First aid for the medicine clerkship. New York: McGraw-Hill, 2002:50.)**

ANSWERS TO CASE 15: Syncope–Heart Block

Summary: An older man presents with a witnessed syncopal episode, which was brief and not associated with seizure activity. He has had decreasing exercise tolerance recently because of weakness and presyncopal symptoms. He is bradycardic, with third-degree atrioventricular block on EKG. Arrows in figure point to P waves.

- **Most likely diagnosis:** Syncope as a consequence of third-degree atrioventricular (AV) block.

- **Next step:** Placement of temporary transcutaneous or transvenous pacemaker and evaluation for placement of a permanent pacemaker.

Analysis

Objectives

1. Know the major causes of syncope and important historical clues to the diagnosis.
2. Understand the basic evaluation of syncope based on the history.
3. Recognize vasovagal syncope and carotid sinus hypersensitivity.
4. Be able to diagnose and know the management of first-, second-, and third-degree AV block.

Considerations

There are two major considerations to the management of this patient: the cause and the management of his AV block. He should be evaluated for myocardial infarction, and structural cardiac abnormalities. If this evaluation is negative, he may simply have conduction system disease as a consequence of aging. Regarding temporary management, atropine or isoproterenol can be used when the conduction block is at the level of the AV node, but in this case, the heart rate is less than 40 bpm, and the QRS borderline is widened, suggesting the defect is below the AV node, in the bundles of His. A pacemaker is likely to be required.

APPROACH TO SYNCOPE

Syncope is a transient loss of consciousness and postural tone with subsequent spontaneous recovery. It is a very common phenomenon, resulting in 5–10% of emergency room visits and resulting hospitalization. The causes are varied, but they all result in transiently diminished cerebral perfusion leading to the loss of consciousness. The prognosis is quite varied, ranging from a benign episode in an otherwise young, healthy person with a clear precipitating event, such as emotional stress, to a more serious occurrence in an older patient with cardiac disease. In the latter syncope has been referred to as "sudden cardiac death, averted." For that reason, higher risk patients routinely undergo hospitalization and sometimes extensive evaluation to determine the cause.

Traditionally, the etiologies of syncope have been divided into neurologic and cardiac. However, this is probably not a useful classification, because neurologic diseases are almost never the cause of syncopal episodes. Syncope is essentially never a result of transient ischemic attacks (TIAs), because syncope reflects global cerebral hypoperfusion, and TIAs are a result of regional ischemia. Vertebrobasilar insufficiency with resultant loss of consciousness is often discussed, yet rarely seen in clinical practice. Seizure episodes are a common cause of transient loss of consciousness, and it is often quite difficult to distinguish seizure episodes from syncopal episodes based on history. To further complicate matters, the same lack of cerebral blood flow that produced the loss of consciousness can lead to post-syncopal seizure activity. But seizures are best discussed elsewhere, so our discussion here is confined to syncope. **The only neurologic diseases that commonly cause syncope** are disturbances in **autonomic function** leading to **orthostatic hypotension as occurs in diabetes, Parkinson, or idiopathic dysautonomia**. For patients in whom a definitive diagnosis of syncope can be ascertained, the causes are usually excess vagal activity, orthostatic hypotension, or cardiac disease—either arrhythmias or outflow obstructions. Table 15–1 lists the most common causes of syncope. By far, the most useful evaluation to try to diagnose the cause of syncope is the patient's history. Because, by definition, the patient was unconscious, the patient may only be able to report preceding and subsequent symptoms, so finding a witness to describe the episode is extremely helpful.

Vasovagal syncope refers to excessive vagal tone causing impaired autonomic responses, that is, a fall in blood pressure without appropriate rise in heart rate or vasomotor tone. This is, by far, the **most common cause of syncope**, and is the usual cause of a "fainting spell" in an otherwise healthy young person. Episodes are often precipitated by physical or emotional stress, or by a painful experience. There is usually a clear precipitating event by history and, often, prodromal symptoms such as nausea, yawning, or diaphoresis. The episodes are brief, lasting seconds to minutes, with a rapid recovery. Syncopal episodes can also be triggered by physiologic activities that increase vagal tone, such as **micturition**, defecation, or coughing in otherwise healthy people.

Carotid sinus hypersensitivity is also **vagally mediated**. This usually occurs in older men, and episodes can be triggered by turning the head to the side, by wearing a tight collar, or even by shaving the neck over the area. Pressure over one or both carotid sinuses causes excess vagal activity with resultant cardiac slowing, and can produce sinus bradycardia, sinus arrest, or even atrioventricular block. Less commonly, carotid sinus pressure can cause a

Table 15-1
CAUSES OF SYNCOPE

Cardiogenic

A. Cardiac arrhythmias
   1. Bradyarrhythmias
      a. Sinus bradycardia, sinoatrial block, sinus arrest, sick-sinus syndrome
      b. Atrioventricular block
   2. Tachyarrhythmias
      a. Supraventricular tachycardia with structural cardiac disease
      b. Atrial fibrillation associated with the Wolff-Parkinson-White syndrome
      c. Atrial flutter with 1:1 atrioventricular conduction
      d. Ventricular tachycardia

B. Other cardiopulmonary etiologies
   1. Pulmonary embolism
   2. Pulmonary hypertension
   3. Atrial myxoma
   4. Myocardial disease (massive myocardial infarction)
   5. Left ventricular myocardial restriction or constriction
   6. Pericardial constriction or tamponade
   7. Aortic outflow tract obstruction (Aortic valvular stenosis, Hypertrophic obstructive cardiomyopathy)

Noncardiogenic

A. Vasovagal (vasodepressor, neurocardiogenic)

B. Postural (orthostatic) hypotension
   1. Drug induced (especially antihypertensive or vasodilator drugs)
   2. Peripheral neuropathy (diabetic, alcoholic, nutritional, amyloid)
   3. Idiopathic postural hypotension
   4. Neurologic disorder (Shy-Drager syndrome)
   5. Physical deconditioning
   6. Sympathectomy
   7. Acute dysautonomia (Guillain-Barré syndrome variant)
   8. **Decreased blood volume (adrenal insufficiency, acute blood loss, etc.)**

C. Carotid sinus hypersensitivity

D. Situational
   1. Cough
   2. Micturition
   3. Defecation
   4. Valsalva

Modified from Daroff RB, Carlson MD. Nervous system dysfunction: syncope. In Braunwald E, Fauci AS, Kasper DL, et al, eds. *Harrison's Principles of Internal Medicine*, 15th ed. New York: McGraw Hill, 2001: 112.

fall in arterial pressure without cardiac slowing. When recurrent syncope as a result of bradyarrhythmias occurs, a demand pacemaker is often required.

Patients with **orthostatic hypotension** typically report symptoms related to position changes such as rising from a seated or recumbent position, and **the postural drop in systolic blood pressure by more than 20 mmHg** can be demonstrated on examination. This can occur because of hypovolemia (hemorrhage, anemia, diarrhea or vomiting, Addison disease), or with adequate circulating volume, but impaired autonomic responses. Probably the most common reason for this autonomic impairment is iatrogenic as a result of antihypertensive or other medications, especially in elderly persons. It can also be caused by autonomic insufficiency seen in diabetic neuropathy, or in a syndrome of chronic idiopathic orthostatic hypotension in older men, or by the primary neurologic conditions mentioned previously. Multiple events that are all unwitnessed or that only occur in periods of emotional upset suggest **factitious** symptoms.

Etiologies of **cardiogenic syncope** include rhythm disturbances and structural heart abnormalities. Certain structural heart abnormalities will cause obstruction of blood flow to the brain, resulting in syncope. These include aortic stenosis, hypertrophic obstructive cardiomyopathy (HOCM), massive pulmonary embolism, or severe pulmonary hypertension. Syncope caused by cardiac outflow obstruction typically presents during or immediately after exertion. An echocardiogram is often obtained to elucidate such abnormalities.

Arrhythmias are the most common cardiac cause of syncope. Sinus bradycardia, AV nodal blocks (see *Heart Block* below), and sick sinus syndrome are bradyarrhythmic causes of syncope. On the other hand, tachyarrhythmias can result from atrial fibrillation or flutter, supraventricular tachycardia (SVT) ventricular tachycardia (VT), or ventricular fibrillation (VF). Often, the rhythm abnormality is apparent by routine EKG, or if it occurs paroxysmally, it can be recorded using a 24-hour Holter monitor or an event monitor. Sometimes evaluation requires invasive electrophysiologic studies to assess sinus node or atrioventricular node function, or to induce supraventricular or ventricular arrhythmias.

Heart Block

There are three types of AV node block, all based on EKG findings. **First-degree AV block** is a prolonged PR interval >200 msec (>1 large box). This is a conduction delay in the AV node. Prognosis is good, and there is usually no need for pacing. **Second-degree AV block** comes in two types. Mobitz type I (Wenckebach) is a progressive **lengthening of the PR interval**, until a dropped beat is produced. The resulting P wave of the dropped beat is not followed by a QRS complex. This phenomenon is caused by abnormal conduction in the AV node, and may be the result of inferior myocardial infarction. Prognosis is good, and there is generally no need for pacing unless symptomatic (i.e., bradycardia, syncope, heart failure, asystole >3 seconds).

On the other hand, **Mobitz type II produces dropped beats without lengthening of the PR interval.** This is usually caused by a block within the bundle of His. Permanent pacing is often indicated in these patients because the Mobitz type II AV block may later progress into complete heart block. **Third-degree AV block** is a complete heart block, where the sinoatrial (SA) node and AV node fire at independent rates. The atrial rhythm is faster than the ventricular escape rhythm. Permanent pacing is indicated in these patients, especially when associated with symptoms such as exercise intolerance or syncope.

Comprehension Questions

[15.1] An 18-year-old girl is brought to the emergency room because she fainted at a rock concert. She apparently recovered spontaneously, did not exhibit any seizure activity, and has no medical history. She has a heart rate of 90 bpm and a blood pressure of 110/70 mmHg. The neurological examination is normal. The pregnancy test is negative. Which of the following is the most appropriate management?

A. Admit to hospital for cardiac evaluation
B. Outpatient echocardiogram
C. 24-hour Holter monitor
D. Reassurance and discharge home

[15.2] A 67-year-old woman has diabetes and mild hypertension. She is noted to have some diabetic retinopathy, and states that she cannot feel her legs. She has recurrent episodes of lightheadedness when she gets up in the morning and comes in because she had fainted this morning. Which of the following is the most likely cause of her syncope?

A. Carotid sinus hypersensitivity
B. Pulmonary embolism
C. Autonomic neuropathy
D. Critical aortic stenosis

[15.3] A 74-year-old man with no prior medical problems faints while shaving. He has a quick recovery and has no neurological deficits. His blood sugar is normal and EKG shows a normal sinus rhythm. Which of the following is the most useful diagnostic test of his probable condition?

A. Carotid massage
B. Echocardiogram
C. CT scan of head
D. Serial cardiac enzymes

[15.4] A 49-year-old man is admitted to the ICU with a diagnosis of an inferior MI. He has a heart rate of 35 bpm, and a blood pressure of 90/50 mmHg. The EKG shows a Mobitz type I heart block. Which of the following is the best next step?

A. Atropine
B. Transvenous pacer
C. Lidocaine
D. Observation

Answers

[15.1] **D.** A young patient without a medical history and with no seizure activity is unlikely to have any serious problems.

[15.2] **C.** This diabetic patient has evidence of micro-vascular disease including peripheral neuropathy, and likely has autonomic dysfunction.

[15.3] **A.** He likely has carotid hypersensitivity; thus, careful carotid massage (after auscultation to ensure no bruits are present) may be attempted to try to reproduce the symptoms.

[15.4] **A.** This patient's bradycardia is severe, probably a result of the inferior MI. Atropine is the agent of choice in this situation. The Mobitz type I block has a good prognosis (versus complete heart block), so that transvenous pacing is not usually required.

CLINICAL PEARLS

❖ Vasovagal syncope is the most common cause of syncope in healthy young people. It often has a precipitating event, prodromal symptoms, and an excellent prognosis.

❖ Carotid sinus hypersensitivity causes bradyarrhythmias in older patients with pressure over the carotid bulb, and sometimes requires a pacemaker.

❖ Syncope caused by cardiac outflow obstruction, such as aortic stenosis, occurs during or after exertion.

❖ Syncope is a very common problem, affecting nearly one-third of the adult population at some point, but a specific cause is identified in less than half of cases.

❖ Permanent pacing is usually indicated for symptomatic bradyarrhythmias (e.g., sick sinus syndrome), Mobitz II atrioventricular block, or third-degree heart block.

REFERENCES

Gregoratos G, Abrams J, Epstein AE, et al. ACC/AHA/NASPE 2002 Guideline Update for Implantation of Cardiac Pacemakers and Antiarrhythmia Devices—Summary article: a report of the American College of Cardiology/American Heart Association Task Force on Practice Guidelines (ACC/AHA/NASPE Committee to Update the 1998 Pacemaker Guidelines). *J Am Coll Cardiol* 2002;40:1703-1709

Daroff RB, Carlson MD. Nervous system dysfunction: syncope. In: Braunwald E, Fauci AS, Kasper KL, et al., eds. Harrison's principles of internal medicine, 15th ed. New York: McGraw-Hill, 2001:111–16.

Josephson ME. Disorders of rhythm: AV conduction disturbances. In: Braunwald E, Fauci AS, Kasper KL, et al., eds. Harrison's principles of internal medicine, 15th ed. New York: McGraw-Hill, 2001:1286–92.

❖ CASE 16

A 28-year-old man comes to the emergency room complaining of 2 days of abdominal pain and diarrhea. He describes his stools as frequent, with 10–12 per day, small volume, sometimes with visible blood and mucus, and preceded by a sudden urge to defecate. The abdominal pain is crampy, diffuse, and moderately severe, and is not relieved with defecation. He has had similar episodes in the past several months of abdominal pain and loose mucoid stools, but they were milder, and resolved within 24–48 hours. He has no other medical history, and takes no medications. He has neither traveled out of the United States nor had contact with anyone with similar symptoms. He works as an accountant and does not smoke or drink alcohol. There is no one in his family with gastrointestinal problems.

On examination, his temperature is 99°F, his heart rate is 98 bpm, and his blood pressure is 118/74 mmHg. He appears uncomfortable, is diaphoretic, and is lying still on the stretcher. His sclerae are clear and his oral mucosa is pink and clear. His chest is clear and his heart is regular without murmurs. His abdomen is soft and mildly distended, with hypoactive bowel sounds, and moderate diffuse tenderness, but no guarding or rebound tenderness.

Laboratory studies are significant for a white blood cell count of 15,800/mm^3 with 82% polymorphonuclear leukocytes, hemoglobin of 10.3 g/dL, and a platelet count of 754,000/mm^3. The HIV assay is negative. Renal function and liver function tests are normal. A plain film radiograph of the abdomen shows a mildly dilated air-filled colon with a 4.5-cm diameter and no pneumoperitoneum or air/fluid levels.

- **What is the most likely diagnosis?**

- **What is your next step?**

ANSWERS TO CASE 16: Ulcerative Colitis

Summary: A young man comes in with a moderate to severe presentation of colitis, as manifested by the crampy abdominal pain with tenesmus, low-volume bloody mucoid stool, and colonic dilatation on x-ray. He has no travel or exposure history to suggest infection. He reports a history of previous similar episodes, which suggests a chronic inflammatory rather than acute infectious process.

- **What is the most likely diagnosis?** Colitis, probably ulcerative colitis.
- **What is your next step?** Admit to the hospital, obtain stool samples to exclude infection, and begin therapy with corticosteroids.

Analysis

Objectives

1. Know the typical presentation of inflammatory bowel disease.
2. Know the differences between Crohn disease and ulcerative colitis.
3. Know the treatment of inflammatory bowel disease.

Considerations

Although the likelihood of infection seems low, it must be excluded, and it is necessary to check for infections such as Entamoeba histolytica, *Salmonella, Shigella,* and *Campylobacter,* as well as *Clostridium difficile,* which can occur in the absence of prior antibiotic exposure. We can rule out radiation colitis because there is no history of abdominal neoplasm followed by radiation. Ischemic colitis would be unusual for a patient of his age. The main consideration in this case would be inflammatory bowel disease (IBD) versus infectious colitis. The absence of travel history, family members ill, and the chronicity of the illness all point away from infection. This leaves us with IBD as the most likely diagnosis and there are plenty of clues in the case to support this, beginning with the age of the patient (28 years old). The abdominal x-ray shows a mildly dilated air-filled colon, which implies that the disease is limited to the colon. The grossly bloody stool is also more often seen with ulcerative colitis than with Crohn disease.

At the moment, the patient does not appear to have any life-threatening complication of colitis, such as perforation or toxic megacolon, but he needs to be monitored closely, and surgical consultation may be helpful. The combination of abdominal pain, bloody diarrhea, and the abdominal x-ray localizing the disease to the colon points to a "colitis."

APPROACH TO COLITIS

This differential diagnosis for colitis includes ischemic colitis, infectious colitis (*C. difficile, E. coli, Salmonella, Shigella, Campylobacter*), radiation colitis and inflammatory bowel disease (IBD: Crohn disease versus ulcerative colitis). Mesenteric ischemia is usually encountered in people older than age 50 years with known atherosclerotic vascular disease or other cause of hypoperfusion. The pain is usually acute in onset following a meal and not associated with fevers. With an infectious etiology, patients often have engaged in foreign travel, the symptoms are acute, or there is a recent use of antibiotics. Also, family members often have with the same symptoms.

IBD is most commonly diagnosed in young patients between the ages of 15 and 25 years. There is also a second peak in the incidence of IBD (usually Crohn disease) between the ages of 60 and 70 years. IBD may present with a low-grade fever. The chronic nature of the patient's disease (several months) is typical for IBD and the hemoglobin of 10.3 g/dL suggests that the patient has likely been slowly losing blood in his stool for at least a few weeks to months. Patients with IBD often present with fatigue and weight loss as well. This patient had diffuse abdominal tenderness, which is consistent with serositis, and it is important to note that Crohn disease may present with right lower quadrant tenderness.

Ulcerative colitis usually presents with grossly bloody stool, whereas Crohn disease often presents with a tender palpable mass in the right lower quadrant. Ulcerative colitis only involves the large bowel, whereas Crohn disease may affect any portion of the gastrointestinal tract, and typically involves the colon and terminal ileum. **Ulcerative colitis** always begins in the rectum and proceeds proximally in a **continuous** pattern and disease is **limited to the colon**. Crohn disease classically involves the terminal ileum but may occur anywhere in the GI tract from the mouth to the anus. Additionally, the pattern of Crohn disease is not contiguous in the GI tract; classically, it has a patchy distribution that is often referred to as "skip lesions." Strictures caused by fibrosis from repeated inflammation may lead to obstruction of the bowel and can lead to crampy abdominal pain with nausea/vomiting and without diarrhea in Crohn disease. **Ulcerative colitis** is characterized by diarrhea and no signs of obstruction. The diagnosis is usually confirmed after colonoscopy with biopsy of the affected segments of bowel and histological examination. In ulcerative colitis, inflammation will be limited to the **mucosa and submucosa**, whereas in **Crohn disease,** the inflammation will be **transmural** (throughout all layers of the bowel). See Tables 16-1 and 16-2 for further clinical features.

Crohn Disease versus Ulcerative Colitis

The treatment of ulcerative colitis can be complex because the pathophysiology of the disease is incompletely understood. Management is aimed at reducing the inflammation. Most commonly, 5-aminosalicylic acid (ASA) compounds are used and are available in oral and rectal preparations. They are used in mid to moderate active disease and in the maintenance of disease to reduce the frequency of flare-ups. These medications are active topically and reduce inflammation at the site of contact. Steroids may be used (PO, PR, or IV) to induce a remission. Once remis-

Table 16-1
COMPARISON OF CROHN DISEASE VERSUS ULCERATIVE COLITIS

	CROHN DISEASE	ULCERATIVE COLITIS
Site of origin	Terminal ileum	Rectum
Pattern of progression	"Skip" lesions/irregular	Proximally contiguous
Thickness of inflammation	Transmural	Submucosa or mucosa
Symptoms	Crampy abdominal pain	Bloody diarrhea
Complications	Fistulas, abscess, obstruction	Hemorrhage, toxic megacolon
Radiographic findings	String sign on barium x-ray	Lead pipe colon on barium x-ray
Risk of colon cancer	Slight increase	Marked increased
Surgery	For complications such as stricture	Curative

Table 16-2
EXTRAINTESTINAL MANIFESTATIONS OF INFLAMMATORY BOWEL DISEASE

	CROHN DISEASE	ULCERATIVE COLITIS
Skin manifestations	Erythema nodosum 15% Pyoderma gangrenosum: rare	Erythema nodosum 10% Pyoderma gangrenosum: 1–12%
Rheumatological	Arthritis (polyarticular, assymmetric): common Ankylosing spondylitis: 10%	Arthritis: less common Ankylosing spondylitis: less common
Ocular	Uveitis: common (photohobia, blurred vision, headache)	Uveitis: common (photophobia, blurred vision, headache)
Hepatobiliary	Cholelithiasis Fatty liver: common Primary sclerosing cholangitis: rare	Fatty liver: common Primary sclerosing cholangitis: rare
Urologic	Nephrolithasis (10–20%) after small bowel resection or ileostomy	

sion is achieved, the steroids should be tapered over 6-8 weeks and stopped. Immune modulators are used in more severe, refractory disease. Such medications include 6-mercaptopurine, azathioprine, methotrexate, and the tumor necrosis factor (TNF) antibody infliximab. Anti-TNF therapy such as infliximab is an important treatment for Crohn disease.

Surgery is indicated for complications of ulcerative colitis. **Total colectomy** is performed in patients with **carcinoma, toxic megacolon perforation, and uncontrollable bleeding**. Surgery is curative for ulcerative colitis if symptoms persist despite medical therapy. There are two very important and potentially life-threatening complications of ulcerative colitis: toxic megacolon and colon cancer. **Toxic megacolon** occurs when the colon dilates to a diameter of >6 cm. It is usually accompanied by **fever, leukocytosis, tachycardia, tenderness over the colon, and hypoactive bowel sounds**. Therapy is designed to reduce the chance of perforation and includes IV fluids, nasogastric tube placed to suction and placing the patient NPO (nothing by mouth). Additionally, IV antibiotics are given in anticipation of possible perforation and IV steroids are given to reduce inflammation. The most severe consequence of toxic megacolon is colonic perforation complicated by peritonitis or hemorrhage.

Patients with ulcerative colitis have a marked increase in the incidence of colon cancer as compared to the general population. The risk of cancer increases over time and is related to disease duration and extent. It is seen in patients with active disease and in patients whose disease has been in remission. The increase in risk usually begins 7–10 years after diagnosis. These cancers are often multifocal and poorly differentiated, unlike the typical colonic adenocarcinoma found in a patient without ulcerative colitis. Yearly colonoscopy is advised in patients with ulcerative colitis, beginning 8 years after diagnosis of pancolitis, and random biopsies should be sent for evaluation. If colon cancer or dysplasia is found, a colectomy should be performed.

Comprehension Questions

[16.1] A 32-year-old woman has a history of chronic diarrhea and gallstones, and now has rectovaginal fistula. Which of the following is the most likely diagnosis?

A. Crohn disease
B. Ulcerative colitis
C. Systemic lupus erythematosus
D. Laxative abuse

[16.2] Which of the following forms of ulcerative colitis has the highest risk of cancer?

A. Proctitis
B. Left-sided colitis
C. Pancolitis
D. Colitis of the rectum and sigmoid colon

[16.3] A 25-year-old male is hospitalized for ulcerative colitis. He has now developed abdominal distension, cecum with a diameter of 14 cm, and transverse colon diameter of 7 cm on x-ray. Which of the following is the best next step?

A. Oral antacids
B. Psychotherapy
C. Antibiotics and prompt surgical consultation
D. Diuretic therapy

[16.4] A 35-year-old woman has chronic abdominal pain and diarrhea, but no weight loss or gastrointestinal bleeding. Colonoscopy with biopsies are normal. What is your most likely diagnosis?

A. Infectious colitis
B. Irritable bowel syndrome
C. Crohn disease
D. Ulcerative colitis

Answers

[16.1] **A.** Fistulae are common with Crohn disease because of its transmural nature, but uncommon in ulcerative colitis.

[16.2] **C.** Pancolitis has the highest risk of malignancy in ulcerative colitis.

[16.3] **C.** With toxic megacolon, antibiotics and surgical intervention are often necessary.

[16.4] **B.** Irritable bowel syndrome is characterized by intermittent diarrhea, crampy abdominal pain, but no weight loss or abnormal blood in the stool.

CLINICAL PEARLS

❖ Ulcerative colitis always involves the rectum and may extend proximally in a continuous distribution.

❖ Crohn disease most commonly involves the distal ileum, but may involve any portion of the GI tract, and has "skip lesions."

❖ Because of transmural inflammation, Crohn disease is often complicated by fistula formation.

❖ Toxic megacolon is characterized by dilatation of the colon along with systemic toxicity; failure to improve with medical therapy may require surgical intervention.

❖ Both ulcerative colitis and Crohn disease can be associated with extraintestinal manifestations such as uveitis, erythema nodosum, pyoderma gangrenosum, arthritis, and primary sclerosing cholangitis.

REFERENCES:

Banerjee S, Peppercorn MA. Inflammatory Bowel Disease. Medical Therapy of Specific Clinical Presentations. Gastroenterol Clin North Am 2002;341:147-166.

Podolsky DK. Medical progress: inflammatory bowel disease. N Engl J Med 2002;342:7.

Stenson WF. Inflammatory Bowel Disease. In: Goldman L, Bennett JC, eds.: Cecil's textbook of medicine, 21st ed., 2000:722-729.

CASE 17

A 54-year-old man with a history of type 2 diabetes and coronary artery disease is admitted to the coronary care unit with worsening angina and hypertension. His pain is controlled with intravenous nitroglycerin, and he is treated with aspirin, beta-blockers to lower his heart rate, and angiotensin-converting enzyme (ACE) inhibitors to lower his blood pressure. The cardiac enzymes are normal. He undergoes coronary angiography, which reveals no significant stenosis. By the next day, his urine output has diminished to 200 mL over 24 hours. The examination at that time reveals that he is afebrile, his heart rate is regular at 56 bpm, and his blood pressure is 109/65 mmHg. His fundus reveals dot hemorrhages and hard exudates, his neck veins are flat, his chest is clear, and his heart rhythm is normal with an S4 gallop and no murmur or friction rub. His abdomen is soft without masses or bruits. He has no peripheral edema or rashes, with normal pulses in all extremities. Current laboratory studies include Na (140 mEq/L), K (5.3 mEq/L), Cl (104 mEq/L), CO_2 (19 mEq/L), and blood urea nitrogen (BUN) (69 mg/dL), and his creatinine has risen to 2.9 mg/dL from 1.6 mg/dL on admission.

- **What is the patient's new clinical problem?**

- **What is your next step to diagnose it?**

ANSWERS TO CASE 17: Acute Renal Failure

Summary: A 54-year-old diabetic male undergoes medical therapy for his angina and hypertension, consisting of oral aspirin, beta-blockers, ACE inhibitor, and intravenous nitroglycerin. He undergoes coronary angiography, which reveals no significant stenosis. His current blood pressure is 109/65 mmHg; the funduscopic examination shows dot hemorrhages and hard exudates, and the remainder of the examination is normal. Laboratory studies include a K (5.3 mEq/L), CO_2 (19 mEq/L), and BUN (69 mg/dL), and his creatinine has risen to 2.9 mg/dL from 1.6 mg/dL on admission. By the next day, his urine output has diminished to 200 mL over 24 hours.

- **New clinical problem:** Acute renal failure (ARF).
- **Next step:** Urinalysis and urine chemistries.

Analysis

Objectives

1. Be familiar with the common causes, evaluation, and prevention of acute renal failure in hospitalized patients.
2. Know how to use the urinalysis and serum chemistry values in the diagnostic approach of ARF so as to be able to categorize the etiology as prerenal, renal, or postrenal.
3. Be familiar with the management of hyperkalemia and indications for acute dialysis.

Considerations

A 54-year-old man with diabetes, retinopathy, and some preexisting kidney disease (admission creatinine of 1.6 mg/dL) develops acute renal failure (ARF) in the hospital, as indicated by the elevated serum creatinine to 2.9 mg/dL and BUN of 69 mg/dL. He has undergone several medical therapies and procedures, all of which might be potentially contributory: acute lowering of his blood pressure, an ACE inhibitor, radiocontrast media, and arterial catheterization with possible atheroemboli. The mortality rate associated with critically ill patients who develop ARF is high; thus, it is essential to identify and treat the underlying etiology of this patient's kidney failure, and take measures to protect the kidneys from further damage.

APPROACH TO ACUTE RENAL FAILURE

Definitions

Acute renal failure: Abrupt decline in glomerular filtration rate (GFR). True GFR is difficult to measure, so we rely on increases in serum creatinine levels to indicate a fall in GFR. Because creatinine is both filtered and secreted by the kidneys, changes in serum creatinine concentrations always lag behind and underestimate the decline in the GFR. In other words, **by the time the serum creatinine rises, there has already been a significant fall in GFR.**

Anuria: Less than 50 mL of urine output in 24 hours. Acute obstruction, cortical necrosis, and vascular catastrophes such as aortic dissection should be considered in the differential diagnosis.

Oliguria: Less than 400 mL of urine output in 24 hours. Physiologically, it is the lowest amount of urine a person on a normal diet can make if severely dehydrated and not retain uremic waste products. **Oliguria is a poor prognostic sign in acute renal failure**. Patients with **oliguric renal failure have higher mortality rates** and less renal recovery than patients who are nonoliguric.

Uremia: Nonspecific symptoms of fatigue, weakness, nausea and early morning vomiting, itchiness, confusion, pericarditis, and coma attributed to the retention of waste products in renal failure, and does not always correlate with the BUN level. A very malnourished patient with renal failure may have a modestly elevated BUN and be uremic. Another patient may have a very elevated BUN and be asymptomatic. Elevated BUN without symptoms is called **azotemia**.

Clinical Approach

The differential diagnosis of ARF proceeds from consideration of three basic pathophysiologic mechanisms: **prerenal failure, postrenal failure, and intrinsic renal failure.** Individuals with **prerenal failure** experience diminished GFR as a result of a marked **decreased renal blood perfusion** so that less glomerular filtrate is formed. Sometimes, the clinical presentation is straightforward, such as volume depletion from gastrointestinal fluid loss or hemorrhage, while at other times, the presentation of patients with prerenal failure can be more confusing. For example, a patient with severe nephrotic syndrome may appear to be volume overloaded because of the massive peripheral edema present, while the effective arterial blood volume may be very low as a consequence of the severe hypoalbuminemia. Yet the mechanism of this individual's ARF is prerenal. Similarly, a patient with severe congestive heart failure may have prerenal failure because of a low cardiac ejection fraction, yet be fluid overloaded with peripheral and pulmonary edema. **The key is to assess "what the kidneys see" versus the remainder of the body.** Medications such as aspirin, nonsteroidal antiinflammatory agents, and ACE inhibitors can alter intrarenal blood flow and result in prerenal failure. See Table 17–1 for an abbreviated listing of etiologies of prerenal failure.

Postrenal failure, also referred to as obstructive nephropathy, implies **blockage of urinary flow.** The site of the obstruction can be anywhere along the urinary system including the intratubular region (crystals), the ureters (stones, extrinsic compression by tumor), the bladder, or the urethra. The patient's symptoms depend on whether on not both kidneys are involved, the

Table 17-1
CAUSES OF PRERENAL ACUTE RENAL FAILURE

- True volume depletion
  Gastrointestinal losses
  Renal losses (diuretics)
- Reduced effective arterial blood volume
  Nephrotic syndrome
  Cirrhosis with portal hypertension
  Severe burns
  Sepsis
  Systemic inflammatory response syndrome (SIRS)
- Medications
  ACE inhibitors
  NSAIDs
- Decreased cardiac output
  Congestive heart failure
  Pericardial tamponade

Table 17-2
CAUSES OF POSTRENAL ACUTE RENAL FAILURE

- Bladder
  Stones
  Hemorrhagic cystitis
  Prostatic hypertrophy or malignancy
  Neurogenic (diabetes, medications)
  Bladder cancer
- Ureteral
  Stones
  Sloughed papillae
  Blood clots
  Malignancy
  Extrinsic compression (tumors, retroperitoneal fibrosis)
- Urethra
  Strictures
  Stones

degree of obstruction, and the time course of the blockage. Usually, **hydronephrosis is noted on renal ultrasound.** Table 17–2 lists common causes of urinary obstruction.

Intrinsic renal failure is caused by disorders that injure the renal glomeruli or tubules directly. These include glomerulonephritis, tubulointerstitial nephritis, and acute tubular necrosis (ATN) from either ischemia or nephrotoxic drugs. Table 17–3 lists major causes of intrinsic acute renal failure.

The evaluation of a patient with ARF starts with a detailed history and physical exam. Does the patient have signs or symptoms of a systemic disease such as heart failure or cirrhosis that could cause prerenal failure? Does the patient have symptoms of a disease such as lupus that could cause a glomerulonephritis? Did the patient receive something in the hospital that could cause acute tubular necrosis (ATN) such as intravenous contrast or an aminoglycoside? Did they become hypotensive from sepsis or from hemorrhage in the operating suite that caused ischemic ATN? Is the patient receiving a cephalosporin and now has allergic interstitial nephritis? In addition to the history and physical examination, the **urinalysis and measurement of urinary electrolytes** are helpful in making a diagnosis.

Urinalysis The urine findings based on testing with reagent paper and microscopic examination help with the diagnosis of ARF (see Table 17–4). In **pre-renal failure**, the urinalysis usually reveals a **high specific gravity**, and **normal microscopic findings**. Individuals with **post-renal failure** typically are **unable to concentrate the urine**, so the urine osmolality is equal to the serum osmolality (**isosthenuria**) and the **specific gravity is 1.010**. The **microscopic findings vary** depending on the cause of the obstruction: hematuria (crystals or stones), leukocytes (prostatic hypertrophy), or normal (extrinsic ureteral compression from a

Table 17-3
CAUSES OF INTRINSIC ACUTE RENAL FAILURE

- Acute Tubular Necrosis
  - Nephrotoxic agents
    - Aminoglycosides
    - Radiocontrast
    - Chemotherapy
  - Ischemic
    - Hypotension
    - Vascular catastrophe
- Glomerulonephritis
  - Post-infectious
  - Vasculitis
  - Immune-complex diseases (lupus, MPGN [mesangioproliferative glomerulonephritis] cryoglobulinemia)
  - Cholesterol emboli syndrome
  - Hemolytic uremic syndrome/thrombotic thrombocytopenic purpura
- Tubulointerstitial nephritis
  - Medications (cephalosporins, methicillin, rifampin)
  - Infection (pyelonephritis, HIV)

Table 17-4
EVALUATION OF ACUTE RENAL FAILURE

ETIOLOGY OF RENAL FAILURE	URINALYSIS	FeNa	U_{Na}
Preerenal failure	Concentrated with normal sediment	<1%	<20 mEq/L
ATN	Isosthenuric with muddy brown granular casts	>1%	>20 mEq/L
Glomerulonephritis	Moderate to severe proteinuria with red blood cells and red blood cell casts	<1%	Variable
Interstitial nephritis	Mild to moderate proteinuria with red and white blood cells and white blood cell casts	>1%	>20 mEq/L
Postrenal failure	Variable depending on cause	<1% (early) >1% (later)	<20 mEq/L (early) >20 mEq/L (later)

tumor). The urinalysis of various intrinsic renal disorders may be helpful. **Ischemic and nephrotoxic ATN** is usually associated with urine that is **isosthenuric,** often with **proteinuria**, and containing **"muddy brown" granular casts** on microscopy. In **glomerulonephritis**, the urine generally reveals moderate to severe **proteinuria**, sometimes in the nephrotic range, and **microscopic hematuria and RBC casts. Tubulointerstitial nephritis** classically produces urine that is **isosthenuric**, has **mild proteinuria**, and on microscopy, reveals **leukocytes, white cell casts, and urinary eosinophils**.

Urinary Electrolytes The measurement of urinary electrolytes and the calculation of the fractional excretion of sodium (FeNa) were devised to differentiate oliguric prerenal failure from oliguric ATN; they are of little use in other circumstances. The FeNa represents the amount of sodium filtered by the kidneys that is not reabsorbed. The **kidneys of a healthy person on a normal diet** usually **reabsorb more than 99% of the sodium that is filtered, with a corresponding FeNa of <1%.** Normally, the excreted sodium represents the dietary intake of sodium, maintaining sodium homeostasis. In prerenal failure, decreased renal perfusion leads to a diminished GFR; if the renal tubular function is intact, the FeNa remains <1%. Furthermore, because the patient has either true volume depletion or "effective" volume depletion, serum aldosterone will stimulate the kidneys to retain sodium and the urinary sodium will be low (<20 mEq/L). On the other hand, in oliguric ATN, the renal failure is caused by tubular injury. Hence, there is **tubular dysfunction** with an associated **inability to reabsorb sodium**, leading to a **FeNa >2%** and a **urinary sodium >20 mEq/L**.

The measurement of FeNa and urinary sodium is less helpful in other circumstances. For example, in nonoliguric ATN, the injury is usually less severe, so that the kidneys may still maintain sodium reabsorption, and be able to produce a FeNa <1%. Diuretic medications, which interfere with sodium reabsorption, are often used in congestive heart failure or nephrotic syndrome. Although these patients may have prerenal failure, the use of diuretics will increase the urinary sodium and FeNa. In acute glomerulonephritis, the kidneys often avidly resorb sodium, leading to very low urinary sodium levels and FeNa. Early in the course of postobstructive renal failure caused by ureteral obstruction, the afferent arteriole typically undergoes intense vasoconstriction, with consequent, low urinary sodium levels. (see Table 17–4).

The **indications for dialysis** in ARF include **fluid overload, for example, pulmonary edema, metabolic acidosis, hyperkalemia, uremic pericarditis, severe hyperphosphatemia, and uremic symptoms.** Because of the risk of fatal cardiac arrhythmias, severe hyperkalemia is considered an emergency, best treated acutely medically and not with dialysis. An urgent EKG should be performed on any patient with suspected hyperkalemia; if the classic peaked or "tented" T-waves are present, intravenous calcium should be immediately administered. Although it will not lower the serum potassium level, the calcium will oppose the membrane effects of the high potassium concentration on the heart, allowing time for other methods to lower the potassium level. One of the most effective methods of treating hyperkalemia is the administration of **intravenous insulin** (usually 10 units), along with 1–2 ampules of 50% glucose solution to prevent hypoglycemia. Insulin drives potassium into cells, lowering levels within 30 minutes. Potassium can also be driven intracellularly with a beta agonist, such as albuterol by nebulizer. In the presence of a severe metabolic acidosis, the administration of intravenous sodium bicarbonate also promotes intracellular diffusion of potassium, albeit less effectively. All three therapies have only a transient effect on serum potassium levels, because the total body potassium balance is unchanged, and the potassium will eventually leak back out of the cells. The definitive treatment of hyperkalemia, removal of potassium from the body, is accomplished by one of three methods: (a) administration of a loop diuretic such as furosemide to increase urinary flow and excretion of potassium, or, if the patient does not make sufficient urine, (b) administration of Kayexalate, a cationic exchange resin that lowers potassium by exchanging sodium for potassium in the colon, or, finally, (c) emergency dialysis.

Comprehension Questions

[17.1] A 63-year-old woman with a prior history of cervical cancer treated with hysterectomy and pelvic irradiation now presents with acute oliguric renal failure. On physical examination, she has normal jugular venous pressure, is normotensive without orthostasis, and has a benign abdominal examination. Her urinalysis shows a specific gravity of 1.010, with no cells or casts on microscopy. The urinary FeNa is 2% and the Na is 35 mEq/L. What is the next step?

A. Bolus of intravenous fluids
B. Renal ultrasound
C. CT scan of the abdomen with intravenous contrast
D. Administration of furosemide to increase her urine output

[17.2] A 49-year-old man with a long-standing history of chronic renal failure as a consequence of diabetic nephropathy is brought to the emergency room for nausea, lethargy, and confusion. His physical examination is significant for an elevated jugular venous pressure, clear lung fields, and harsh systolic and diastolic sound heard over the precordium. His serum chemistries reveal that K is 5.1 mEq/L, CO_2 is 17 mEq/L, BUN is 145 mg/dL, and creatinine is 9.8 mg/dL. What is the most appropriate therapy?

A. Administer IV insulin and glucose
B. Administer IV sodium bicarbonate
C. Administer IV furosemide
D. Urgent hemodialysis

[17.3] A 62-year-old diabetic male underwent an abdominal aortic aneurysm repair 2 days ago. He is being treated with gentamicin for a urinary tract infection. His urine output has fallen to 300 mL/24 h, and his serum creatinine has risen from 1.1 mg/dL (admission) to 1.9 mg/dL. Which of the following laboratories would be most consistent with a prerenal etiology of his renal insufficiency?

A. FeNa of 3%
B. Urinary sodium level of 10 mEq/L
C. Central venous pressure reading of 10 mmHg
D. Gentamicin trough level of 4 mcg/mL

Answers

[17.1] **B.** Renal ultrasound is the next appropriate step to assess for hydronephrosis and to evaluate for bilateral ureteral obstructions, which are common sites of metastases of cervical cancer. Her physical examination and urine studies are inconsistent with hypovolemia, so that intravenous infusion is unlikely to improve her renal function. Use of loop diuretics may increase her urine output somewhat, but does not help to diagnose the cause of her renal failure or to improve her outcome. Further imaging may be necessary after the ultrasound, but use of intravenous contrast at this point may actually worsen her renal failure.

[17.2] **D.** The patient has uremia, hyperkalemia, and (likely) uremic pericarditis, which may progress to life-threatening cardiac tamponade unless the underlying renal failure is treated with dialysis. As for the other treatments, insulin plus glucose would treat hyperkalemia, and bicarbonate would help with both metabolic acidosis and hyperkalemia, but in this patient, his potassium and bicarbonate are only mildly abnormal, and not immediately life-threatening. Furosemide will not help, as he does not have pulmonary edema.

[17.3] **B.** Prerenal insufficiency connotes insufficient blood volume, typically with FeNa of <1% and urinary sodium <20 mEq/L. Supporting information would be a low central venous pressure reading (normal central venous pressure is 4–8 mmHg). The gentamicin level of 4 ?g/mL is elevated (normal is <2 mcg/mL) and may predispose to kidney damage.

CLINICAL PEARLS

- ❖ The two main causes of renal failure in hospitalized patients are prerenal azotemia and acute tubular necrosis.
- ❖ In the anuric patient, one must quickly determine if the kidneys are obstructed or if the vascular supply is interrupted.
- ❖ The treatment of prerenal renal failure is volume replacement; for postrenal failure, relief of the obstruction.
- ❖ The main causes of postrenal failure are obstruction caused by prostatic hypertrophy in men, ureteral obstruction caused by pelvic malignancy in women, or kidney stones (both genders).
- ❖ Uremic pericarditis is an indication for urgent hemodialysis. Other indications include hyperkalemia, metabolic acidosis, severe hyperphosphatemia, and volume overload when refractory to medical management.
- ❖ Hyperkalemia is treated initially with calcium to stabilize cardiac membranes, insulin and beta-agonists to redistribute potassium intracellularly (sodium bicarbonate if there is a severe metabolic acidosis), and then either with loop diuretics, a potassium exchange resin, or hemodialysis to remove excess potassium from the body.
- ❖ Indications for dialysis: AEIOU (acidosis, electrolyte disturbances, ingestions, overload, uremia).
- ❖ Treatment of hyperkalemia: C BIG K (calcium, bicarbonate/beta-agonist, insulin, glucose, Kayexalate).

REFERENCES

Brady HR, Brenner BM. Acute Renal Failure. In: Braunwald E, Fauci AS, Kasper KL, et al., eds. Harrison's principles of internal medicine, 15th ed. New York: McGraw-Hill, 2001:1541–1551.

CASE 18

A 27-year-old woman presents to the emergency room complaining of retrosternal chest pain for the past 2 days. The pain is constant, not associated with exertion, is worsened when she takes a deep breath, and is relieved by sitting up and leaning forward. She denies any shortness of breath, nausea, or diaphoresis. She has never had symptoms like this before, has had no recent strain or trauma, and has no significant medical history. Her review of systems is positive only for occasional achiness of her hands, which she attributes to her work in a chicken-processing plant, and for which she takes acetaminophen.

On examination, her temperature is 99.4°F, her heart rate is 104 bpm, and her blood pressure is 118/72 mmHg. She is sitting forward on the stretcher, with shallow respirations. Her conjunctivae are clear and her oral mucosa is pink, with two aphthous ulcers. Her neck veins are not distended; her chest is clear to auscultation and is mildly tender to palpation. Her heart is regular, with a harsh leathery sound over the apex heard during systole and diastole. Her abdominal exam is benign, and her extremities show warmth and swelling of the PIP joints of both hands.

Laboratory studies are significant for a white blood cell (WBC) count of $2100/mm^3$ with a differential of 66% polymorphonuclear leukocytes (%Polys), 30% lymphocytes, 4% monocytes, a hemoglobin concentration of 10.4 g/dL with mean corpuscular volume (MCV) of 94, and a platelet count of $98,000/mm^3$. Her blood urea nitrogen (BUN) and creatinine are normal. Urinalysis shows 10–20 WBCs, and 5–10 RBCs per high-powered field (hpf), and a urine drug screen is negative.

Chest x-ray is read as normal with a normal cardiac silhouette, and no pulmonary infiltrates or effusions. EKG is shown in Figure 18–1.

- **What is the most likely diagnosis?**

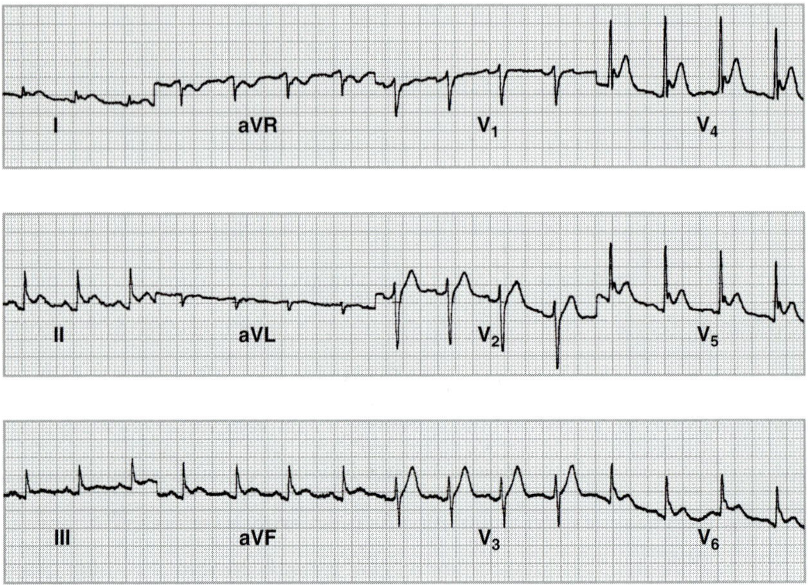

Figure 18–1. EKG. **(Reproduced with permission from Stead, First aid for the medicine clerkship. New York: McGraw-Hill, 2002.)**

ANSWERS TO CASE 18: Acute Pericarditis Caused by SLE

Summary: A young woman presents with nonexertional pleuritic chest pain that is relieved with sitting forward. In addition, she has a pericardial friction rub, and EKG changes consistent with acute pericarditis. She has no radiographic evidence of a large pericardial effusion, and no clinical signs of cardiac tamponade. Regarding the etiology of her pericarditis, she has pancytopenia and an active urinary sediment, which could be caused by infection, but may also represent a connective tissue disease such as systemic lupus erythematosus (SLE).

◆ **Most likely diagnosis:** Acute pericarditis as a consequence of systemic lupus erythematosus.

Analysis

Objectives

1. Know the clinical and EKG features of pericarditis and be able to recognize a pericardial friction rub.
2. Know the causes of pericarditis and its treatment.
3. Know the diagnostic criteria for systemic lupus erythematosus.
4. Know the major complications of SLE and its treatment.

Considerations

In patients with chest pain, one of the primary diagnostic considerations is always myocardial ischemia or infarction. This is particularly true when the EKG is abnormal with changes that may represent myocardial injury, such as ST elevation. However, other conditions may produce ST elevation, such as acute pericarditis. EKG findings can help distinguish between these two diagnoses.

APPROACH TO ACUTE PERICARDITIS

Acute pericarditis is an inflammation of the pericardial sac surrounding the heart. It can result from a multitude of disease processes, but the most common causes are listed in Table 18–1.

There is a wide spectrum of clinical presentations, from subclinical or inapparent inflammation, to the classic presentation of acute pericarditis with chest pain, to subacute or chronic inflammation, persisting weeks to months. Most patients with acute pericarditis will seek medical attention because of **chest pain**. The classic description is a sudden onset of substernal chest pain, which worsens on inspiration and with recumbency, that often radiates to the trapezius ridge, and is improved by sitting and leaning forward. Other clinical features will vary according to the cause of the pericarditis, but most patients are thought to have viral infection, and often present with low-grade fever, malaise, or upper respiratory illness (URI) symptoms.

A **pericardial friction rub** is pathognomonic and virtually 100% specific of acute pericarditis. The sensitivity of this sign varies, though, since friction rubs tend to come and go over hours. Classically, a rub is harsh, high-pitched,

Table 18-1

COMMON CAUSES OF ACUTE PERICARDITIS

Idiopathic pericarditis: specific diagnosis unidentified, presumably either viral or autoimmune and requires no specific management
Infectious: viral, bacterial, tuberculous, parasitic
Vasculitis: autoimmune diseases, postradiation therapy
Hypersensitivity/ immunologic reactions, e.g., Dressler syndrome
Diseases of contiguous structures, e.g., during transmural myocardial infarction
Metabolic disease, e.g., uremia, Gaucher disease
Trauma: penetrating or nonpenetrating chest injury
Neoplasms: usually thoracic malignancies such as breast, lung, or lymphoma

Adapted from Spodick DH. Current Concepts and Practice. JAMA 2003.

scratchy sound, with variable intensity, usually best heard at the left sternal border. It can have one, two, or three components: presystolic (correlating with atrial systole) systolic, and diastolic. The large majority of rubs are triphasic (all three components) or biphasic, having a systolic and either an early or late diastolic component. In these cases, it is usually easy to diagnose the pericardial friction rub and acute pericarditis. When the rub is monophasic (just a systolic component), it is often difficult to distinguish a pericardial friction rub from a harsh murmur, making bedside diagnosis difficult and uncertain. In these cases, one should look for EKG evidence of pericarditis (see Table 18–2) and perform serial examinations, because the rub may vary with time.

The classic EKG findings in **acute pericarditis** as seen in our patient include **diffuse ST-segment elevation,** in association with PR-segment depression. The opposite findings (PR elevation and ST depression) are often seen in leads aVR and V1. Because of the presentation with chest pain and ST-segment elevation on EKG, acute pericarditis may be confused with acute myocardial infarction. This is potentially a serious problem, in that if the patient is treated with **thrombolytics** for infarction, the patient may develop **pericardial hemorrhage and cardiac tamponade**. Several clinical features can help to differentiate the two: acute ischemia is more likely to have a gradual onset of pain with crescendo pattern, it is usually described as a heavy pressure or squeezing sensation rather than the sharp pain of pericarditis, it does not typically vary with respiration, and it is relieved with nitrates, whereas the pain of pericarditis is not. In addition, several EKG features can help to make the distinction: the ST-segment elevation of myocardial infarction should be localized to a vascular territory, whereas that of pericarditis involves nearly all the leads. In addition, PR depression is not a typical feature of ischemia.

Table 18-2
PERICARDITIS VERSUS MYOCARDIAL INFARCTION

EKG	ACUTE PERICARDITIS	ACUTE MI
ST segment elevation	Diffuse: in limb leads as well as V2-V6	Regional (vascular territory), for example, inferior, anterior, or lateral
PR-segment depression	Present	Usually absent
Reciprocal ST-segment depression	Absent	Typical (example: ST-segment depression inferiorly with anterior ischemia [ST elevation])
QRS complex changes	Absent	Loss of R-wave amplitude and development of Q waves

If the EKG reveals arrhythmias or conduction abnormalities, it is much more likely to represent ischemia rather than pericarditis.

Most patients with acute viral or idiopathic pericarditis have excellent prognoses, and treatment is mainly symptomatic with aspirin or another NSAID such as indomethacin, for relief of chest pain. Some authors favor ibuprofen with colchicine, and use of corticosteroids for refractory symptoms. In most patients, symptoms typically resolve within days to 2–3 weeks. Any form of pericarditis can cause pericardial effusion and bleeding; however, the most serious consequence would be cardiac tamponade. It is a common misconception that a pericardial friction rub cannot coexist with an effusion (this is very common in uremic pericarditis). Therefore, it is important to monitor these patients for signs of developing hemodynamic compromises, such as cardiac tamponade.

Our patient is very young and has no significant previous medical history. The presence of the symmetric arthritis, as well as laboratory findings suggest a systemic disease, such as systemic lupus erythematosus (SLE), as the cause of her pericarditis. SLE is a systemic inflammatory disease that mainly affects women. It is characterized by autoimmune multiorgan involvement, such as pericarditis, nephritis, pleuritis, arthritis, and skin disorders. To diagnose SLE, the patient has to meet 4 of 11 criteria listed in Table 18–3 (96% sensitive and 96% specific).

Our patient has serositis (pericarditis), oral ulcers, hematologic disorders (leukopenia, lymphopenia, thrombocytopenia), arthritis and renal involvement

Table 18-3
DIAGNOSTIC CRITERIA FOR SLE

1. Malar rash: fixed erythema, flat or raised over the malar area, that tend to spare nasolabial folds
2. Discoid rash: erythematous raised patches with adherent keratotic scaling and follicular plugging
3. Photosensitivity: skin rash as a result of exposure to sunlight
4. Oral or vaginal ulcers: usually painless
5. Arthritis: nonerosive, involving two or more peripheral joints with tenderness, swelling, and effusion
6. Serositis: usually pleuritis or pericarditis
7. Renal involvement: persistent proteinuria or cellular casts
8. Neurologic disorder: seizure or psychosis
9. Hematologic disorder: hemolytic anemia or leukopenia ($<4000/\text{mm}^3$) on two or more occasions, or lymphopenia $<1500/\text{mm}^3$) on two or more occasions, or thrombocytopenia ($<100{,}000/\text{mm}^3$)
10. Immunologic disorder: positive LE (lupus erythematosus) cell preparation or positive anti-dsDNA (anti-double-stranded DNA) or positive anti-Sm (anti-Smith antibody)
11. Antinuclear antibody (ANA): positive ANA

(hematuria)—she clearly meets the criteria for SLE. Although the patient in the scenario is like most lupus patients in that she sought medical attention because of the pain of arthritis or serositis, both of these problems are generally manageable or self-limited: the arthritis is generally nonerosive and nondeforming, and the serositis usually resolves spontaneously without sequelae. The major complication of SLE is usually related to the renal involvement, which can cause hypertension, chronic renal failure, nephrotic syndrome, or end-stage renal disease. In the past, the renal disease was the most common cause of death of SLE patients, but it can now be treated with powerful immunosuppressants such as high-dose corticosteroids, or cyclophosphamide. Other serious complications of lupus include central nervous system disorders, which are highly variable and unpredictable, and can include seizures, psychosis, stroke syndromes, and cranial neuropathies. In addition to renal failure and CNS involvement, the most common causes of death in SLE patients are infection (often related to the immunosuppression used to treat the disease) and vascular disease, for example, myocardial infarction.

Comprehension Questions

[18.1] A 48-year-old man is admitted to the hospital for chest pain. On examination, a pericardial friction rub is noted. He has end-stage renal disease as a consequence of diabetes. Which of the following is the best treatment?

A. NSAIDs
B. Dialysis
C. Steroids
D. Kayexalate

[18.2] Which of the following is the most likely outcome following an episode of acute pericarditis?

A. Myocardial infarction
B. Tamponade
C. Constrictive pericarditis
D. Recovery without sequelae

[18.3] A 25-year-old woman with symmetric arthritis of the proximal interphalangeal (PIP) and metacarpophalangeal (MCP) joints also is noted to have thrombocytopenia, hematuria, and a pleural effusion. Which of the following is the most likely diagnosis?

A. Systemic lupus erythematosus
B. Rheumatoid arthritis
C. Gout
D. Reiter syndrome

Answers

[18.1] **B.** Dialysis is the best treatment for pericarditis associated with renal failure.

[18.2] **D.** Acute pericarditis usually resolves without sequelae.

[18.3] **A.** SLE is associated with symmetric arthritis and serositis (usually pleuritis or pericarditis).

CLINICAL PEARLS

❖ Acute pericarditis is characterized by pleuritic chest pain, a pericardial friction rub, and EKG findings of diffuse ST elevation and PR depression.

❖ Pericardial friction rub does not exclude a pericardial effusion; patients with acute pericarditis should be monitored for development of effusion and tamponade.

❖ Treatment of pericarditis is directed at the underlying cause; for example, for uremic pericarditis, urgent dialysis is necessary. For viral or inflammatory causes, treatment is NSAIDs or corticosteroids for refractory cases.

❖ Systemic lupus erythematosus can be diagnosed if a patient has four of the following features: malar rash, discoid rash, photosensitivity, oral ulcers, arthritis, serositis, renal disease, neurologic manifestations, hematologic cytopenias, immunologic abnormalities (e.g., false-positive Venereal Disease Research Laboratory [VDRL] test), and positive ANA.

❖ The major morbidity and mortality of SLE is as a consequence of renal disease, CNS involvement, or infection.

REFERENCES

Philip J Gentlesk PJ., Acute Pericarditis.http://www.emedicine.com/med/topic1781.htm. (December 4, 2003)

Spodick DH. Acute Pericarditis: Current Concepts and Practice. JAMA 2003;289:1150-1153.

Hahn BH. Systemic Lupus Erythematosus. In: Braunwald E, Fauci AS, Kasper KL, et al., eds. Harrison's Principles of Internal Medicine, 15th ed. New York: McGrraw-Hill, 2001:1922-1928.

CASE 19

A 27-year-old man presents to the outpatient clinic complaining of 2 days of facial and hand swelling. He first noticed swelling around his eyes 2 days ago, along with difficulty putting on his wedding ring because of swollen fingers. Additionally, he noticed that his urine appears reddish-brown and that he has had less urine output over the last several days. He has no significant past medical history and his only medication is ibuprofen that he took for fever and a sore throat 2 weeks previously, which has since resolved. On examination, he is afebrile, with a heart rate of 85 bpm and a blood pressure of 172/110 mmHg. He has periorbital edema, his funduscopic exam is normal without arteriovenous nicking or papilledema. His chest is clear to auscultation, his heart is regular with a nondisplaced point of maximal impulse (PMI), and he has no abdominal masses or bruits. He does have edema of his feet, hands, and face. A dipstick urinalysis in the clinic shows specific gravity of 1.025 with 3+ blood and 2+ protein, but it is otherwise negative.

- **What is the most likely diagnosis?**
- **What is your next diagnostic step?**

ANSWERS TO CASE 19: Acute Glomerulonephritis, Poststreptococcal Infection

Summary: A 27-year-old man complains of several days of facial and hand swelling, decreased urine output, and reddish-brown urine. He took ibuprofen for fever and a sore throat 2 weeks previously. He is afebrile, hypertensive with a blood pressure of 172/110 mmHg, and has periorbital edema, but a normal funduscopic examination. His cardiac, pulmonary, and abdominal examinations are normal but he does have edema of his feet, hands, and face. A dipstick urinalysis in the clinic shows specific gravity of 1.025 with 3+ blood and 2+ protein.

- **Most likely diagnosis:** Acute glomerulonephritis.
- **Next diagnostic step:** Examine a fresh spun urine specimen to look for red blood cell (RBC) casts or dysmorphic red blood cells.

Analysis

Objectives

1. Be able to differentiate glomerular from nonglomerular bleeding.
2. Understand the clinical features of glomerulonephritis.
3. Know how to evaluate and treat a patient with glomerulonephritis.
4. Be familiar with the evaluation of a patient with nonglomerular hematuria.

Considerations

A young man without a significant medical history now presents with new onset of hypertension, edema, and hematuria following an upper respiratory tract infection. He has no history of renal disease, does not have manifestations of chronic hypertension, and has not received any nephrotoxins. He does not have symptoms of systemic diseases such as systemic lupus erythematosus. The presentation of acute renal failure, hypertension, edema, and hematuria in a young man with no significant medical history is highly suggestive of glomerular injury (glomerulonephritis). He likely has acute glomerulonephritis, either postinfectious (streptococcal) or IgA nephropathy. The reddish-brown appearance of the urine could represent hematuria, which was later suggested by dipstick urinalysis (3+ blood); hence, microscopic examination of the urine for RBC is very important. Together, the history and exam suggest that our patient is likely to have acute glomerulonephritis, either primary glomerulonephritis (GN) of unknown etiology (no concomitant systemic disease is mentioned) or secondary GN as a result of recent upper respiratory infection (postinfectious GN). The next logical step in diagnosing GN should be to examine the precipitate of a freshly spun urine sample for active sediment (cellular components, red cell cast, dysmorphic red cells). If present, these are signs of inflammation and establish the diagnosis of acute glomerulonephritis. Although likely to be present, these markers do not distinguish among the distinct immune-mediated causes of GN, and merely allow us to give the diagnosis of acute GN (primary or secondary). Further evaluation with serological markers such as complement levels and antistreptolysin-O (ASO) titers (see Table 19–1) may help to further classify the GN.

APPROACH TO SUSPECTED GLOMERULONEPHRITIS

Hematuria

The term hematuria describes the presence of blood in the urine. Although direct visualization of a urine sample (gross hematuria) or dipstick examination (positive blood) can be helpful, the **diagnosis of hematuria is made by microscopic confirmation of the presence of red blood cells** (microscopic hematuria). The first step in evaluating a patient who complains of red-dark urine is to differentiate between true hematuria (presence of RBCs in urine) and pigmented urine (red/dark urine). The breakdown products of muscle cells and red blood cells (myoglobin and hemoglobin, respectively) are heme-containing compounds capable of turning the color of urine dark red or brown in the absence of true hematuria (red blood cells). A dipstick urinalysis positive for blood without the presence of RBC (negative microscopic cellular sediment) is suggestive of hemoglobinuria or myoglobinuria.

After confirmation, the etiology of the hematuria should be determined. **Hematuria** can be classified into two broad categories: **intrarenal or extrarenal** (see Table 19–2). The history and physical examination are very helpful in the evaluation (age, fever, pain, family history). Laboratory analysis and imaging studies are often necessary, and considering the potential clinical

Table 19-1
SEROLOGIC MARKERS OF GLOMERULONEPHRITIS

Complement levels (C3, C4): low in complement-mediated GN (SLE, MPGN, infective endocarditis, poststreptococcal/postinfectious GN, cryoglobulin-induced GN)
Antineutrophil cytoplasmic antibody levels (p-ANCA and c-ANCA): positive in Wegener, microscopic polyangiitis, Churg-Strauss
ANA: positive in SLE (anti-dsDNA, anti-Smith)
Antiglomerular basement membrane antibody levels (anti-GBM): positive in anti-GBM GN and Goodpasture
ASO titers: elevated in poststreptococcal GN (postinfectious GN)
Blood cultures: positive in infective endocarditis
Cryoglobulin titers: positive in cryoglobulin-induced GN
Hepatitis serologies: Heptatitis C and Heptatitis B associated with cryo-induced GN

Table 19-2
COMMON CAUSES OF HEMATURIA

Intrarenal Hematuria	
	Kidney trauma
	Renal stones and crystals
	Glomerulonephritis
	Infection (pyelonephritis)
	Neoplasia (renal cell carcinoma)
	Vascular injury (vasculitis, renal thrombosis)
Extrarenal Hematuria	
	Trauma (e.g., Foley placement)
	Infections (urethritis, prostatitis, and cystitis)
	Nephrolithiasis (ureteral stones)
	Neoplasia (prostate and bladder)

implications, the etiology of hematuria should be pursued in all cases of hematuria. First, examination of the cellular urine sediment can help to differentiate glomerular from nonglomerular hematuria. The presence of **dysmorphic/fragmented RBC or red cell casts** is indicative of **glomerular origin** (glomerulonephritis); renal biopsy may offer further confirmation if indicated. Second, the urine Gram stain and culture can aid in the diagnosis of infectious hematuria. Third, the urine sample should be sent for cytologic evaluation when the diagnosis of malignancy is suspected. Lastly, renal imaging via ultrasound or intravenous pyelogram (IVP) can help in the visualization of the renal parenchyma and vascular structures; cystoscopy may be used to assess the bladder; and abdominal CT or MRI may be done to assess mass effect and surrounding structures.

However, a complete workup for hematuria is rarely needed because the initial evaluation of the patient and urinalysis often lead to the appropriate diagnosis.

Glomerular Disease

Rarely do patients with glomerular disease present according to the description in textbooks. In clinical medicine, glomerulopathies are encountered mainly in the form of two distinct syndromes: nephritic or nephrotic (or, more often, as an overlap of the two syndromes). **Nephritis** (nephritic syndrome) is defined as an **inflammatory** renal syndrome that presents as hematuria, edema, hypertension, and a low degree of proteinuria (<3.5 g/24 h). **Nephrosis** (or the nephrotic syndrome), is a **noninflammatory** (no active sediment in the urine) glomerulopathy. Glomerular injury may result from a variety of insults and present either as the sole clinical finding in a patient (primary renal disease), or as part of a complex syndrome of a systemic disorder (secondary glomerular disease). Although all glomerular disorders are often given the all encompassing name of *glomerulonephritis,* this term specifically describes an inflammatory intraglomerular process associated with cellular proliferation which results in hematuria and renal failure (*nephritis* or nephritic syndrome) and excludes the nonproliferative, noninflammatory glomerulopathies (i.e., *nephrosis* or nephrotic syndrome). For the purpose of this discussion, *glomerulonephritis* (GN) includes only the inflammatory glomerulopathies.

The Nephritic Syndrome

The presentation of acute renal failure with associated hypertension, hematuria, and edema is consistent with acute glomerulonephritis (GN). Acute renal failure, as manifested by a decrease in urine output and azotemia, results from impaired urine production and ineffective filtration of nitrogenous waste by the glomerulus, respectively. The glomerular apparatus (endothelial and epithelial components) is responsible for the ultrafiltration of blood in the kidney and the initial formation of what will later became the urine. Glomerular injury leads to impaired/ineffective filtration of sodium, glucose, nitrogenous products, and amino acids/proteins and its consequent clinical manifestations. Common signs suggesting an inflammatory glomerular cause of renal failure (i.e., acute *glomerulonephritis*) include hematuria (caused by ruptured capillaries in the glomerulus), proteinuria (caused by altered permeability of the capillary walls), edema (caused by salt and water retention), and hypertension (caused by fluid retention and disturbed renal homeostasis of blood pressure). The presence of this constellation of signs in a patient makes the diagnosis of glomerulonephritis very likely. However, it is important to note that often patients present with an overlap syndrome, sharing signs of both nephritis and nephrosis. Moreover, the presence of hematuria in itself is not pathognomonic for GN, because there are multiple causes of hematuria of nonglomerular origin. Therefore, confirmation of the presumptive diagnosis of acute glomerulonephritis requires microscopic examination of a urine sample from the suspected patient. The presence of red cell casts (inflammatory cast) or dysmorphic RBCs (caused by filtration through damaged glomeruli) in a sample of spun urine establishes the diagnosis of GN.

Acute glomerulonephritis is a condition characterized by an inflammatory attack of the glomerular apparatus. The different types of GN have a variety of causes, outcomes, and responses to treatment. Once the presumptive diagnosis of acute GN is made, they can be broadly classified as either *primary* (present clinically as a renal disorder) or *secondary* (renal injury caused by a systemic disease). In the case of primary glomerular disorders, the inciting cause is rarely known (no associated systemic disease) and the pathophysiology is often poorly understood (e.g., IgA nephropathy or membranoproliferative glomerulonephritis [MPGN]). In general, primary glomerulonephritis is named by the histopathological appearance and clinical manifestation of the injured kidney (mesangioproliferative GN, membranoproliferative GN, fibril-

Table 19-3
CLASSIFICATION OF GLOMERULONEPHRITIS BASED ON CLINICAL PRESENTATION

Primary renal disorders (based on histopathology)
Membranoproliferative glomerulonephritis (MPGN, types I and II)
Mesangioproliferative glomerulonephritis (MSGN)
Crescentic glomerulonephritis
Immune deposit (Anti-GBM)
Pauci-immune (ANCA)
Fibrillary glomerulonephritis
Proliferative glomerulonephritis (IgA nephropathy)
Secondary renal disorders (based on clinical presentation)
Lupus nephritis
Postinfectious glomerulonephritis (poststreptococcal GN)
Hepatitis C/hepatitis B-related glomerulonephritis (cryo-GN)
Vasculitis-related glomerulonephritis (Wegener, Churg-Strauss, polyarteritis nodosa microscopic polyangiitis, Henoch-Schönlein purpura)
Infective endocarditis-related glomerulonephritis

lary GN, crescentic GN, rapidly progressive GN) (see Table 19–3). In the case of the secondary GN, the inflammatory systemic disorder causes glomerular injury and presents with the clinical manifestations of acute GN (e.g., SLE, hepatitis C, HIV and a variety of vasculitis) (see Table 19–3). The secondary GN may further be classified by their histopathological appearance. Because the etiology of inflammation and the degree of cellular proliferation varies widely among the different GN, the glomerulonephritis can alternatively be classified by the mechanism of immune-mediated injury to the glomeruli. In this classification, the injury pattern of all glomerulonephritis generally falls under three categories: complement-mediated GN, antibody-mediated GN, or non-antibody and complement-mediated (ANCA-mediated) GN, also known as pauci-immune GN. Glomerular injury occurs via circulating immune complexes (antibody and complement-mediated) that precipitate on the glomeruli, or by direct attack on the glomerular membranes (antibody-, complement-, and ANCA-mediated). This injury pattern can be visualized via immunofluorescence for specific staining patterns (IgG, IgA) and under electron microscopy of the injured glomeruli for characteristic deposit patterns (linear, granular, pauci-immune, etc.).

Therefore, it is easy to see that while the diagnosis of primary versus secondary GN can be made simply by obtaining a detailed medical history, physical exam, and routine lab tests, the classification of a specific GN into a given immune-mediated category requires further microscopic analysis, blood tests, and, sometimes, a kidney biopsy.

Clinical Approach to Glomerulonephritis

The approach to the patient with glomerular disease should be systematic and undertaken in a stepwise fashion. The history should be approached meticulously looking for evidence of preexisting renal disease, systemic disease, and exposure to nephrotoxins. Likewise, the physical examination should assess for blood pressure, evidence of hypertension, presence of edema, renal and vascular bruits, and evidence of systemic disease. The urine should be analyzed for hematuria and sediment. Proteinuria should be categorized as nephrotic (>3.5 g/24 h) versus nephritic range (<3.5 g/24 h). When erythrocyte casts, or dysmorphic red cells are seen in the urine, a diagnosis of GN can be made. Although likely to be present, these markers do not distinguish among the distinct immune-mediated causes of GN and merely allow us to give the diagnosis of acute GN (primary or secondary). Serological markers of systemic diseases should be obtained if indicated (see Figure 19–1) in order to further classify the GN. The serological workup of GN should be guided by the history and physical exam and the clinical suspicion for an individual entity to exist.

Once the appropriate serologic tests have been reviewed, a kidney biopsy may be required. A biopsy sample may be examined under the light microscope in order to determine the primary histopathological injury to the nephron (MPGN, crescentic GN, etc.); further examination of an immunofluorescent stained sample for immune recognition (IgG, IgA, IgM, C3, C4, or pauci-immune staining) of the affected glomerular membrane (capillary, epithelial, etc.) and under electron microscopy for characteristic patterns of immune deposition (granular, linear GN) may provide a definitive diagnosis of the immune-mediated injury to the glomeruli. Figure 19–1 is an algorithmic approach to the patient with acute glomerulonephritis.

Treatment of Glomerulonephritis It is difficult to predict the prognosis and outcome of most glomerulonephritis. While some are self limiting and largely asymptomatic (such as IgA-associated), others may progress to end stage renal failure (ANCA-mediated GN) without treatment. Unfortunately, as is the case with a number of immune-mediated disorders, treatment is currently limited to supportive therapy (hemodialysis for renal failure, antihypertensive medications and diuretics for edema) with or without immunosuppressive drugs. When appropriate, the underlying disease should be treated (infective endocarditis, hepatitis, SLE, or vasculitis). The use of steroids and cyclophosphamide has been advocated in the treatment of ANCA-induced GN, while other antibody-mediated GNs might require plasmapheresis in order to eliminate the inciting antibody/immune complex. Although the diagnosis of acute glomerulonephritis may be straightforward, the ensuing therapy is often frustrating and ineffective and leaves the clinician at the mercy of supportive measures.

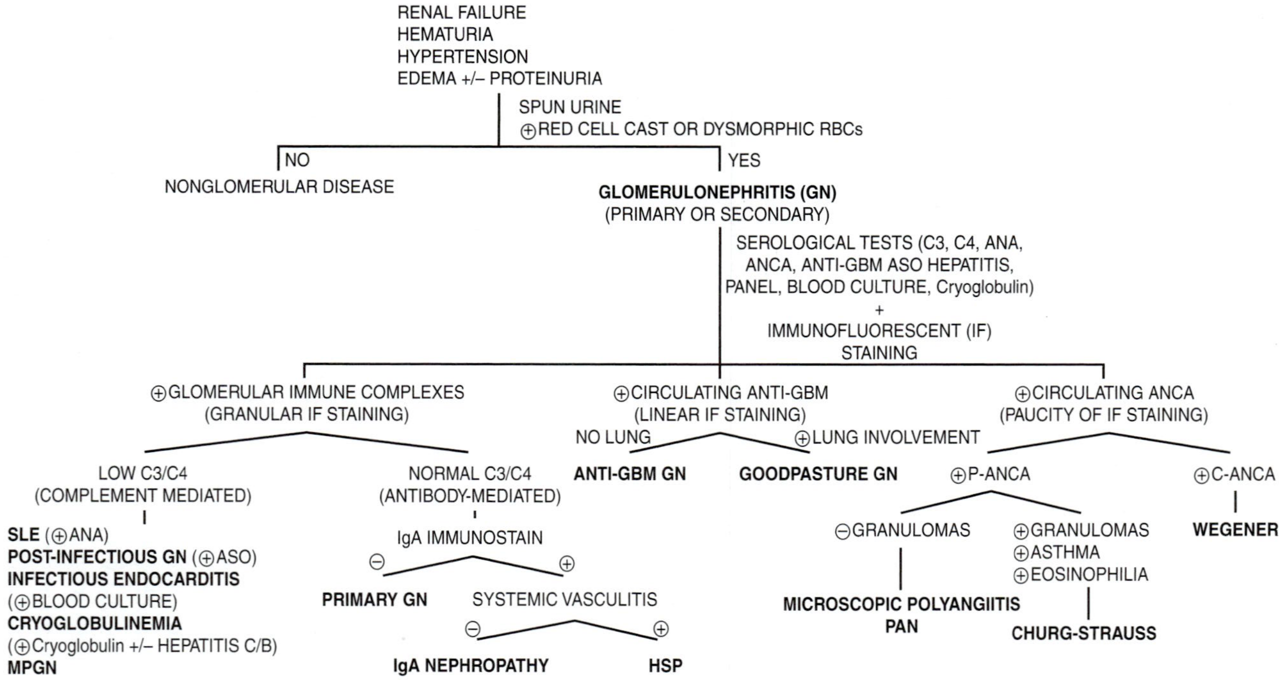

Figure 19–1. Algorithm approach to the patient with acute glomerulonephritis. Abbreviations: ANA = antinucleurantibody; ANCA = antineutrophil cytoplasmic antibody; ASO = antistreptolysin-O; c-ANCA = cytoplasmic antineutrophil cytoplasmic antibody; GBM = glomerular basement membrane; HSP = Henoch-Schönlein purpura; IF staining = immunofluorescent staining; MPGN = membranoproliferative glomerulonephritis; PAN = periarteritis nodosa; p-ANCA = perinuclear antineutrophil cytoplasmic antibody; SLE = systemic lupus erythematosus

Comprehension Questions

[19.1] An 18-year-old marathon runner has been training during the summer. He is brought to the emergency room disoriented after collapsing on the track. His temperature is 102°F. A Foley catheter is placed and reveals reddish urine with 3+ blood on dip stick and no cells seen microscopically. Which of the following is the most likely explanation for his urine?

A. Underlying renal disease
B. Prerenal azotemia
C. Myoglobinuria
D. Glomerulonephritis

[19.2] Which of the following laboratory findings is most consistent with poststreptococcal glomerulonephritis?

A. Elevated serum complement levels
B. Positive antinuclear antibody titers
C. Elevated ASO titers
D. Positive blood cultures
E. Positive cryoglobulin titers

[19.3] A 22-year old man complains of acute hemoptysis over the past week. He denies smoking or pulmonary disease. His blood pressure is 130/70 mmHg, and his physical examination is normal. His urinalysis also shows microscopic hematuria and red blood cell casts. Which of the following is the most likely etiology?

A. Metastatic renal cell carcinoma to the lungs
B. Acute tuberculosis of the kidneys and lungs
C. Systemic lupus erythematosus
D. Goodpasture disease (antiglomerular basement membrane)

Answers

[19.1] **C.** This individual is suffering from heat exhaustion, which can lead to rhabdomyolysis. The myoglobin, which is broken down, enters the serum and is filtered through the kidneys, leading to a reddish appearance and positive dipstick reaction. Microscopic analysis of the urine will likely demonstrates no red cells.

[19.2] **C.** The antistreptolysin-O titers are typically elevated, and serum complement levels are decreased in poststreptococcal GN.

[19.3] **D.** Goodpasture (antiglomerular basement membrane) disease typically affects young males, who present with hemoptysis and hematuria. Antibody against the type IV collagen, expressed in the pulmonary alveolar and glomerular basement membrane, lead to the pulmonary and renal manifestations. Hypertension is typically absent. After the initial clinical signs, renal insufficiency usually progresses rapidly. Anti-GBM antibodies are almost always present; the gold standard for diagnosis is renal biopsy.

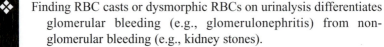

CLINICAL PEARLS

- Finding RBC casts or dysmorphic RBCs on urinalysis differentiates glomerular bleeding (e.g., glomerulonephritis) from non-glomerular bleeding (e.g., kidney stones).
- Glomerulonephritis is characterized by hematuria, edema, and hypertension caused by volume retention.
- Gross hematuria following a upper respiratory illness suggests either IgA nephropathy or poststreptococcal glomerulonephritis.
- Antibiotic therapy for streptococcal pharyngitis prevents rheumatic fever, but not glomerulonephritis.
- Patients with nonglomerular hematuria and no evidence of infection should undergo investigation with imaging (ultrasound or IVP) or cystoscopy to evaluate for stones or malignancy.

REFERENCES

Brady HR, O'Meara YM, Brenner BM. The Major Glomerulopathies. In: Braunwald E, Fauci AS, Kasper KL, et al., eds. Harrison's principles of internal medicine, 15th ed. New York: McGraw-Hill, 2001:1580-1590.

Greenberg A, ed. Primer on kidney diseases, 2nd ed. National Kidney Foundation, New York: Academic Press, 1998.

Hricik DE, Chung-Park M, Sedor JR, et al. Glomerulonephritis. N Engl J Med 1998;339:888–899.

Johnson RJ, Freehally J, eds. Comprehensive clinical nephrology. St. Louis: CV Mosby, 2000.

Sabatine MS, ed. Pocket medicine: the MGH handbook of internal medicine. Philadelphia: Lippincott, Williams & Wilkins, 2000.

CASE 20

A 48-year-old Hispanic woman presents to your office complaining of persistent swelling of her feet and ankles, so much so that she cannot put on her shoes. She first noted mild ankle swelling about 2–3 months ago and borrowed a few diuretic pills from a friend, which seemed to help, but now she has run out. She also reports that she has gained 20–25 pounds over the last few months, despite regular exercise and trying to adhere to a healthy diet. Her past medical history is significant for type 2 diabetes, for which she takes a sulfonylurea she buys in Mexico. She neither sees a doctor regularly nor monitors her blood glucose at home. She denies dysuria, urinary frequency, or urgency, but does report that her urine has appeared foamy. She had no fevers, joint pain, skin rashes, or GI symptoms.

Her physical examination is significant for mild periorbital edema, multiple hard exudates, and dot hemorrhages on funduscopic examination, and pitting edema of her hands, feet, and legs. Her chest is clear, her heart is regular without murmurs, and her abdominal exam is benign. She has diminished sensation to light touch in her feet and legs to mid-calf. A urine dipstick obtained in the office shows 2+ glucose, 3+ protein, and negative leukocyte esterase, nitrates, and blood.

- **What is the most likely diagnosis**

- **What is the best intervention to slow disease progression?**

ANSWERS TO CASE 20: Nephrotic Syndrome, Diabetic Nephropathy

Summary: A 48-year-old woman with long-standing diabetes now presents with edema, and significant proteinuria on a urine dipstick. She has diabetic retinopathy, some peripheral neuropathy, and no other findings suggestive of any other systemic disease.

- **Most likely diagnosis:** Nephrotic syndrome as a consequence of diabetic nephropathy.
- **Best intervention:** Angiotensin-converting enzyme (ACE) inhibitors.

Analysis

Objectives

1. Recognize the clinical features and complications of nephrotic syndrome.
2. Know the most common causes of nephrotic syndrome.
3. Understand the natural history of diabetic renal disease and how to diagnose and manage it.
4. Learn the principles of treatment of nephrotic syndrome.

Considerations

Patients develop significant proteinuria as a result of glomerular damage, which can result from many systemic diseases. It is important to screen for diseases such as HIV, autoimmune diseases, and malignancy by history, physical examination, and sometimes laboratory investigation to determine the underlying cause and appropriate treatment of the renal manifestations.

Definition

Nephrotic syndrome: Urine protein excretion >3.5 g/24 h, serum hypoalbuminemia (<3 g/dL), and edema.

APPROACH TO NEPHROTIC SYNDROME

Normally, the kidneys do not excrete appreciable amounts of protein (<150 mg/d) because serum proteins are excluded from the urine by the glomerular filter both by their large size and their net negative charge. Thus, the appearance of significant proteinuria heralds glomerular disease, with disruption of its normal barrier function. Proteinuria in excess of 3–3.5 g of protein/1.73 m^2 body surface area (normal adult male BSA) per day is considered to be in the nephrotic range. The key feature of nephrotic syndrome is the heavy proteinuria, which leads to loss of albumin and other serum proteins. The hypoalbuminemia and hypoproteinemia results in a decreased intravascular oncotic pressure leading to tissue edema, which usually starts in dependent areas such as the feet, but may progress to involve the face, hands, and, ultimately, anasarca, or whole-body edema. The decreased oncotic pressure also triggers the liver to start lipoprotein synthesis and thus leads to hyperlipidemia.

Patients typically present to the doctor complaining of the edema and have the laboratory features described above. Urinalysis usually shows few or no cellular elements, and may have waxy casts and oval fat bodies (which look similar to "Maltese crosses" under polarized light) if there is hyperlipidemia.

In adults, one-third of patients with nephrotic syndrome have a systemic disease that involves the kidneys, such as diabetes or lupus, and the remainder have a primary renal disease, with one of four pathologic lesions: minimal change disease, membranous nephropathy, focal segmental glomerulosclerosis (FSGS), or membranoproliferative glomerulonephritis (MPGN). Thus, a new diagnosis of nephrotic syndrome warrants further investigation into an underlying systemic disease. Common testing includes serum glucose and glycosylated hemoglobin to be evaluated for diabetes, antinuclear antibody (ANA) to screen for systemic lupus erythematosus, serum and urine protein electrophoresis to look for multiple myeloma, or amyloidosis, and viral serologies, because HIV and viral hepatitis can cause nephrosis. Less-common causes include various cancers, medications such as NSAIDs, heavy metals such as mercury, or hereditary renal conditions. Of these, diabetes mellitus is by far the most common, as in the patient presented in this scenario.

Patients with nephrotic syndrome usually undergo renal biopsy, especially if the underlying diagnosis is unclear, or if there is a possibility of a treatable or reversible condition. Patients with advanced diabetes who have heavy proteinuria and microvascular disease, such as retinopathy, are presumed to have diabetic nephropathy. They typically do not undergo renal biopsy because the nephrotic proteinuria represents irreversible glomerular damage.

Treatment of nephrotic syndrome consists of treatment of the underlying disease, if present, as well as management of the edema, and trying to limit the progression of the renal disease. For edema, all patients need strict **salt restriction**, but most patients will also need **diuretics**. Because both thiazide and loop diuretics are highly protein bound, there is reduced delivery to the kidney, and often very large doses are required to manage the edema. Counterintuitively for a patient with hypoproteinemia, dietary protein restriction is usually recommended. It is thought that high protein intake only causes heavier proteinuria, which can have an adverse effect on the renal function. Additionally, use of **ACE inhibitors** may reduce proteinuria and is useful in the management of many patients with nephrotic syndrome.

Besides the edema, patients with nephrotic syndrome have other consequences of renal protein-wasting. They have **decreased levels of antithrombin III and proteins C and S**, and are often **hypercoagulable**, with formation of venous thromboemboli, including renal vein thrombosis. Patients with evidence of thrombus formation require anticoagulation, often for life. Other complications include hypogammaglobulinemia with **increased infection risk** (especially pneumococcal infection), iron deficiency anemia caused by hypotransferrinemia, and vitamin D deficiency because of loss of vitamin D-binding protein.

In the progression of diabetic nephropathy, initially the glomerular filtration rate (GFR) is elevated and then declines over time. Prior to the decline in GFR, the earliest stages of diabetic nephropathy can be detected as **microalbuminuria.** This is defined as a urine albumin excretion of between 30 and 300 mg/d. It is possible to measure this in a random urine sample rather than a timed collection, because a ratio of albumin in mg:creatinine in g of 30–300 usually correlates with the total excretion described. When albuminuria exceeds 300 mg/d, it is detectable on ordinary urine dipsticks, and the patient is said to have **overt nephropathy.**

After the development of microalbuminuria, most patients will remain asymptomatic but the glomerulopathy will continue to progress over the subsequent 5–10 years until overt nephropathy develops. At this point, many patients have some edema, and nearly all of them have developed hypertension. The presence of hypertension will markedly accelerate the decline of renal function. Untreated, patients then progress to **end-stage renal disease (ESRD),** requiring dialysis or transplant, within a 5–15-year period.

The development of nephropathy and proteinuria is very significant in that it is associated with a much higher risk of cardiovascular disease, which is the leading cause of death for patients with diabetes. By the time patients with diabetes develop ESRD and require dialysis, the average life expectancy is less than 2 years.

Thus, the development of microalbuminuria in diabetic patients is extremely important because of the progressive disease it heralds, and because it is potentially reversible, or at least its progression to overt proteinuria can be slowed via medications. **ACE inhibitors slow the progression of renal disease** and should be initiated even when patients are normotensive. Tight **glycemic control** with a goal hemoglobin A_{1c} of <6.5–7.0 has also been shown to slow or prevent the progression of microvascular complications of diabetes such as retinopathy and nephropathy. If overt nephropathy and hypertension have developed, **blood pressure control** with a goal of <130/85 mmHg is essential to slow progression.

In addition, because cardiovascular disease is the major killer of patients with diabetes, aggressive risk factor reduction should be attempted, including smoking cessation, and reduction of hypercholesterolemia. In the newest recommendations regarding management of cholesterol, patients with diabetes are now regarded as the highest risk category, along with patients who already have established coronary artery or other atherosclerotic vascular disease, and should be treated with diet and statins to a goal low-density lipoprotein (LDL) cholesterol of <100 mg/dL.

Comprehension Questions

[20.1] A 49-year-old woman with type 2 diabetes presents to your office for new onset swelling in her legs and face. She has no other medical problems and says that at her last ophthalmologic appointment she was told that the diabetes had started to affect her eyes. She takes glyburide daily for her diabetes. Physical exam is normal except pitting edema of bilateral upper and lower extremities, hard exudates and dot hemorrhages on funduscopic exam, and diminished sensation to the mid shin bilaterally. Her urine analysis shows 3+ protein and 2+ glucose (otherwise negative). What is the best treatment for this patient?

A. Have the patient return in 6 weeks and check a repeat urine analysis at that time
B. Start metoprolol
C. Change the glyburide to glipizide and have the patient return for follow up in 6 weeks
D. Start lisinopril
E. Refer the patient to a cardiologist

[20.2] Which of the following disease states is not known to be a common cause of nephrotic syndrome?

A. Amyloidosis
B. Urinary stones
C. Diabetes
D. Focal segmental glomerulosclerosis
E. Systemic lupus erythematosus

[20.3] What is the best screening test for early diabetic nephropathy?

A. Urine microalbuminuria
B. Dipstick urinalysis
C. Renal biopsy
D. Fasting blood glucose
E. 24-Hour urine collection for creatinine clearance

[20.4] A 58-year-old man with type 2 diabetes is normotensive but has a persistent urine albumin to creatinine ratio of 100, but no proteinuria on urine dipstick. What is the best management for this patient?

A. Start ACE inhibitor
B. High-protein diet
C. Switch from oral agent to insulin
D. Refer to ophthalmologist for examination

Answers

[20.1] **D.** Beta-blockers are a good first-choice agent for a patient with hypertension and no comorbidities but in a patient with diabetes and nephropathy, the benefit of an ACE inhibitor for decreasing proteinuria makes this the best choice for initial treatment of the patient described in the clinical vignette. Changing from one sulfonylurea to another is of no benefit because all are equally efficacious, and there is no indication for a referral to a cardiologist based on the information provided in the vignette.

[20.2] **B.** Of all of the causes listed in the answer choices, urinary stones are not a common cause of nephrotic syndrome. The six most common causes of nephrotic syndrome include diabetes mellitus, membranous glomerulonephritis, FSGS, MPGN, minimal change disease, and amyloidosis. Other causes can include toxins such as lead, gold, and heroin, infections such as HIV, hepatitis, streptococcus, and syphilis, and multisystem disorders such as lupus, Henoch-Schönlein purpura, sarcoidosis, Sjögren syndrome, and rheumatoid arthritis. A new diagnosis of nephrotic syndrome warrants further investigation into its etiology.

[20.3] **A.** Although a 24-hour urine collection for creatinine may be useful in assessing declining GFR, it is not the best screening test in the diagnosis of early diabetic nephropathy. In the outpatient setting, a dipstick urinalysis is readily available, but will only detect patients with overt nephropathy (proteinuria >300 mg/d). Thus, a random urinary albumin to creatinine ratio of 30–300 is the best test to screen for early diabetic nephropathy. A fasting blood glucose may aid in the diagnosis of diabetes but not nephropathy. Finally, although most patients with nephrotic syndrome require a renal biopsy for diagnosis, a patient with worsening renal function who has had long-standing diabetes is assumed to have renal disease secondary to diabetic nephropathy, and the majority of these patients do not get a renal biopsy.

[20.4] **A.** The albumin to creatinine ratio of 100 is indicative of microalbuminuria. Screening for microalbuminuria is very important because it is the one aspect of the disease that is reversible and that physicians can target therapy at to blunt progression to overt renal failure. Disease progression is slowed with ACE inhibitors, blood pressure control, limiting dietary protein intake, losing weight, and improving glycemic control.

CLINICAL PEARLS

Nephrotic syndrome is characterized by >3.5 g proteinuria/24 h, hypoalbuminemia and edema. Often, hypercoagulability and hyperlipidemia are present.

Nephrotic syndrome can be a result of a primary renal disease, but is often a manifestation of a systemic disease such as diabetes, HIV infection, an autoimmune disease, or a malignancy.

Patients with diabetes should be screened for microalbuminuria (albumin excretion 30–300 mg/d), and if present, treatment should be initiated with an ACE inhibitor, even if the patient is normotensive.

Patients with diabetic nephropathy and proteinuria have very high risk for cardiovascular disease, so aggressive risk factor reduction, such as use of statins, is important.

REFERENCES:

Brady HR, O'Meara YM, Brenner BM. Glomerulopathies Associated with Multisystem Diseases. In: Braunwald E, Fauci AS, Kasper KL, et al., eds. Harrison's Principles of Internal Medicine, 15th ed. New York: McGraw-Hill, 2001:1590-1598.

Foggensteiner L, Mulroy S, Firth J. Management of diabetic nephropathy. J R Soc Med 2001;94(5):210–217.

CASE 21

A 48-year-old man comes to your office complaining of severe right knee pain for 8 hours. He states that the pain, which started abruptly at 2 A.M., waking him from sleep, is quite severe, so painful that even the weight of the bed sheets on his knee was unbearable. By the morning, the knee had become warm, swollen, and tender. He explains that he prefers to keep his knee bent, and extending his leg to straighten the knee causes the pain to worsen. He has never had pain, surgery, or injury to his knees. A year ago, he did have some pain and swelling at the base of his great toe on the left foot, which was not as severe as this episode, and resolved in 2 or 3 days after taking ibuprofen. His only prior medical history is hypertension, which is controlled with hydrochlorothiazide. He works as a financial analyst; he is married, does not smoke, but does drink one or two drinks after work one to two times a week.

On examination, his temperature is 100.6°F, his heart rate is 104 bpm, and his blood pressure is 136/78 mmHg. His head and neck examination is unremarkable, his chest is clear, and his heart is tachycardic but regular, with no gallops or murmurs. His right knee is swollen, with a moderate effusion, and appears erythematous, warm, and very tender to palpation. He is unable to fully extend the knee because of pain. He has no other joint swelling, pain, or deformity, and no skin rashes.

- **What is the most likely diagnosis?**
- **What is your next step?**
- **What is the best initial treatment?**

ANSWERS TO CASE 21: Acute Monarticular Arthritis—Gout

Summary: A 48-year-old hypertensive man complains of the acute onset of severe right knee pain for 8 hours duration. He denies previous pain, surgery, or injury to his knees. One year ago, he had great toe pain and swelling for several days that resolved with ibuprofen. He takes hydrochlorothiazide, and occasionally drinks alcohol. On examination, his temperature is 100.6°F, his heart rate is 104 bpm, and his blood pressure is 136/78 mmHg. His right knee is swollen, with a moderate effusion, and appears erythematous, warm, and very tender to palpation. He is unable to fully extend the knee because of pain. He has no other joint swelling, pain, or deformity, and no skin rashes.

◆ **Most likely diagnosis:** Acute monarticular arthritis, likely crystalline or infectious, most likely gout because of history.

◆ **Next step:** Aspiration of the knee joint to send fluid for cell count, culture, and crystal analysis.

◆ **Best initial treatment:** If the joint fluid analysis is consistent with infection, he needs drainage of the infected fluid by aspiration, and administration of antibiotics. If it is suggestive of crystal-induced arthritis, he can be treated with colchicine, NSAIDs, or corticosteroids.

Analysis

Objectives

1. Be familiar with the use of synovial fluid analysis to determine the etiology of arthritis.
2. Know the stages of gout and the appropriate treatment for each stage.
3. Know about the similarities and differences between gout and pseudogout.

Considerations

A middle-aged man presents with an acute attack of monarticular arthritis, as evidenced by the knee effusion, limitation of range of motion, and signs of inflammation: low-grade fever, erythema, warmth, and tenderness. The two most likely causes are either infection, for example, *Staphylococcus aureus,* or crystalline arthritis, such as gout or pseudogout. If the patient is at risk, gonococcal arthritis is also a possibility. The previous less-severe episode involving his first metatarsophalangeal joint sounds like podagra, the most common presentation of gout. The previous attack of arthritis in the first metatarsal phalangeal joint and the very rapid onset of severe symptoms during the current attack are consistent with acute gouty arthritis. In this patient, the attack could have been precipitated by the use of alcohol, which increases uric acid production, and his use of thiazide diuretics, which decrease renal excretion of uric acid.

Although the first attack was typical of gout, which makes this episode very likely to also be acute gouty arthritis, the current presentation is also entirely consistent with bacterial infection. Untreated septic arthritis could lead to rapid destruction of the joint, so joint aspiration and empiric antibiotic therapy are appropriate until his cultures and crystal analysis are available.

APPROACH TO MONARTICULAR ARTHRITIS

Almost any joint disorder may begin as monarthritis, or inflammation of a single joint; however, the primary concern is always **infectious arthritis**, because it may lead to **joint destruction, and resultant severe morbidity**. For that reason**, acute monarthritis should be considered a medical emergency** and investigated and treated aggressively.

Monarthritis may be a result of infection (e.g., bacterial, fungal, Lyme disease, tuberculosis) or crystal-induced arthritis (e.g., pseudogout and gout), or, less often, it may be the presentation of a systemic disease typically associated with polyarticular disease, such as rheumatoid arthritis or systemic lupus erythematosus. It may also be a result of noninflammatory causes such as trauma or osteoarthritis.

Accurate diagnosis starts with good history and physical examination supplemented by additional diagnostic testing such as **synovial fluid analysis, radiographs**, and occasionally **synovial biopsy**. A history of prior episodes of arthritis suggests crystalline disease or other noninfectious arthropathies. Patients with crystal-induced arthritis may give a history of previous recurrent, self-limited episodes. Precipitation of an attack by surgery or some other stress can occur with both crystalline disorders, but **gout is far more common than pseudogout.** The clinical course can also provide some clues to the etiology: septic arthritis usually worsens unless treated; osteoarthritis worsens with physical activity.

The location of joint involvement may be helpful. **Gout** most commonly involves the **first metatarsophalangeal joint (podagra), ankle, midfoot, or knee**. Pseudogout most commonly affects the large joints such as the knee, and may also affect the wrist or the first metatarsophalangeal joint (hence, the name pseudogout). In **gonococcal** arthritis, there are often **migratory arthralgias and tenosynovitis**, often involving the wrist and hands, associated with **pustular skin lesions**, before progressing to a purulent monarthritis or oligoarthritis. Nongonococcal causes of septic arthritis often involve large weight-bearing joints such as the knee or hip.

The basic approach in physical examination is to differentiate arthritis from inflammatory conditions adjacent to the joint, such as cellulitis or bursitis. **True arthritis** is characterized by **swelling and redness around the joint, and painful limitation of motion in all planes**, during **active and passive motion**. **Joint movement that is not limited by passive motion** suggests **a soft-tissue disorder such as bursitis** rather than an arthritis.

Diagnostic arthrocentesis is usually necessary when evaluating an acute monarthritis, and is always essential when infection is suspected. Synovial fluid analysis helps to differentiate between inflammatory and noninflammatory causes of arthritis. Fluid analysis typically includes gross examination, cell count and differential, Gram stain and culture, and crystal analysis. Table 21–1 shows the typical results that can help one distinguish between noninflammatory conditions such as osteoarthritis, inflammatory arthritis such as crystalline disease, and septic arthritis, which is most often a bacterial infection.

Normal joints contain a small amount of fluid that is essentially acellular. Noninflammatory effusions should have a white blood cell count <1000–2000/mm^3 with less than 25–50% polymorphonuclear cells. **If the fluid is inflammatory, the joint should be considered infected until proven otherwise**, especially if the patient is febrile.

Crystal analysis requires the use of a polarizing light microscope. Monosodium urate crystals, the cause of **gout**, are **needle-shaped**, typically **intracellular** within a polymorphonuclear cell, and are **negatively birefringent, appearing yellow** under the polarizing microscope. Calcium pyrophosphate dehydrate (CPPD) crystals, the cause of **pseudogout**, are **short and rhomboid**, and are **weakly positively birefringent**, appearing blue under polarized light. **Even when crystals are seen, infection should be excluded when the synovial fluid is inflammatory!** Crystals and infection may coexist in the same joint, and chronic arthritis or previous joint damage, such as occurs in gout, may predispose that joint to hematogenous infection.

In septic arthritis, the Gram stain and culture of the synovial fluid is positive in 60–80% of the cases. False-negative results may be related to prior antibiotic use or fastidious microorganisms. For example, in **gonococcal arthritis, joint fluid cultures are typically negative, while cultures of blood or the pustular skin lesions may be positive**. Sometimes, the diagnosis rests upon demonstration of gonococcal infection in another site, such as urethritis, with the typical arthritis–dermatitis syndrome. **Synovial biopsy** may be required when the cause of monarthritis remains unclear. It is **usually necessary to diagnose arthritis caused by tuberculosis or hemochromatosis.**

Plain radiographs are usually unremarkable in cases of inflammatory arthritis, the typical finding being soft-tissue swelling. **Chondrocalcinosis** or linear calcium deposition in joint cartilage suggests pseudogout. They are often found when evaluating for fracture in patients with a history of trauma.

Generally, patients require initiation of treatment before all test results are available. When septic arthritis is suspected, the clinician should culture the joint fluid and start antibiotic therapy; the antibiotic choice should be initially based on the Gram stain, and when available, on the culture results. If the Gram stain is negative, the clinical picture should dictate antimicrobial selection. For example, if the patient has the typical presentation of **gonococcal arthritis, intravenous ceftriaxone** is the usual initial therapy, usually with rapid improvement in symptoms. Nongonococcal septic arthritis is usually caused by Gram-positive organisms, most often ***S. aureus***, so treatment would involve an **antistaphylococcal penicillin such as nafcillin**, or vancomycin when methicillin-resistance is suspected. **It is essential to drain the purulent**

Table 21-1
JOINT ASPIRATE CHARACTERISTICS

GROSS EXAMINATION	NORMAL	NONINFLAMMATORY	INFLAMMATORY	SEPTIC
Volume (knee)	<1 mL	Often >1mL	Often >1mL	Often >1mL
Viscosity	High	High	Low	Variable
Color	Colorless to straw	Straw to yellow	Yellow	Variable
Clarity	Transparent	Transparent	Translucent	Opaque
Leukocytes/mm^3	<200	50–1000	2000–75,000	Often >100,000
Polymorphonuclear cells	<25%	<25%	Often >50%	>85%
Culture results	Negative	Negative	Negative	Often positive
Glucose	Nearly equal to blood	Nearly equal to blood	<50 mg/dL lower than blood	<50 mg/dL lower than blood

Source: Koch AE. Approach to the patient with pain in one or a few joints. In Kelly's textbook of internal medicine. New York; Williams and Wilkins; 2000: 1322

joint fluid, usually by repeated percutaneous aspiration. Open surgical drainage or arthroscopy is required when joint fluid is loculated, or when shoulders, hips, or sacroiliac joints are involved.

Gout classically is progresses through four stages.

Stage 1 is **asymptomatic hyperuricemia.** Patients have elevated uric acid levels without arthritis or kidney stones. The majority of patients with hyperuricemia never develop any symptoms, but the higher the uric acid level, and the longer the duration of hyperuricemia, the greater the likelihood of the patient developing gouty arthritis.

Stage 2 is **acute gouty arthritis**, which most often involves the acute onset of severe **monarticular pain**, often occurring at night, in the first metatarsophalangeal (MTP) joint, ankle, or knee, with rapid development of joint swelling and erythema, and sometimes associated with systemic symptoms such as fever and chills. This usually follows decades of asymptomatic hyperuricemia. Attacks may last hours, or up to 2 weeks.

Stage 3 is **intercritical gout**, or the period between acute attacks. Patients are generally completely asymptomatic, but monosodium urate crystals and elevated cell counts can often be found in synovial fluid, perhaps indicating ongoing subclinical inflammation. The vast majority of patients will have another acute attack within 1–2 years.

Sage 4 is **chronic tophaceous gout**, which usually occurs after 10 or more years of acute intermittent gout. In this stage, the intercritical periods are no longer asymptomatic; the involved joints now have chronic swelling and discomfort, which worsens over time. Patients also develop subcutaneous tophaceous deposits of monosodium urate.

In general, **asymptomatic hyperuricemia requires no specific treatment**. Lowering the urate level does not necessarily prevent the development of gout, and most of these patients will never develop any symptoms. Acute gouty arthritis is treated with therapies to reduce the inflammatory reaction to the presence of the crystals, all of which are most effective if started early in the attack**. Potent NSAIDs, such as indomethacin, are the mainstay of therapy.** Alternatively, oral colchicine may be taken every hour until the joint symptoms abate, but dosing is limited by gastrointestinal side effects such as nausea or diarrhea. Individuals affected by acute joint pain with **renal insufficiency**, for which **NSAIDs or colchicine** is relatively **contraindicated**, usually benefit **from corticosteroid intraarticular injection or oral therapy.** Steroids should only be used if infection has been excluded. Treatment to lower uric acid levels is inappropriate during an acute episode, as any sudden increase or decrease in urate levels may precipitate further attacks.

During intercritical gout, the focus is shifted to prevention of further attacks by lowering uric acid levels. Dietary restriction is mainly aimed at avoiding organ-rich foods such as liver, and the avoidance of alcohol. Patients taking thiazide diuretics should be switched to another antihypertensive if possible. Urate lowering can be accomplished by therapy to increase uric acid excretion by the kidney, such as probenecid. Uricosuric agents such as this are ineffective in patients with renal failure, however, and are contraindicated in patients with a history of uric acid kidney stones. In these patients, allopurinol may be used to diminish uric acid production. In either case, urate lowering can precipitate acute attacks, so initial prophylaxis with daily low-dose colchicine is usually necessary.

Patients with tophaceous gout are managed as above during acute attacks, and treated with allopurinol to help tophaceous deposits resolve. Surgery may be indicated if the mass effect of tophi causes nerve compression, joint deformity, or chronic skin ulceration with resultant infection.

Patients with pseudogout are treated similarly for acute attacks (NSAIDs, colchicine, systemic or intraarticular steroids). Prophylaxis with colchicine may be helpful in patients with chronic recurrent attacks, but there is no effective therapy to prevent CPPD crystal formation or deposition.

Comprehension Questions

[21.1] A previously healthy 18-year-old college freshman presents to the student health clinic complaining of pain on the dorsum of her left wrist and in her right ankle, fever, and a pustular rash on the extensor surfaces of both her forearms. She has mild swelling and erythema of her ankle, and pain on passive flexion of her wrist. Less than 1 mL of joint fluid is aspirated from her ankle, which shows 8000 polymorphonuclear cells (PMNs)/high-power field (hpf), but no organisms on Gram stain. Which of the following is the best initial treatment?

A. Indomethacin orally
B. Intravenous ampicillin
C. Colchicine orally
D. Intraarticular prednisone
E. Intravenous ceftriaxone

[21.2] What diagnostic test is most likely to give the diagnosis in the case above [21.1]?

A. Crystal analysis of the joint fluid
B. Culture of joint fluid
C. Blood culture
D. Cervical culture

[21.3] A 30-year-old man is noted to have an acutely swollen and red knee. Joint aspirate reveals numerous leukocytes and polymorphonuclear leukocytes, but no organisms on Gram stain. Analysis shows few negatively birefringent crystals. Which of the following is the best initial treatment?

A. Oral corticosteroids
B. Intraarticular corticosteroids
C. Intravenous antibiotic therapy
D. Oral colchicine

Answers

[21.1] **E.** The patient described best fits the picture of disseminated gonococcal infection. She has the rash, which is typically located on extensor surfaces of distal extremities. Pain on passive flexion of her wrist indicates likely tenosynovitis of that area. The fluid is inflammatory, but gonococci are typically not seen on Gram stain. Ceftriaxone is the usual treatment of choice for gonococcal infection. Nafcillin would be useful for staphylococcal arthritis, which would be more likely if she were older, had some chronic joint disease like rheumatoid arthritis, or were immunocompromised. Gonococcal arthritis is the most common cause of infectious arthritis in patients under 40 years of age. Indomethacin or colchicine would be useful if she had a crystalline arthritis, but that is unlikely in this clinical picture. Intraarticular prednisone is contraindicated while infectious arthritis is a possibility.

[21.2] **D.** Synovial fluid cultures are usually sterile in gonococcal arthritis (in fact, the arthritis is more likely caused by immune complex deposition than by actual joint infection), and blood cultures are positive <50% of the time. Diagnosis is more often made by finding gonococcal infection in a more typical site, such as urethra, cervix, or pharynx.

[21.3] **C.** Corticosteroids should not be used until infection is ruled out. The inflammatory arthritis as shown by the joint aspirate Gram stain is suspicious for infection, even with a no organisms seen on Gram stain. Also, the presence of a few crystals does not eliminate an infection.

CLINICAL PEARLS

- ❖ In the absence of trauma, acute monarthritis is most likely to be caused by septic or crystalline arthritis.
- ❖ In a febrile patient with a joint effusion, diagnostic arthrocentesis is mandatory. Inflammatory fluid, that is, a white blood cell (WBC) count >2000/mm^3, should be considered infected until proven otherwise.
- ❖ Gonococcal arthritis usually presents as a migratory tenosynovitis, often involving the wrists and hands, with few vesicopustular skin lesions. Nongonococcal septic arthritis is most often caused by *S. aureus* and most often affects large weight-bearing joints.
- ❖ Monosodium urate crystals in gout are needle-shaped and negatively birefringent (yellow) under the polarizing microscope. Calcium pyrophosphate dihydrate crystals in pseudogout are rhomboid and positively birefringent (blue).
- ❖ Treatment of gout depends on the stage: NSAIDs, colchicine, or steroids for an acute gouty arthritis, and urate lowering with probenecid or allopurinol during the intercritical period.

REFERENCES

Ruddy S, Harris ED Jr, Sledge CB, eds. Kelley's textbook of rheumatology, 6th ed. Philadelphia: WB Saunders, 2001: Chapters 26, 42, 89.

Klippel JH. Rheumatology, 2nd ed. London, UK: Mosby International, 1998: Chapters 2.1–10, 3.1–6.

Klippel JH, Crofford L, eds. Primer on the rheumatic diseases, 12th ed. Atlanta: Arthritis Foundation, 2001: Chapters 12, 13, 15.

CASE 22

A 32-year-old nurse presents to your office with a complaint of intermittent episodes of pain, stiffness, and swelling in both hands and wrists for about 1 year. The episodes last for several weeks and then resolve. More recently, she noticed similar symptoms in her knees and ankles. Joint pain and stiffness are making it harder for her to get out of bed in the morning and are interfering with her ability to perform her duties at work. The joint stiffness usually lasts for several hours before improving. She also reports malaise and easy fatigability for the past few months but denies fever, chills, skin rashes, and weight loss. On physical exam, this is a well-developed woman with a blood pressure of 120/70 mmHg, a heart rate of 82 bpm, and a respiratory rate 14 breaths per minute. Her skin does not reveal any rashes. The head, neck, cardiovascular, chest, and abdominal exams are normal. There is no hepatosplenomegaly. The joint examination reveals the presence of bilateral swelling, redness and tenderness of most proximal interphalangeal joints, metacarpophalangeal (MCP) joints, the wrists, and the knees. Laboratories show a mild anemia with a hemoglobin of 11.2 g/dL, a hematocrit of 32.5%, a mean corpuscular volume (MCV) of 85.7 fL, a white blood cell (WBC) count of 7.9/mm^3 with a normal differential, and a platelet count of 300,000/mm^3. The urinalysis is clear with no protein and no red blood cells (RBCs). The erythrocyte sedimentation rate (ESR) is 45 mm/h, and the kidney and liver function tests are normal.

- **What is your most likely diagnosis?**

- **What is your next diagnostic step?**

ANSWERS TO CASE 22: Rheumatoid Arthritis

Summary: This is a 32-year-old woman with a 1-year history of joint pain, stiffness, and swelling in both hands and knees. She also has increased fatigue. The joint examination reveals the presence of bilateral swelling, redness and tenderness of most proximal interphalangeal joints, MCP joints, the wrists, and the knees. She has a mild anemia with a hemoglobin of 11.2 g/dL, an MCV of 85.7 fL, and a WBC 7.9/mm^3 with a normal differential. The urinalysis, renal, and liver function tests are normal. The ESR is 45 mm/h.

- **Most likely diagnosis:** Rheumatoid arthritis.
- **Next diagnostic step:** Rheumatoid factor and antinuclear antibody titer.

Analysis

Objectives

1. Discern between the clinical presentation of the rheumatoid arthritis and other symmetric polyarthritis syndromes.
2. Learn about the clinical course and treatment of rheumatoid arthritis.

Considerations

This patient's history offers a fairly straightforward etiology for her joint pain, even if the presence of a symmetric polyarthritis should bring to mind other diseases, such as systemic lupus erythematous. Systemic lupus erythematosus (SLE) usually causes a leukopenia or thrombocytopenia; skin rashes (such as the malar rash) are common. Rheumatoid arthritis is a systemic autoimmune disorder of unknown etiology. Its major distinctive feature is a chronic symmetric and erosive synovitis of peripheral joints. Rheumatoid synovium is characterized by massive expansion of stromal connective-tissue cells, primarily fibroblast-like cells and new blood vessels. This process causes the manifestations of rheumatoid arthritis, which are swelling, pain, and stiffness of the affected joints. The diagnosis of rheumatoid arthritis is based on the presence of a combination of clinical findings and laboratory abnormalities. The majority of patients have elevated titers of serum rheumatoid factor.

APPROACH TO SYMMETRIC ARTHRITIS

Symmetric polyarthritis may be the feature of many causes such as SLE or postviral infection, which is usually self-limited. **Rheumatoid factors** are **immunoglobulins** that react to the **F_C portion of IgG molecules**. The usual serologic tests employed in clinical laboratories detect IgM rheumatoid factor. Anemia of chronic disease may be present. Radiologic findings in rheumatoid arthritis, such as erosion of periarticular bone and cartilage destruction with loss of joint space, may help the diagnosis. Usually, though, the typical x-ray findings don't develop until later in the disease process after a diagnosis has been made on a clinical ground. Joint deformities in rheumatoid arthritis occur from several different mechanisms, all related to synovitis and pannus formation with resulting cartilage destruction and erosion of periarticular bone. The structural damage to the joint is irreversible and worsens with disease progression. Multiple different joints may be affected, such as hand, foot, ankle, hip, shoulders, elbow, and cervical spine.

There are also several **extraarticular manifestations in rheumatoid arthritis**. Most individuals will experience generalized malaise or fatigue. There are skin manifestations such as the appearance of **rheumatoid nodules** over pressure points and over the tendons. Extraarticular manifestation of rheumatoid arthritis also include vasculitic lesions with the development of ischemic ulcers, which implies systemic involvement; ocular manifestations with symptoms of **keratoconjunctivitis sicca** (Sjögren syndrome); respiratory manifestations caused by **interstitial lung disease**; cardiac manifestations; and several neurological manifestations, such as myelopathy, related to cervical spine instability. Although not common, the continuous bone erosion may result in an atlantoaxial subluxation with cervical dislocation and spinal cord compression. Entrapment neuropathy may develop, such as carpal tunnel syndrome. The hematologic manifestations include anemia, typically anemia of chronic disease. At this stage in the disease process, our patient is presenting with joint complaints, fatigue, and malaise. No other extraarticular manifestations have developed yet. At the very onset of rheumatoid arthritis, the characteristic symmetric inflammation of the joints and the typical serologic findings may not be evident. Therefore, initially it may be harder to distinguish rheumatoid arthritis from other conditions, such as lupus. Usually, the development of extraarticular phenomenon will allow the physician to make a more specific diagnosis.

Lupus, which may present with a symmetric polyarthritis is usually characterized by the presence of other symptoms, such as malar rash, symptoms related to serositis (pleuritis and pericarditis), renal disease with proteinuria or hematuria, CNS manifestation, as well as pronounced hematologic disorders, such as hemolytic anemia or leukopenia or lymphopenia or thrombocytopenia. Rheumatic fever, which could cause symmetric polyarthritis, is an acute febrile illness lasting only 6–8 weeks. In psoriatic arthritis the pattern of joint involvement varies widely. The vast majority of patients have peripheral joint involvement with more than five involved joints. Others have a pauciarticular asymmetric arthritis or exclusive distal interphalangeal involvement. Inflammation is not limited to the joints but also occurs at the periosteum, along tendons, and at the insertion points into the bone resulting in the development of "sausage digits," which are typical of psoriatic arthritis (and Reiter syndrome). Although the arthritis can precede the development of a skin rash, the definite diagnosis of psoriatic arthritis cannot be made without the evidence of skin or nail changes typical of psoriasis. Laboratory abnormalities are mild and nonspecific. The psoriatic synovium has many similarities to the synovium in rheumatoid arthritis with lymphocyte and plasma cell infiltrate and microvascular changes. X-ray findings include distal interphalangeal erosive disease with, in severe cases, osteolysis and joint destruction.

Degenerative joint disease may affect multiple joints, but it occurs in an older age group, is usually not associated with inflammation or constitutional symptoms, and tends not to be episodic. Also, in **osteoarthritis** the hand joints most commonly involved are the **distal interphalangeal joints where the formation of Heberden nodes** can be noted (see Figure 22–1). On x-rays, the typical findings are joint space narrowing, subchondral polysclerosis, marginal osteophyte formation, and cyst formation. Crystal-induced arthritis, such as gout and pseudogout, can be ruled out as well because of the completely different clinical presentation.

Virtually all patients with **rheumatoid arthritis** are affected in the **wrist, the MCP joints**, and **the proximal interphalangeal** (PIP) joints, while the distal interphalangeal joints (DIP) are usually spared. **Ulnar deviation of the MCP joints** is often associated with **radial deviation of the wrists**; **swan-neck deformities** can develop as well as the **boutonnière deformity (see Figure 22–2)**. The swan-neck deformity results from contracture of the interosseous and flexor muscles and tendons, which causes a flexion contracture of the MCP joint, hypertension of the PIP joint, and flexion of the distal interphalangeal joint. In the boutonnière deformity, there is a flexion of the PIP and hyperextension of the DIP joints. These findings are typical of advanced rheumatoid arthritis. The combination of **rheumatoid arthritis, splenomegaly, leucopenia, lymphadenopathy**, and **thrombocytopenia** is called **Felty syndrome**. Felty syndrome is most common with severe nodule-forming rheumatoid arthritis.

Treatment

Several drugs are currently used in the treatment of rheumatoid arthritis (RA). Corticosteroids have an immediate and dramatic effect on joint symptoms, but they do not alter the natural progression of the disease. **DMARDs** (disease-modifying antirheumatic drugs) may have favorable impact on the natural course of the disease, reducing joint inflammation, disease activity, and improving functional status in people with RA. **DMARDs include methotrexate, hydroxychloroquine, sulfasalazine, oral and parenteral gold, penicillamine, azathioprine, cyclophosphamide, and cyclosporine.** There is no consensus as to which drug should be used in what order. The treatment should be individualized and the use of less-toxic drugs is preferred initially, except in patients with very aggressive disease or life-threatening complications such as vasculitis. More recently, tumor necrosis factor (TNF) antagonists (etanercept and infliximab) have been found to reduce disease activity within weeks, unlike other DMARDs that may take several months to act.

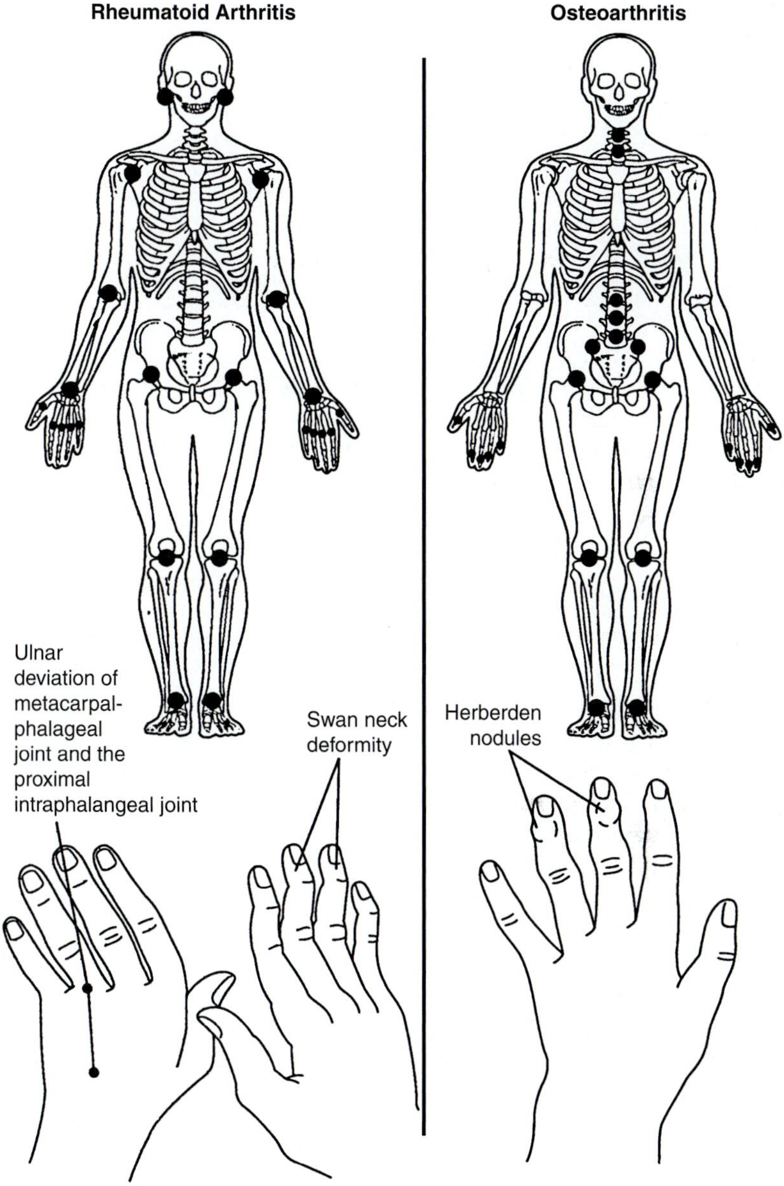

Figure 22–1. Rheumatoid arthritis versus osteoarthritis.

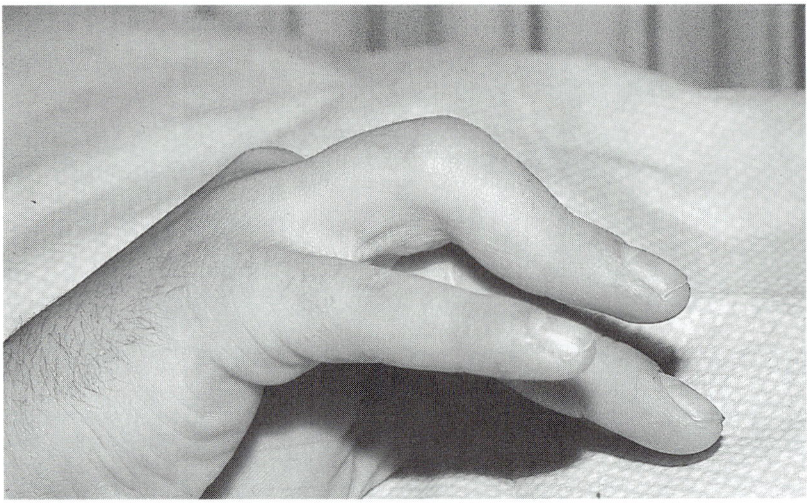

A

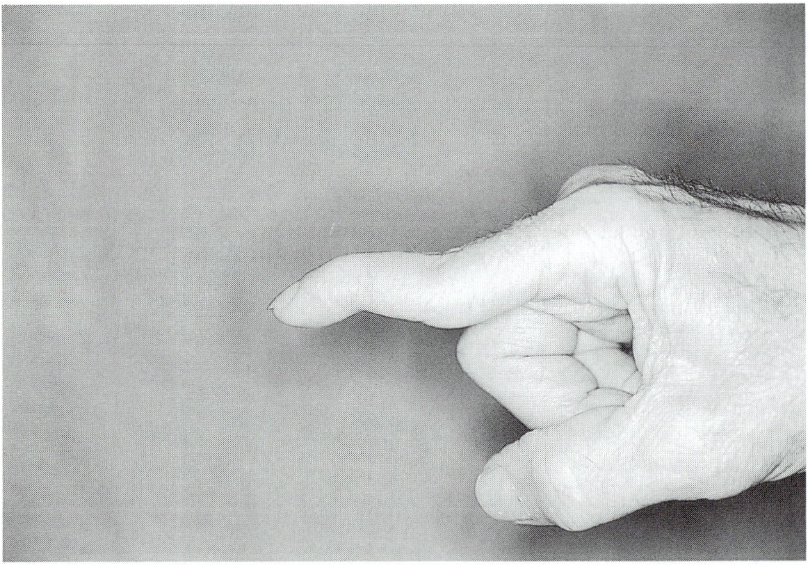

B

Figure 22–2. Boutonnière (A) and swan-neck (B) deformities. **(Reproduced with permission from Knoop KJ, Stack LB, Storrow AB, eds. Atlas of emergency medicine. New York: McGraw-Hill, 1997:291.)**

Comprehension Questions

[22.1] A 72-year-old man develops severe pain and swelling in both knees, shortly after undergoing an abdominal hernia repair surgery. Physical examination shows warmth and swelling of both knees with large effusions. Arthrocentesis of the right knee reveals the presence of intracellular and extracellular *weakly positive birefringent crystals* in the synovial fluid. Gram stain is negative. The most likely diagnosis is:

A. Gout.
B. Septic arthritis.
C. Calcium oxalate deposition disease.
D. Reactive arthritis.
E. Pseudogout.

[22.2] A 65-year-old man with a history of chronic hypertension, diabetes mellitus, and degenerative joint disease presents with acute onset of severe pain of the MTP joint and swelling of the left first toe. Physical examination shows exquisite tenderness of the joint, with swelling, warmth, and erythema. There is no history of trauma or other significant medical problems. Synovial fluid analysis and aspiration is most likely to show:

A. Hemorrhagic fluid.
B. Needle-shaped, negatively birefringent crystals.
C. Gram-negative organisms.
D. Noninflammatory fluid.
E. Rhomboidal, positively birefringent crystals.

[22.3] A 17-year-old sexually active man presents with a 5-day history of fever, chills, and persistent left ankle pain and swelling. On physical examination, maculopapular and pustular skin lesions are noted on the trunk and extremities. He denies any symptoms of genitourinary tract infection. Synovial fluid analysis is most likely to show:

A. WBC 75,000/mm^3 with 95% polymorphonuclear leukocytes.
B. RBC 100,000/mm^3, WBC 1,000/mm^3.
C. WBC 48,000/mm^3 with 80% lymphocytes.
D. WBC 500m/m^3 with 25% polymorphonuclear leukocytes.

[22.4] A 22-year-old man presents with complaints of low back pain for 3–4 months and stiffness of the lumbar area, which worsen with inactivity. He reports difficulty in getting out of bed in the morning and may have to roll out sideways, trying not to flex or rotate the spine to minimize pain. An L-S spine x-ray film would most likely show:

A. Degenerative joint disease with spur formation.
B. Sacroiliitis with increased sclerosis around the sacroiliac joints.
C. Vertebral body destruction with wedge fractures.
D. Osteoporosis with compression fractures of L3-L5.
E. Diffuse osteonecrosis of the L-S spine.

Answers

[22.1] **E.** Pseudogout is diagnosed by positive birefringent crystals.

[22.2] **B.** This is most likely gout, and the synovial fluid is likely to show **needle-shaped, negatively birefringent crystals.**

[22.3] **A.** This history is suggestive of gonococcal arthritis, and the rash is suggestive of disseminated gonococcal disease. The synovial fluid would most likely show an acute inflammatory exudate, WBC 72,000/mm^3 with 75% polymorphonuclear cells.

[22.4] **B.** A young man is not likely to have osteoporosis, osteoarthritis, or compression fractures. His morning stiffness, which worsens with rest, suggests an inflammatory arthritis, such as ankylosing spondylitis, which would include sacroiliitis with increased sclerosis around the sacroiliac joints.

CLINICAL PEARLS

❖ Rheumatoid arthritis is a chronic sytemic inflammatory disorder characterized by the insidious onset of symmetric polyarthritis and extraarticular symptoms.

❖ Rheumatoid factor (RF) is found in the serum of 85% of patients with rheumatoid arthritis.

❖ In nearly all patients with rheumatoid arthritis, the wrist, the MCP, and the PIP joints are affected, while the DIP are spared.

❖ DIP joints and large weight-bearing joints are most commonly involved in osteoarthritis.

❖ The typical x-ray findings in rheumatoid arthritis, periarticular bone erosion (loss of joint space) may not develop until later in the disease process, when the diagnosis has already been made on clinical grounds.

REFERENCES

Lipski PE. Rheumatoid Arthritis. In: Braunwald E, Fauci AS, Kasper KL, et al., eds. Harrison's principles of internal medicine, 15th ed. New York: McGraw-Hill, 2001;1928-2937.

CASE 23

A 36-year-old man comes to the office complaining of 7–10 days of low-grade fevers with fatigue, myalgias, and headaches, which he attributes to the "flu." This morning, when he awoke, he noticed that he had weakness of the right side of his face. He denies cough, congestion, sore throat, abdominal pain, diarrhea, or any urinary symptoms. He has had a mildly pruritic rash near his waist for the last several days, which he thought was "jock itch." He works as a Wall Street commodities broker, is married, and is monogamous. He recently accompanied his son on a weekend Boy Scout camping trip in New Jersey but he does not recall any bites or injury.

On physical examination, his temperature is 100.8°F, with a heart rate of 94 bpm, and a blood pressure of 128/79 mmHg. He is alert, talkative, and appears comfortable. He has drooping of the right corner of his mouth, and inability to elevate his eyebrow on the right. His conjunctivae are clear and he has no oral lesions. His neck is somewhat stiff when passively flexed. His chest is clear and his heart is regular without murmurs. His abdominal exam is benign, without liver or splenic enlargement. He has a 10-cm × 6-cm raised erythematous annular plaque with partial central clearing at his waistline (see Figure 23–1). He has no joint swelling or erythema, and except for the facial weakness, he has no focal neurologic deficits.

- **What is the most likely diagnosis?**

- **What is the most appropriate next step?**

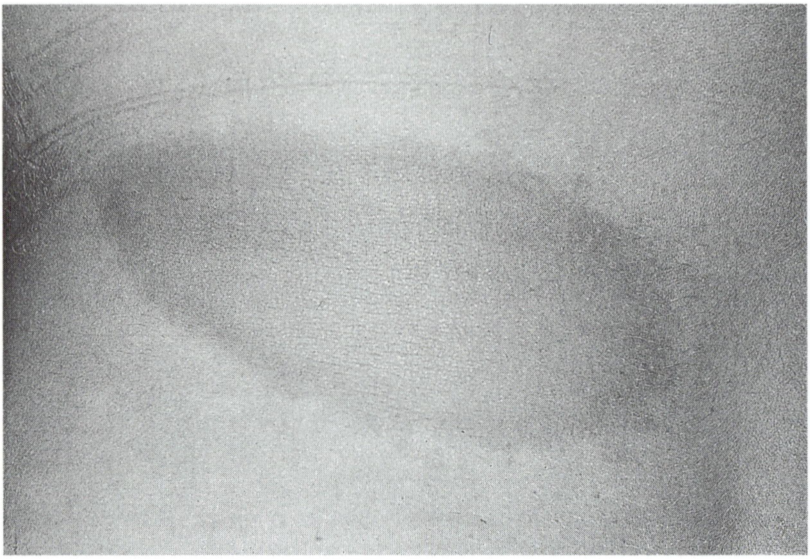

Figure 23–1. Skin rash. **(Reproduced with permission from Fitzpatrick TB, Johnson RA, Wolff K, et al. Color atlas and synopsis of clinical dermatology. 3rd ed. New York: McGraw-Hill, 1997:679.)**

ANSWERS TO CASE 23: Lyme Disease

Summary: A young man presents with a peripheral facial nerve palsy, occurring in the setting of a febrile illness associated with arthralgias, myalgias, neck stiffness, and an erythematous annular plaque at his waistline. He was recently on a camping trip, but shows no specific tick or other arthropod exposure. The rash is consistent with erythema migrans, the distinctive lesion of early Lyme disease, and all of the clinical features are consistent with that disease.

- **Most likely diagnosis:** Lyme disease, probably early disseminated stage.
- **Most appropriate next step:** Lumbar puncture to evaluate for meningitis and look for antibody production against *Borrelia burgdorferi.*

Analysis

Objectives

1. Understand the distinctive features of common diseases that present with fever and a rash.
2. Know the clinical features and phases of Lyme disease.
3. Learn the appropriate treatment for Lyme disease based on the stage of disease.

Considerations

This patient has fever, headache, stiff neck, and an acute neurologic deficit. It is essential to exclude serious CNS pathology, such as meningitis or Guillain-Barré syndrome, which necessitates a lumbar puncture. The **diagnosis of Lyme disease is made on clinical grounds**, and the use of serologic testing is only done for confirmation. Treatment is primarily undertaken to prevent late chronic cardiac and neurologic sequelae.

APPROACH TO SUSPECTED LYME DISEASE

The evaluation of the patient who presents with fever and a rash is a very common problem that often frustrates and confuses beginning clinicians, partly because of their unfamiliarity with many typical rash patterns, and partly because the rash may be an incidental nonspecific finding (as in miliaria or heat rash), may be a sign of serious, even fatal illness (as in the purpuric rash of meningococcemia), or it may be the pathognomonic finding that yields the diagnosis, as in the case of the **erythema migrans rash of Lyme disease**. Table 23–1 illustrates some important clinical features of systemic febrile syndromes associated with rash.

Lyme disease is diagnosed by the clinical presentation of the patient and can be verified by serologies at the earliest 6 weeks after the initial infection; thus, the patient's history is the key to the diagnosis. Lyme disease can present in three different stages; early localized (stage 1), early disseminated (stage 2), and late disease (stage 3). The **early localized stage** occurs **within the first month of the tick bite**. It presents with the **classic erythema migrans**; an expanding lesion that may or may not have a central clearing. It occurs most commonly around the belt line or the axilla because the ticks favor these areas. The erythema migrans is most often asymptomatic and can therefore be overlooked by the patient, although it sometimes is associated with burning, itching, or pain. In the first stage of the illness, the patient may also complain of a viral-like syndrome with fatigue, headaches, myalgias, and arthralgias. The physical exam during this stage may or may not show the skin lesion, as well as generalized lymphadenopathy or organomegaly.

The **early disseminated (second stage)** disease occurs **days to months after the initial tick bite** and there may be additional skin lesions similar to the primary skin lesion. There may be systemic symptoms of headache, mild neck stiffness, malaise, fatigue, fever, and chills. Commonly, there is also **migratory musculoskeletal pain without joint inflammation** that can last from hours to days and can affect one or two locations at time. This stage may also include cardiac or neurological manifestations. The **cardiac manifestations** of the disease may include conduction disturbances, myocarditis, or pericarditis. This problem will usually resolve within weeks without any antibiotics; however, in some instances, it can progress to cardiomyopathy (this most often occurs in Europe) or permanent heart block. The neurologic manifestations can occur in 10% of untreated patients after several weeks to months. They can present as cranial nerve palsies, most commonly facial nerve palsy that may be bilateral. **Meningitis** with a lymphocytic pleocytosis and elevated protein in the cere-

Table 23-1
DIFFERENTIAL DIAGNOSIS OF RASH AND FEVER

	LYME DISEASE	RHEUMATIC FEVER	ROCKY MOUNTAIN SPOTTED FEVER	TOXIC SHOCK SYNDROME	MEASLES
Organism	*Borrelia burgdorferi*	Group A streptococcus	*Rickettsia rickettsii*	*Staphylococcus aureus*	Paramyxovirus
Characteristic rash	Erythema migrans: papule that expands to an *annular lesion* with a *central clearing* a.k.a. "bull's eye". Usually occurs at the belt line or the axilla.	Erythema marginatum: nonpruritic, erythematous papules occurring in polycyclic waves over the trunk, *sparing the face*	Rash begins on *wrists and ankles* and spreads *centripetally*. Appears on palms and soles later.	Diffuse *erythema involving the palms* followed by *desquamation* after 7–10 days.	Discrete lesions that become confluent as the *rash proceeds from the hairline down, but spares the palms and the soles.*
Clinical features	• Initially viral-like syndrome • Cardiac and neurological manifestations if no initial treatment • Migratory oligoarticular (knee) or polyarticular arthritis weeks to months later	• Streptococcal pharyngitis • Migratory polyarthritis • Carditis—cardiac valvular and muscle damage • Rheumatic heart disease (10–20 years after original attack)	• Headache, myalgias, abdominal pain • 40% mortality if not treated	• Fever >102°F, hypotension, multiorgan dysfunction • Menstruating woman with tampon placed for a long period of time • Wound or skin infections	• Cough, conjunctivitis, coryza, severe prostration • Koplik spots: 1–2-mm bluish lesions with an erythematous halo on buccal mucosa pathognomonic for measles

		• Chorea—abrupt, purposeless, non-rhythmic, involuntary movements. • Subcutaneous nodules			
Treatment	• Doxycycline (first line) • Amoxicillin	• Anti-inflammatory agents, usually aspirin • Corticosteroids if carditis present • Penicillin for pharyngitis	• Doxycycline (first-line) • Tetracycline	• Penicillin or oxacillin plus clindamycin	• Supportive therapy • Antibiotics for otitis and pneumonia

(Sources: Kaye ET, Kaye KM. Fever and rash. Braunwald E, Fauci AS, Kaspar KL, et al., eds. Harrison's principles of internal medicine, 15th ed. New York: McGraw-Hill. 2001;p95–102.

brospinal fluid or a mild encephalitis is also possible. There may also be a sensory radiculoneuropathy. In Asia and Europe, the first characteristic neurological sign is radicular pain followed by the development of cerebrospinal fluid (CSF) pleocytosis, which is known as Bannwarth syndrome.

The third stage of the disease represents late or persistent infection. This occurs months to years after initial infection, usually when the initial presentation of the disease was not recognized nor treated with medications. The common presentation is that of generalized musculoskeletal pain and a migratory polyarthritis which may mimic juvenile rheumatoid arthritis in 50% of the cases. There are also intermittent attacks of oligoarthritis most often involving the knees which can last from weeks to months within the involved joint. Aspiration of joint fluid shows about 25,000 white blood cells per mm^3 with a predominance of polymorphonuclear leukocytes. This may develop into a chronic inflammatory joint disease lasting 5–8 years, especially if no treatment is given. Late neurological manifestations or tertiary borreliosis in the form of subtle encephalitis, neurocognitive dysfunction, or peripheral neuropathy occur in this stage.

Treatment of Lyme disease is with antibiotics. It is important to recognize the illness in the early phase to avoid progression to the later and more chronic stages. Most patients with Lyme disease, including those with skin or joint manifestations can be treated with oral antibiotics, preferably **doxycycline** 100 mg twice daily. Other choices include **amoxicillin** 500 mg three times daily, **cefuroxime** 500 mg twice daily, or **erythromycin** 250 mg four times daily. The treatment period is usually **1 month**. In more severe manifestations of the disease, such as **third-degree heart block or neurological** manifestations, an **intravenous** delivery of antibiotics is preferred, usually ceftriaxone 2 g daily, cefotaxime 2 g every 8 hours, or penicillin G 5 million units every 6 hours. Again, the treatment is to be given for a period of 1 month.

Comprehension Questions

[23.1 to 23.3] Match the Lyme disease stage (A to D) to the clinical manifestations [23.1–23.3].

A. First stage (localized infection)
B. Second stage (disseminated infection)
C. Third stage (persistent infection)
D. Not consistent with Lyme disease

[23.1] A 35-year-old woman with heart rate of 54 bpm, slightly irregular, with 2° AV block on EKG.

[23.2] A 22-year-old man who has facial weakness on the right, headache and fever

[23.3] A 28-year-old man who complains of 2 weeks of headache, fatigue, myalgias, and a rash along the belt line.

[23.4] A 45-year-old woman complains of near syncope. Her heart rate is noted to be 50 bpm. On EKG, third- degree heart block is noted. She had been in good health, but spent time camping in the woods of New Hampshire and had numerous tick bites 6 months previously. Which of the following is the best treatment for this condition?

A. Oral doxycycline
B. Intravenous lidocaine
C. Oral amoxicillin
D. Intravenous ceftriaxone

Answers

[23.1] **B.** Heart block occurs in about 8% of patients in the second stage (early disseminated) of Lyme barreliosis.

[23.2] **B.** Fluctuating symptoms of meningitis with facial nerve palsy are often seen in early disseminated stage. Facial weakness and cardiac heart block are both within the second (early disseminated) stage of the disease.

[23.3] **A.** The first stage of Lyme disease is the acute symptoms of headache, fatigue, low-grade fever, myalgias, and the typical erythema migrans rash along the axilla or belt line.

[23.4] **D.** Intravenous antibiotics are indicated with severe disease such as neurological or severe cardiac disease.

CLINICAL PEARLS

❖ The diagnosis of Lyme disease is made on clinical grounds; serologic testing is only confirmatory, that is a positive serologic test in an asymptomatic patient is not meaningful.

❖ Erythema migrans, particularly with the classic "bull's-eye" lesion, is the only pathognomonic feature of Lyme disease.

❖ The treatment of Lyme disease is oral doxycycline or amoxicillin for early localized disease.

❖ Intravenous cephalosporins are used to treat early disseminated or late disease.

REFERENCES

Kaye ET, Kaye KM. Fever and a Rash. In: Braunwald E, Fauci AS, Kasper KL, et al., eds. Harrison's principles of internal medicine, 15th ed. New York: McGraw-Hill, 2001:95-102.

Sigal LH. Lyme Disease. In: Klippel JH, Weyand CM, Wormann RL,eds. Primer on the rheumatic diseases, 11th ed. Atlanta: The Arthritis Foundation, 1997:204-207.

CASE 24

An obese 35-year-old housekeeper presents with low back pain, requesting an x-ray. She has had this pain off and on for several years, however, for the past 2 days it is worse than it has ever been. It started after she vigorously vacuumed a rug, is primarily on the right lower side, radiates down her posterior right thigh to her knee, but is not associated with any numbness or tingling. It is relieved by laying flat on her back with her legs slightly elevated, and lessened somewhat when she takes ibuprofen 400 mg. Except for moderate obesity and difficulty maneuvering onto the exam table because of pain, her exam is fairly normal. The only abnormalities you note are a positive straight leg raise test, with raising the right leg eliciting more pain than the left. Her strength, sensation, and deep tendon reflexes in all extremities are normal.

- **What is your diagnosis?**
- **What is your next step?**

ANSWERS TO CASE 24: Low Back Pain

Summary: An obese 35-year-old woman with acute worsening of chronic low back pain, complains of shooting pain down her right leg. Her physical exam is normal.

- **Most likely diagnosis:** Musculoskeletal low back pain, possible sciatica without neurological deficits.
- **Next step:** Encourage continuation of usual activity, avoiding twisting motions or heavy lifting. Use of NSAIDs on a scheduled basis; you could also recommend muscle relaxants, although these drugs may cause sleepiness. Massage might also be helpful. Follow up in 4 weeks. Long-term advice includes weight loss and back-strengthening exercises.

Analysis

Objectives

1. Learn the historical and physical exam findings that help to distinguish benign musculoskeletal low back pain from more serious causes of low back pain.
2. Understand the variety of treatment options and their effectiveness in low back pain.
3. Learn the judicious use of laboratory and imaging tests in evaluating low back pain.

Considerations

This young patient with chronic back pain has an acute exacerbation with pain radiating down her leg, which may indicate possible sciatic nerve compression. She has no other neurological abnormalities, such as sensory deficits, motor weakness, or "red flags" of more serious etiologies of back pain, which if present would demand a more urgent evaluation. Thus, this individual has a good prognosis for recovery with conservative therapy, perhaps time being the most important factor. If she does not improve after 6 weeks, then imaging studies can be considered.

APPROACH TO LOW BACK PAIN

Definitions

Sciatica: Pain in the distribution of the lumbar or sacral nerve roots, with or without motor or sensory deficits.

Spondylolisthesis: An anterior displacement an upper vertebral body on the lower body, which can cause symptoms and signs of spinal stenosis. This condition can result from spondylolysis or from degenerative disk disease in the elderly.

Spondylolysis: A defect in the pars interarticularis, either congenital or secondary to a stress fracture.

Clinical Approach

Low back pain is experienced by two-thirds of all adults at some point in their lives. Approximately 2% of adults miss work each year because of low back pain. This complaint is most common in adults in their working years, usually affecting patients between 30 and 60 years of age. Although it is common in workers required to perform lifting and twisting, it is also a common complaint in those who sit or stand for prolonged periods of time. Low back pain is a recurrent disease, that tends to be mild in younger patients, often resolving by 2 weeks, but can be more severe and prolonged as the patient ages. It is one of the most common reasons for young adults to seek medical care, second only to upper respiratory infections, and millions of health care dollars are expended on this problem each year. In evaluating patients with low back pain, the clinician needs to exclude potentially serious conditions such as **malignancy, infection**, and dangerous neurologic processes such as **spinal cord compression or cauda equina syndrome**. Individuals without these conditions are initially managed with conservative therapy. Nearly all patients recover spontaneously within 4–6 weeks; only 3–5% remain disabled for longer than 3 months. If patients do not improve within 4 weeks with conservative management, they should receive further evaluation to rule out systemic or rheumatic disease and to clarify the anatomic cause, especially patients with localized pain, nocturnal pain, or sciatica.

The potential causes of back pain are legion (see Table 24–1). Pain can emanate from the bones, ligaments, muscles, nerves, or, rarely, it can be a result of referred pain from a visceral organ or other structure. Back pain with **radiation down the back of the leg** suggests **sciatic nerve root compression**, generally caused by a herniated intervertebral disc at the **L4-L5** or **L5-S1** levels. Patients typically report aching pain in the buttock and paresthesias radiating into the posterior thigh and calf or lateral foreleg. When pain radiates below the knee, it is more likely to indicate a true radiculopathy than radiation only to the posterior thigh; a history of persistent leg numbness or weakness further increases the likelihood of neurologic involvement.

Most cases are idiopathic, and this group, in general, is referred to as musculoskeletal low back pain**. Imaging studies and other diagnostic tests are generally not helpful in managing these cases**. Studies show that the history and physical exam can help separate the majority of patients with simple and self-limited musculoskeletal back pain from the minority with more serious underlying causes. Finding "red-flag" symptoms can help the physician use diagnostic tests in a more judicious manner (Table 24–2). When the patient has worrisome symptoms or signs, in most cases, the most effective initial evaluation is plain anteroposterior and lateral radiographs of the involved area of the spine, a sedimentation rate, and a complete blood count. More expen-

Table 24-1
ETIOLOGIES OF LOW BACK PAIN

CAUSES OF LOW BACK PAIN	INCIDENCE
Musculoskeletal low back or leg pain	97%
Lumbar sprain or strain	70%
Degenerative disk disease	10%
Herniated disk	4%
Spinal stenosis	3%
Trauma	1%
Congenital disease, i.e., kyphoscoliosis	<1%
Referred or visceral pain	2%
Pelvic disease	
Renal disease	
Aortic aneurysm	
Gastrointestinal disease	
Nonmechanical low back pain	1%
Neoplasia	
Infection	
Inflammatory arthritis	
Paget disease	

(Adapted with permission from Deyo RA. Low back pain. N Engl J Med 2001; 344(5): 365)

sive tests, such as MRI, should be reserved for those cases in which surgery is being considered, because it is not required to make most diagnoses.

It is rare that the patient can recall a precipitating event. Patients often have a history of recurrent episodes of low back pain. Psychological causes have not been consistently related to low back pain; however, there does seem to be an association with job satisfaction. During the physical exam, palpable point tenderness over the spinous processes may indicate a destructive lesion of the spine itself; however, those with musculoskeletal back pain most often have tenderness in the muscular paraspinal area. Strength, sensation, and reflexes should be assessed, especially in those with complaints of radicular, or radiating pain.

Table 24-2
"RED FLAG" SIGNS AND SYMPTOMS OF LOW BACK PAIN

New onset of pain in a patient older than 50 or younger than 20 years
Fever
Unintentional weight loss
Severe nighttime pain or pain worse in supine position
Bowel or bladder incontinence
History of cancer
Immunosuppression (chemotherapy or HIV)
Saddle anesthesia
Major motor weakness

Straight-leg-raising testing, in which the examiner, holding the patients ankle, passively elevates the patient's leg to 45 degrees, is helpful if it elicits pain in the lower back. However, it is **not a very sensitive or specific test.** The Patrick maneuver, in which the patient externally rotates the hip, flexes the knee, and crosses the knee of the other leg with the ankle (like a number 4) while the examiner simultaneously presses down on the flexed knee and the opposite side of the pelvis, can help distinguish pain emanating from the sacral-iliac joint.

Treatment In treating idiopathic low back pain, various modalities have been shown to be equally effective in the long run. Randomized, controlled trials have shown that encouraging the patient to continue their **usual activity is superior to recommendations of bedrest**. Patients without disability and without evidence of nerve root compression probably can maintain judicious activity rather than be sent for bedrest. Bedrest is probably only appropriate for individuals with severe pain or with neurological deficits. The patient should be instructed to position himself so as to minimize pain; this usually consists of lying supine with the upper body slightly elevated and with a pillow under the knees. Nonsteroidal antiinflammatory medications (on a scheduled rather than on an as-needed basis), nonaspirin analgesics, and muscle relaxants may help in the acute phase. Because most cases of disk herniation with radiculopathy will resolve spontaneously within 4–6 weeks without surgery, this is the initial regimen recommended for these patients as well. Narcotic analgesics are also an option in cases of severe pain; however, because idiopathic low back pain is often a chronic problem their prolonged use beyond the initial phase is discouraged. Chiropractors, physical therapists, massage therapists, and acupuncture have been studied (in trials of varying quality) with results comparable to traditional approaches. **Referral** to a surgeon may be considered for those patients with radicular pain with or without neuropathy that **doesn't resolve with 4–6 weeks of conservative management**.

Comprehension Questions

[24.1] A 35-year-old obese hotel housekeeper presents with 1 week of lower back pain. Her history and exam are without "red flags" and completely normal, except for her weight. Which of the following is the best next step?

A. Regular doses of a nonnarcotic analgesic
B. Six weeks of bedrest
C. MRI of the lumbar spine
D. Plain film x-ray of lumbosacral spine

[24.2] A 32-year-old woman from Nigeria presents with a 12-week history of persistent lower lumbar back pain, associated with a low-grade fever and night sweats. She denies any extremity weakness or HIV risk factors. Her exam is normal except for point tenderness over the spinous processes of L4-L5. What is the most likely diagnosis?

A. *Staphylococcus aureus* osteomyelitis
B. Tuberculous osteomyelitis
C. Given her age, idiopathic low back pain
D. Metastatic breast cancer
E. Multiple myeloma

[24.3] A 70-year-old woman presents with a 4-week history of low back pain, generalized weakness, and a 15-pound weight loss over the last 2 months. Her past medical history is unremarkable, and her exam is normal except that she is generally weak. Initial labs reveal an elevated sedimentation rate, a mild anemia, a creatinine of 1.8 mg/dL, and a calcium level of 11.2 mg/dL. What is the most likely diagnosis?

A. Osteoporosis with compression fractures
B. Renal failure with osteodystrophy
C. Multiple myeloma
D. Lumbar strain
E. Osteomyelitis

Answers

[24.1] **A.** Bedrest has not been shown to improve outcome in idiopathic low back pain when compared to encouraging usual activities that don't exacerbate the pain. Imaging is not necessary with uncomplicated back pain.

[24.2] **B.** The patient's country of origin, the chronic and slowly progressive nature of the pain in association with fever, and night sweats, are highly suggestive of tuberculous osteomyelitis of the spine, or Pott disease. Bacterial osteomyelitis presents more acutely, often with high, spiking fevers. Metastatic breast cancer and multiple myeloma are extremely rare in this age group. The fevers, night sweats, and persistent and progressive nature of her back pain make a musculoskeletal cause unlikely.

[24.3] **C.** This patient has many red flags in her presentation: her age, new onset pain, and history of weight loss. The elevated calcium and mild renal failure are classic for multiple myeloma. Plain radiographs of the spine and, more likely, of the skull, may illustrate the punched out lytic bone lesions often seen in this disease.

CLINICAL PEARLS

- ❖ In 90% of patients, acute low back pain, even with sciatic nerve involvement, resolves within 4–6 weeks.
- ❖ Analgesics such as NSAIDs or narcotics, as well as muscle relaxants, along with trying to maintain some level activity, are helpful in managing acute low back pain; bedrest does not help.
- ❖ Pain that interferes with sleep, significant unintentional weight loss, or fever suggest an infectious or neoplastic cause of back pain.
- ❖ Imaging studies such as MRI are only of use if surgery is being considered (persistent pain and neurological symptoms after 4–6 weeks of conservative care in patients with herniated disks) or if a neoplastic or inflammatory cause of back pain is being considered.

REFERENCES

Deyo RA, Weinstein JN. Low back pain. N Engl J Med 2001;344(5):363–70.

Jarvik JG, Deyo RA. Diagnostic evaluation of low back pain with emphasis on imaging. Ann Intern Med 2002;137:586–97.

CASE 25

A healthy 52-year-old man presents to the doctor's office complaining of increasing fatigue for the past 4–5 months. He exercises every day but lately he has noticed becoming short of breath while jogging. He denies orthopnea, paroxysmal nocturnal dyspnea (PND), or swelling in his ankles. The patient reports occasional joint pain for which he uses over-the-counter ibuprofen. He denies bowel changes, melena, or bright red blood per rectum, but reports vague left-side abdominal pain for a few months off and on, not related to food intake. The patient denies fever, chills, nausea, or vomiting. He has lost a few pounds intentionally with diet and exercise.

On examination, his weight is 205 pounds and he is afebrile. There is slight pallor of the conjunctiva, skin, and palms. No lymphadenopathy is noted. Chest is clear to auscultation bilaterally. Cardiovascular system: regular rate and rhythm, with no rub or gallop. There is a II/IV systolic ejection murmur. His abdomen is soft, nontender, and without hepatosplenomegaly. Bowel sounds are present. He has no extremity edema, cyanosis, or clubbing. His peripheral pulses are palpable and symmetric. A hemoglobin level is 9.2 g/dL.

- **What is the most likely diagnosis?**

- **What is your next diagnostic step?**

ANSWERS TO CASE 25: Iron-Deficiency Anemia

Summary: A healthy 52-year-old man complains of a 4–5 month history of increasing exercise intolerance, but denies orthopnea, PND, or swelling in his ankles. The patient uses ibuprofen. He denies bowel changes, melena, or bright red blood per rectum, but reports vague left-side abdominal pain. On examination, he weighs 205 pounds and has slight pallor of the conjunctiva, skin, and palms. He has a II/IV systolic ejection murmur; otherwise the examination is normal. His hemoglobin level is 9.2 g/dL.

- **Most likely diagnosis:** Iron-deficiency anemia as a result of chronic blood loss.

- **Next diagnostic step:** Analyze the complete blood count (CBC), particularly the mean corpuscular volume (MCV), to determine if the anemia is microcytic, normocytic, or macrocytic; assess the leukocyte count and platelet count.

Analysis

Objectives

1. Understand that iron-deficiency anemia is the most common cause of anemia.
2. Know the diagnostic approach to anemia.
3. Be familiar with the treatment of iron-deficiency anemia.

Considerations

This 52-year-old man presents to the doctor's office with a complaint of fatigue and dyspnea on exertion for the few months prior to the office visit. His physical examination is significant only for pallor. The serum hemoglobin level confirms anemia. The next step would be to characterize the anemia as microcytic, which would be consistent with iron deficiency, and confirmed with further testing for TIBC and ferritin. The most likely source of blood loss in male patients is the gastrointestinal tract; therefore, finding iron-deficiency anemia should suggest the presence of a possible GI source of bleeding, colon cancer being the most serious possibility. This patient is using ibuprofen, which may predispose to erosive gastritis. Once iron-deficiency anemia is confirmed, a thorough evaluation of the GI tract, including upper and lower endoscopy is needed.

APPROACH TO SUSPECTED IRON-DEFICIENCY ANEMIA

Definitions

Anemia: Decreased red blood cell mass, leading to less oxygen-carrying capacity. Hemoglobin levels <13 g/dL in men and <12 g/dL in women are generally used.

Iron studies: Ferritin is a marker of iron stores, but also is an acute-phase reactant, which is decreased in iron deficiency, but increased with chronic disease. Total iron-binding capacity is an indirect measure of transferrin saturation levels, and is increased in iron deficiency.

Mean corpuscular volume (MCV): Average red blood cell volume. This offers a method of categorizing anemias as microcytic (MCV <80 fL), normocytic (80–100 fL), or macrocytic (>100 fL).

Reticulocyte: A new red blood cell that is usually 1–1.5 days old.

Reticulocyte count: The fraction of red blood cells consisting of reticulocytes indirectly indicates the bone marrow activity of the erythrocyte line. It is usually expressed as a percentage, and normally is 1%. Corrected reticulocyte count accounts for anemia.

Clinical Approach

Iron Deficiency Although anemia may be caused by disorders of bone marrow production, red cell maturation, or increased destruction, iron deficiency is the most common cause of anemia in the United States, affecting all ages and both genders. Iron is essential to the synthesis of hemoglobin. The normal daily intake of elemental iron is about 15 mg of which only 1–2 mg is absorbed. The daily iron losses are about the same, but menstruation adds approximately 30 mg of iron lost each month. The primary etiology for iron-deficiency anemia is blood loss (see Table 25–1). **In men, the most frequent cause is chronic GI tract occult bleeding**. In women, menstrual loss may be the main mechanism, but other sites must be considered. Supplemental iron is needed during pregnancy because there is a transfer of iron from the mother to the developing fetus. Iron deficiency may also be a result of increased iron requirements, diminished iron absorption, or both. Iron deficiency can develop during the first 2 years of life if dietary iron is inadequate for the demands of rapid growth. Adolescent girls may become iron deficient from inadequate diet plus the added loss from menstruation. The growth spurt in adolescent boys may also produce a significant increase in demand for iron. Other possible causes of anemia are decreased iron absorption after gastrectomy and upper bowel malabsorption syndrome, but such mechanisms are rare when compared to blood loss.

When the iron loss exceeds intake, iron deposits are progressively depleted. The hemoglobin and serum iron levels may remain normal in the initial stages, but the **serum ferritin** (iron stores) will start to fall. As the serum iron levels fall, the percent of transferrin saturation falls, and the **total iron-binding capacity will increase**, leading to a progressive decrease in iron available for the red blood cell formation. At this point, anemia will develop initially with normal-appearing red blood cells. As the iron deficiency becomes more severe, microcytosis and hypochromia will develop. Later in the disease process, iron deficiency will affect other tissues, resulting in a variety of symptoms and signs.

Typical symptoms of anemia include fatigue, shortness of breath, dizziness, headache, palpitations, and impaired concentration. Additionally, patients with chronic severe iron deficiency may develop **cravings for dirt or paint (pica) or**

Table 25-1
COMMON CAUSES OF IRON-DEFICIENCY ANEMIA

Blood loss
- Gastrointestinal blood loss
  - Esophageal varices
  - Peptic ulcer disease
  - Gastritis, e.g., NSAID induced
  - Small bowel polyp or carcinoma
  - Colonic angiodysplasia
  - Colon cancer
  - Inflammatory bowel disease, e.g., ulcerative colitis
  - Hookworm infestation
- Uterine blood loss
  - Menstruation/menorrhagia
  - Uterine fibroids
- Other blood loss
  - Chronic hemodialysis
  - Surgical blood loss
  - Repeated blood donation or phlebotomy
  - Paroxysmal nocturnal hemoglobinuria

Malabsorption
- Gastrectomy
- Celiac disease
- Inflammatory bowel disease, e.g., Crohn disease

Inadequate dietary intake/increased physiological demands
- Infancy/adolescence
- Pregnancy
- Vegetarian diet

ice (pagophagia). **Glossitis**, cheilosis or koilonychia may develop and in rare advanced cases, dysphagia, associated with a postcricoid **esophageal web (Plummer-Vinson syndrome)**. When the anemia develops over a long period of time, the typical symptoms of fatigue and shortness of breath may not be evident. Many patients with iron-deficiency anemia may be asymptomatic. The lack of symptoms reflects the very slow development of iron deficiency and the ability of the body to adapt to lower iron reserves and anemia.

Evaluation of Anemia Once anemia is discovered, a CBC with differential, platelets, and red blood cell indices are helpful in narrowing the differential diagnosis. The first step is to look at the **MCV** to classify the common causes of the common causes of anemia (Table 25–2). Iron deficiency usually leads to a microcytic anemia. The red blood cell distribution width (RDW) is a calculated index that quantitates the variation in the size of red blood cells. RDW is a quantitative

Table 25-2
CLASSIFICATION OF ANEMIA BY MCV

Microcytic (low MCV)
Iron deficiency
Thalassemia
Sideroblastic anemia
Lead poisoning
Normocytic (normal MCV)
Acute blood loss
Hemolysis
Anemia of chronic disease
Anemia of renal failure
Myelodysplastic syndromes
Macrocytic anemia (high MCV)
Folate deficiency
Vitamin B_{12} deficiency
Drug toxicity, e.g., zidovudine
Alcoholism/chronic liver disease

measure of anisocytosis that helps to distinguish uncomplicated iron deficiencies from uncomplicated thalassemia. An increased RDW associated with microcytic anemia is suggestive of iron-deficiency anemia, because the bone marrow produces erythrocytes of various sizes. A normal RDW in the presence of microcytic anemia may be more suggestive of chronic disease, thalassemia, or even iron deficiency associated with anemia of a chronic disease. A detailed history, physical exam, and further laboratory data may be necessary to achieve a final diagnosis.

The **reticulocyte count** is another important parameter to help in the differential diagnosis of anemia. A new red blood cell remains a reticulocyte for 1–1.5 days, after which the RBC circulates for about 120 days. The blood normally contains about one reticulocyte per 100 red blood cells (RBCs). The reticulocyte count, usually reported as a percentage of reticulocytes per 100 RBCs, may be falsely elevated in the presence of anemia. Therefore, a corrected reticulocyte percentage is calculated by multiplying the reported reticulocyte count by the patient's hematocrit divided by 45 (normal hematocrit). The reticulocyte may also be converted to an absolute number by multiplying the reported reticulocyte count by the RBC count and dividing by 100. The absolute reticulocyte count is normally 50,000–70,000 reticulocytes/mm^3. If the **reticulocyte count is low**, causes of **hypoproliferative bone marrow** disorders should be suspected. A **high reticulocyte count** may reflect **acute blood losses**, **hemolysis**, or a response to therapy for anemia.

Iron studies are very helpful to confirm a diagnosis of iron deficiency anemia and to help in the differential diagnosis with other types of anemia such as anemia of chronic disease and sideroblastic anemia (Table 25–3). **Serum**

Table 25-3
DIFFERENT ANEMIAS WITH CHARACTERISTICS AND LAB STUDIES

TESTS	IRON DEFICIENCY	INFLAMMATION	THALASSEMIA	SIDEROBLASTIC ANEMIA
Smear	Micro/hypo	Normal micro/hypo	Micro/hypo with targeting	Variable
SI	<30	<50	Normal to high	Normal to high
TIBC	>360	<300	Normal	Normal
Percent saturation	<10	10-20	30-80	30-80
Ferritin (μg/L)	<15	30-200	50-300	50-300
Hemoglobin pattern	Normal	Normal	Abnormal	Normal

NOTE: SI, serum iron; TIBC, total iron-binding capacity
Reproduced with permission from Adamson JW. Iron Deficiency and Other Hypoproliferative Anemias. Braunwald E, Fauci AS, Kasper KL, et al., Harrison's principles of internal medicine, 15th ed. New York: McGraw-Hill, 2001: 663.

ferritin concentration is a reliable indication of iron deficiency. Serum **ferritin values are increased with chronic inflammatory disease**, malignancy, or liver injury; therefore, serum ferritin concentration may be above normal when iron deficiency exists with chronic diseases, such as rheumatoid arthritis, Hodgkin disease, or hepatitis, among many other disorders. Measurement of serum iron concentration, serum TIBC, and calculation of percent saturation of transferrin has been widely used for diagnosis of iron deficiency. **True iron deficiency** is strongly suspected on the basis of **low serum iron level** and **normal or high binding capacity,** which will result in a low calculated saturation. In anemia of **chronic disease, serum iron concentration is low, but usually the total iron-binding capacity is also reduced;** therefore, percent transferrin saturation typically is normal in anemia of chronic disease. **Chronic disease typically causes elevation in serum ferritin concentration**. When chronic disease and iron-deficiency anemia coexist, serum ferritin concentration may be normal. Sideroblastic anemia is commonly microcytic and hypochromic. The iron studies in **sideroblastic anemia** include **increases in serum iron and serum ferritin concentration and saturation of transferrin**. An important clue to the presence of sideroblastic anemia is the presence of **stippled RBCs** in the peripheral blood smear. Iron stain in the bone marrow reveals pathognomonic feature of engorged mitochondria in the developing RBCs called **ringed sideroblasts.**

Evaluating the peripheral blood smear for specific abnormalities in RBC morphology may be very useful for determining the etiology of anemia. In iron-deficiency anemia, the peripheral blood smear shows RBCs smaller than normal (microcytes) and hypochromia.

Although the treatment of iron deficiency is straightforward, finding the underlying etiology is paramount. Treatment of iron-deficiency anemia is by iron-replacement therapy, typically with **oral ferrous sulfate 325 mg two or three times daily**. Correction of anemia usually occurs **within 6 weeks,** but therapy should continue for at least 6 months to replenish the iron stores. A number of patients may develop gastrointestinal side effects, such as constipation, nausea, abdominal cramping. Taking the iron with meals may help with tolerance but can reduce absorption. Parenteral iron therapy is indicated in rare instances, such as in patients with a poor absorption state or with excessive intolerance to oral therapy. Caution must be taken with parenteral iron because **anaphylaxis** may occur.

Comprehension Questions

[25.1] A 25-year-old man with a history of a duodenal ulcer is noted to have a hemoglobin level of 10 g/dL. Which of the following is most likely to be seen on laboratory investigation?

A. Reticulocyte count of 4%
B. Elevated total iron-binding capacity (TIBC)

C. Normal serum ferritin
D. MCV of 105 fL

[25.2] A 22-year-old woman is pregnant and at 14 weeks gestation. Her hemoglobin level is 9 g/dL. She asks why she could have iron deficiency when she is no longer menstruating. Which of the following is the best explanation?

A. Occult gastrointestinal blood loss
B. Expanded blood volume and transport to the fetus
C. Hemolysis
D. Iron losses as a result of relative alkalosis of pregnancy

[25.3] A 35-year-old man has undertaken a self-imposed diet for 3 months. Previously, he had been healthy, but now complains of fatigue. His hemoglobin level is 10 g/dL and his MCV is 105 fL. Which of the following is the most likely etiology of his anemia?

A. Iron deficiency
B. Folate deficiency
C. Vitamin B_{12} deficiency
D. Thalassemia
E. Sideroblastic anemia

Match the following laboratory parameters (A to E) to the clinical picture (25.4 to 25.6).

	MCV	Ferritin	TIBC	RDW
A.	Elevated	Decreased	Elevated	Decreased
B.	Decreased	Decreased	Elevated	Increased
C.	Normal	Elevated	Normal	Normal
D.	Decreased	Increased	Normal	Normal
E.	Elevated	Increased	Decreased	Increased

[25.4] A 20-year-old woman with heavy menses.

[25.5] A 34-year-old man of Mediterranean descent with a family history of anemia.

[25.6] A 50-year-old man with severe rheumatoid arthritis.

Answers

[25.1] **B.** Chronic gastrointestinal blood loss leads to low ferritin levels reflecting diminished iron stores, elevated TIBC, and low iron saturation. There is a microcytic anemia (low MCV) with a low reticulocyte count.

[25.2] **B.** Iron deficiency occurs in pregnancy as a result of the expanded blood volume and active transport of iron to the fetus.

[25.3] **B.** Macrocytic anemia is usually a result of folate or vitamin B_{12} deficiency. Because vitamin B_{12} stores last for nearly 10 years, a diet of several months would more likely cause folate deficiency. Folate is found in green leafy vegetables.

[25.4] **B.** This laboratory finding is diagnostic of iron-deficiency anemia (microcytic, low ferritin, high TIBC, high RDW).

[25.5] **D.** Thalassemia usually leads to a microcytic anemia with uniform red cell size (normal RDW) and excess iron stores.

[25.6] **C.** Chronic disease generally leads to a normocytic anemia with elevated ferritin level (acute-phase reactant).

CLINICAL PEARLS

❖ Anemia is a clinical finding, not a diagnosis, and requires some investigation to determine the underlying etiology.

❖ Iron-deficiency anemia in men or postmenopausal women is primarily a result of gastrointestinal blood losses; therefore, finding iron-deficiency anemia in this patient population warrants a thorough GI workup.

❖ Iron-deficiency anemia in women of reproductive age is most often caused by menstrual blood loss.

❖ The fecal occult blood testing (FOBT) is negative in about 50% of patients with GI cancer. Therefore, a negative FOBT in the presence of iron-deficiency anemia should not discourage you from pursuing a thorough GI workup.

❖ The mean corpuscular volume, RDW, and the reticulocyte index are important parameters in the evaluation of anemia.

REFERENCES

Adamson JW. Iron Deficiency and Other Hyproproliferative Anemias. In: Braunwald E, Fauci AS, Kasper KL, et al, (eds). Harrison's principles of internal medicine, 15th ed. New York: McGraw Hill, 2001;660-666.

CASE 26

A 61-year-old man comes to the emergency room complaining of 3 days of worsening abdominal pain. The pain is localized to the left lower quadrant of his abdomen. It began as an intermittent crampy pain and now has become steady and moderately severe. He feels nauseated, but has not vomited. He had a small loose stool at the beginning of this illness, but has not had any bowel movements since. He has never had symptoms like this before, nor any gastrointestinal illnesses.

On examination, his temperature is 100.2°F, with a heart rate of 98 bpm and a blood pressure of 110/72 mmHg. He has no pallor or jaundice. His chest is clear and his heart is regular without murmurs. His abdomen is mildly distended with hypoactive active bowel sounds and marked left lower quadrant tenderness with voluntary guarding. Rectal examination reveals tenderness, and his stool is negative for occult blood.

Laboratory studies are significant for a white blood cell (WBC) count of 11,800/mm^3 with 74% polymorphonuclear leukocytes (%Polys), 22% lymphocytes, and a normal hemoglobin and hematocrit. A plain film of the abdomen shows no pneumoperitoneum and a nonspecific bowel gas pattern.

◆ **What is the most likely diagnosis?**

◆ **What is the most appropriate next step?**

ANSWERS TO CASE 26: Acute Sigmoid Diverticulitis

Summary: A 61-year-old man has 3 days of new-onset, worsening, left lower quadrant abdominal pain. He feels nauseated, and has not had any bowel movements since the illness began. His temperature is 100.2°F and he has no pallor or jaundice. His abdomen is mildly distended with hypoactive active bowel sounds, and marked left lower quadrant tenderness with voluntary guarding. Rectal examination reveals tenderness, and his stool is negative for occult blood. The WBC count is 11,800/mm^3 with 74%Polymorphonuclear cells, 22% lymphocytes, and a normal hemoglobin and hematocrit. A plain film of the abdomen shows no acute changes.

- **Most likely diagnosis:** Acute sigmoid diverticulitis.
- **Most appropriate next step:** Admit to the hospital for intravenous antibiotics and monitoring. CT scan of the abdomen will be very useful to confirm the diagnosis and to exclude pericolic abscess or other complications, such as fistula formation.

Analysis

Objectives

1. Understand the complications of diverticular disease.
2. Understand the appropriate therapy of acute diverticulitis, which is dependent on the age of the patient and the severity of the disease presentation.
3. Learn the complications of diverticulitis and the indications for surgical intervention.

Considerations

This is an older patient with new-onset, progressively severe, lower abdominal pain. It is on the left side, suggesting diverticulitis as a diagnosis. The pattern of the pain suggests a bowel process because he has had nausea, no bowel movement, and pain that was initially crampy and intermittent but is now steady. The low-grade temperature is consistent with acute sigmoid diverticulitis, which is likely to improve with antibiotic therapy. Because the clinical presentation is similar, it is important to evaluate the patient for colon cancer with perforation, once all signs of inflammation have subsided. The abdominal film reveals no free air under the diaphragm. Ischemic colitis is another diagnostic consideration in an older patient, but it is usually associated with signs of bleeding, whereas diverticulitis is not.

APPROACH TO SUSPECTED DIVERTICULITIS

Definitions

Colonic diverticulum: herniation of the mucosa and submucosa through a weakness of the muscle lining of the colon.

Diverticulitis: Inflammation of the colonic diverticulum, typically on the left colon, such as the sigmoid.

Diverticulosis: The presence of diverticular disease in the colon with uninflamed diverticula.

Clinical Approach

Diverticulosis is extremely common, affecting 50–80% of people older than age 80 years. Diverticula are, in fact, *pseudo*diverticula through a weakness in the muscle lining, typically at areas of vascular penetration to the smooth muscle. Therefore, their walls do not contain the muscle layers surrounding the colon. They are typically 5–10 mm in diameter, and occur mainly in the distal colon in western societies. The development of diverticula has been linked to insufficient dietary fiber leading to alteration in colonic transit time and increased resting colonic intraluminal pressure. The majority of patients will remain asymptomatic. However, some patients will have chronic symptoms resembling those of irritable bowel syndrome (nonspecific lower abdominal pain aggravated by eating with relief upon defecation, bloating, and constipation or diarrhea). They may even present with acute symptoms that could be confused with acute diverticulitis, but without evidence of inflammation upon further workup. This entity has been named "painful diverticular disease without diverticulitis." **Complications of diverticulosis** include **acute diverticulitis, hemorrhage, and obstruction**.

Diverticular hemorrhage, one of the most common causes of lower GI bleeding in patients older than age 40 years, typically presents as **painless passage of bright red blood**. Generally, the hemorrhage is **abrupt in onset and abrupt in resolution**. The diagnosis may be established by finding diverticula on endoscopy without other pathology. Most diverticular hemorrhages are self-limited, and treatment is supportive, with intravenous fluid or blood replacement as needed. Treatment of diverticulosis consists of dietary measures with increased fiber. Avoidance of foods with small seeds (such as strawberries) is traditionally advised although data to support this recommendation is scant. For patients with recurrent or chronic bleeding, resection of the affected colonic segment may be indicated.

Acute diverticulitis is the **most common complication of diverticulosis**, developing in approximately 20% of all patients with diverticula. Patients often present with acute abdominal pain and signs of peritoneal irritation localizing to the left lower quadrant, and is often thought of presenting like "left-sided appendicitis." Inspissated stool particles (fecaliths), appear to obstruct the diverticular neck, setting up for more inflammation and diminished venous outflow, as well as bacterial overgrowth, which ultimately leads to abrasion and perforation of the thin diverticular wall. It is classified to four stages according to the extent of the inflammation and perforation (Table 26–1).

Diagnosis Patients usually present with visceral pain that localizes later to the **left lower quadrant**, and that is associated with fever, nausea, vomiting,

Table 26-1
STAGES OF DIVERTICULITIS

Stage I	Small, confined pericolic abscess
Stage II	Distant abscess (retroperitoneal or pelvic)
Stage III	Generalized suppurative peritonitis from rupture of abscess (noncommunicating with bowel lumen)
Stage IV	Fecal peritonitis caused by a free communicating perforation

or constipation. A right lower quadrant presentation would not exclude this diagnosis because ascending colon or cecal diverticulitis can occur. If a **colovesical fistula** is present, the patient may present with **pneumaturia** or **fecaluria** (a virtually pathognomic finding). On examination, the patient may have localized left lower quadrant tenderness or more diffuse abdominal tenderness with peritoneal irritation signs, such as guarding or rebound tenderness. The differential diagnoses include painful diverticular disease without diverticulitis, acute appendicitis, Crohn disease, colon carcinoma, ischemic colitis, irritable bowel syndrome, and gynecologic disorders such as ruptured ovarian cyst, endometriosis, ectopic pregnancy, or pelvic inflammatory disease.

Plain film radiographs, including abdominal erect and supine films with a chest x-ray, are routinely performed but are usually not diagnostic. They help in identifying the patients with pneumoperitoneum and assess their cardiopulmonary status, especially in patients with other comorbid conditions. Contrast enemas are contraindicated for fear of perforation and spillage of contrast into the abdominal cavity, a catastrophic complication. Endoscopy is also relatively contraindicated in the acute phase and is usually reserved to at least 6 weeks after the resolution of the attack, and is performed then to primarily exclude colonic neoplasia. **CT scan** is typically considered the **preferred modality of choice for diagnosing diverticulitis** if there is a high pretest probability from clinical suspicion. Findings consistent with diverticulitis include the presence of pericolic fat stranding, thickening of the bowel wall to more than 4 mm, or the finding of a peridiverticular abscess.

Therapy Factors that advocate for **inpatient** therapy include the need for narcotics to control pain; the presence of peritoneal signs; the presence of comorbid illnesses; the inability to tolerate oral liquids; or the presence of any of the complications that may potentially require surgical intervention (abscess or peritonitis). Indications for **emergent surgical intervention** include **generalized peritonitis, uncontrolled sepsis, perforation, and clinical deterioration**. In the absence of acute complications, **elective resection** is undertaken later in cases of complications including fistula formation and where there are recurrent episodes of diverticulitis.

Individuals treated as outpatients should be put on a broad-spectrum antibiotic regimen that covers abdominal Gram-negative rods and anaerobes, such as trimethoprim/sulfamethoxazole, *or* ciprofloxacin with metronidazole *or* clindamycin with gentamicin. Patients should be also on a clear liquid diet and have a close followup.

The treatment priorities in hospitalized patients are intravenous hydration, correction of electrolyte imbalances, and bowel rest (nothing by mouth). Some recommended broad-spectrum intravenous antibiotic regimens include standard triple therapy (ampicillin, an aminoglycoside, and metronidazole) and beta-lactamase inhibitor combinations (ampicillin-sulbactam or ticarcillin-clavulanate), among others. More empiric agents, such as imipenem or meropenem, are usually reserved for more severe and complicated cases. Pain, fever, and leukocytosis are expected to diminish with appropriate management in the first few days of treatment, at which point the dietary intake may be advanced gradually. Further imaging may be indicated to identify complications (Table 26–2) for the patient who persists with fever or pain.

Comprehension Questions

[26.1] A 55-year-old woman undergoes a barium enema for colon screening and multiple diverticula are noted. Which of the following is the most common complication of diverticula of the colon in this patient?

A. Toxic megacolon
B. Inflammation
C. Hemorrhage
D. Fistula formation

[26.2] A 78-year-old is noted to have fever and chills, decreased mentation, and tachycardia and RLQ abdominal tenderness and guarding. Which of the following is the most likely diagnosis?

A. Ruptured diverticulitis
B. Meningitis
C. Ruptured appendicitis
D. Ischemic bowel
E. Urosepsis

[26.3] A 58-year-old male presents to the emergency room with a temperature of 102°F, abdominal pain localizing to the left lower quadrant, and mild rebound tenderness. Which of the following diagnostic tests is the best next step?

A. Barium enema
B. Lower endoscopy
C. CT imaging of the abdomen
D. Laparoscopic examination

Table 26-2
COMPLICATIONS OF DIVERTICULITIS

COMPLICATION	CHARACTERISTICS	TREATMENT
Abscess	Suspected in patients with a tender mass on examination, persistent fever and leukocytosis in spite of adequate therapy, or a suggestive finding on imaging studies.	Conservative management for small pericolic abscesses. CT-guided percutaneous drainage or surgical drainage for other abscesses depending on the size, content, location, and peritoneal contamination.
Fistulas	Majority is colovesical with male predominance (because of bladder protection by the uterus in females). Others include colovaginal, coloenteric, colouterine, and coloureteral. Colocutaneous fistulas are extremely rare.	Single-stage surgery with fistula closure and primary anastomosis.
Obstruction	Either acutely or chronically. Ileus or pseudo-obstruction is more likely than complete mechanical obstruction. Small bowel obstruction may occur if a small bowel loop was incorporated in the inflamed mass.	Usually amenable to medical management. If not, prompt surgical intervention is required.
Strictures	Occur as a result of recurrent attacks of diverticulitis. Insidious onset colonic obstruction is likely. Colonoscopy is important for an accurate diagnosis and to exclude a stenosing neoplasm as the cause of the stricture.	A trial of endoscopic therapy (bougienage, balloon, laser, electrocautery, or a blunt dilating endoscope) reasonably can be attempted. Surgery is indicated if neoplasm could not be excluded or if such trial has failed.

Answers

[26.1] **B.** Diverticulitis is the most common complication of colonic diverticula.

[26.2] **C.** The most common cause of an acute abdomen at any age is appendicitis.

[26.3] **C.** CT imaging is the modality of choice in evaluating diverticulitis. Barium enema and endoscopy tend to increase intraluminal pressure and can worsen diverticulitis or lead to colonic rupture.

CLINICAL PEARLS

❖ Acute diverticulitis usually presents with left lower quadrant pain, fever, leukocytosis, and constipation, and often with signs of peritoneal inflammation.

❖ A patient with mild diverticulitis can be treated as an outpatient with oral antibiotics; more severe cases require hospital admission for intravenous broad-spectrum antibiotics, bowel rest, and fluids.

❖ Diverticulitis can be complicated by perforation with peritonitis, pericolic abscess, fistula formation, often to the bladder, and strictures with colonic obstruction.

REFERENCES

Isselbacher KJ, Epstein A. Diverticular, Vascular and Other Disorders of the Intestine and Peritoneum. In: Braunwald E, Fauci AS, Kasper KL, et al., eds. Harrison's principles of internal medicine, 15th ed. New York: McGraw-Hill, 2001;1695-1703.

Ferzoco LB, Raptopoulos V, Silen W. Acute Diverticulitis. N Engl J Med 1998;338(21):1521–1526.

Stollman N, Raskin J. Diverticular Disease of the Colon. J Clin Gastroenterol 1999;29(3):241–52.

CASE 27

A 54-year-old man presents to the emergency department complaining of 24 hours of fevers with shaking chills. He is currently being treated for non-Hodgkin lymphoma. His most recent chemotherapy was 6 days previously; he is receiving CHOP (cyclophosphamide, adriamycin, vincristine, and prednisone). He denies any cough or dyspnea, headache, abdominal pain, or diarrhea. He has had no sick contacts or recent travel. On physical examination, he is febrile to 103°F, tachycardic with a heart rate of 122 bpm, a blood pressure of 118/65 mmHg, and a respiratory rate of 22 breaths per minute. He is ill appearing; his skin is warm and moist but without any rashes. He has no oral lesions, his chest is clear to auscultation, his heart is tachycardic but regular with a soft systolic murmur at the left sternal border, and his abdominal exam is benign. The perirectal area is normal, digital rectal exam is deferred, but his stool is negative for occult blood. He has a tunneled vascular catheter at the right internal jugular vein with erythema overlying the subcutaneous tract, but no purulent discharge at the catheter exit site. His laboratory studies reveal a total white blood cell count of 1100 cells/mm^3 with a differential of 10% neutrophils, 16% band forms, 70% lymphocytes, and 4% monocytes (absolute neutrophil count is 286). The chest radiograph is normal.

- **What is the most likely diagnosis?**

- **What are your next therapeutic steps?**

ANSWERS TO CASE 27: Neutropenic Fever, Line Sepsis

Summary: A 54-year-old man with non-Hodgkin lymphoma is receiving immunosuppressive chemotherapy. He now presents with fever. He has no respiratory or abdominal symptoms, a clear chest x-ray, and an absolute neutrophil count of 286/mm^3. He has redness and purulence along the tract of the vascular catheter.

- **Most likely diagnosis:** Neutropenic fever and infected vascular catheter.

- **Next steps:** After drawing blood cultures, the patient should have broad-spectrum intravenous antibiotic administration, including coverage for Gram-positive organisms such as *Staphylococcus* species. The vascular catheter should be removed, if possible.

Analysis

Objectives

1. Be familiar with the possible sources of infection in a neutropenic patient.
2. Learn the management of a patient with neutropenic fever.
3. Be able to diagnose and treat a catheter-related infection.
4. Understand the techniques to prevent infection in immunosuppressed patients, including granulocyte colony-stimulating factor (G-CSF) and vaccination of household contacts.

Considerations

This patient is being treated for a hematological malignancy with combination chemotherapy, which has a common side effect of leukopenia and, especially, neutropenia. Generally, the nadir of the white cell count occurs 10–14 days after the chemotherapy. This patient certainly has neutropenia, defined as an absolute neutrophil count of less than 500 cells/mm^3. Fever in this condition is life-threatening, and immediate antibiotic coverage is paramount. Neutropenic patients are at risk for a variety of bacterial, fungal, or viral infections, but the most common sources of infection are Gram-positive bacteria from the skin, or Gram-negative bacteria from the bowel. Infection of the indwelling catheter, as in this individual, is common. Rapid institution of empiric antibiotic therapy is critical while attempts to find a source of infection are in progress. Because the tract of the catheter is infected, the line usually needs to be removed.

APPROACH TO NEUTROPENIC FEVER

Definitions

CVC: Central venous catheter.

Fever: Single oral temperature measurement of ≥38.3°C (101°F) or a temperature of ≥38.0°C (100.4°F) for ≥1 hour.

Mucositis: Breakdown of skin and mucosal barriers as a result of chemotherapy or radiation. Mucositis can result in bacteremia or fungemia.

Neutropenia: Neutrophil count of <500 cells/mm^3 or a count of <1000 cells/mm^3 with a predicted decrease to <500 cells/mm^3.

Clinical Approach

Fever in a neutropenic patient with cancer should be considered a medical emergency. Approximately 5–10% of cancer patients will die from neutropenia-associated infection; furthermore, individuals with a hematologic malignancy (leukemias or lymphomas) are even at greater risk of sepsis as a result of lymphocyte or granulocyte dysfunction, or because of abnormal immunoglobulin production. Chemotherapy often causes further bone marrow suppression and neutropenia. The incidence of an occult infection in a neutropenic patient increases with the **severity and duration of the neutropenia** (>7–10 days). Some neutropenic patients (such as the elderly or those receiving corticosteroids) may not be able to mount a febrile response to infection; thus, **any neutropenic patient showing signs of clinical deterioration should be suspected of having sepsis.**

The typical signs and symptoms of infection noted in immunocompetent patients are a result of the host's inflammatory response and may be minimal or absent in neutropenic patients. Soft-tissue infections may have diminished or absent induration, erythema, or purulence; pneumonia may not show a discernible infiltrate on a chest radiograph; meningitis may not reveal cerebrospinal fluid (CSF) pleocytosis; and urinary tract infection may be present without pyuria.

Empirical antibiotic therapy should be administered promptly to all neutropenic patients at the onset of fever. Historically, Gram-negative bacilli, mainly enteric flora were the most common pathogens in these patients. Because of their frequency, and because of the high rate of mortality associated with Gram-negative septicemia, empiric coverage for Gram-negative bacteria, including *Pseudomonas aeruginosa,* is almost always indicated for neutropenic fever. Currently, as a consequence of frequent use of CVCs, Gram-positive bacteria now account for 60–70% of microbiologically documented infections. Other clues that the infection is likely to be a Gram-positive organism include the presence of obvious soft-tissue infection such as cellulitis or mucositis, which causes breaks in the mucosal barriers and allows oral flora to enter the blood stream. If any of these factors are present, an appropriate agent, such as vancomycin, should be added to the regimen. If patients continue to be febrile despite antibacterial therapy, empiric antifungal therapy with either fluconazole or amphotericin B should be considered. Figure 27–1 shows a useful algorithm for patient management.

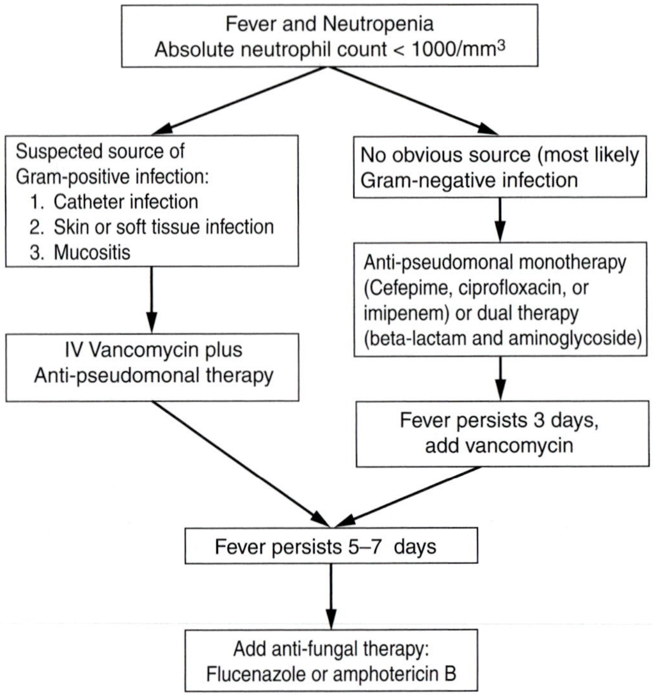

Figure 27–1. Algorithm of a suggested approach to neutropenic fever.

Central venous catheters are in widespread use, and are a common site of infection in hospitalized patients and in those receiving outpatient infusion therapy. Infection may occur as a consequence of contamination by Gram-positive skin flora, or by hematogenous seeding, usually by enteric Gram-negative organisms or *Candida* species. Erythema, purulent drainage, and induration are evidence of infection. A variety of central venous catheters are frequently used, with differing rates of infection.

The two main decisions impacting suspected catheter-related infection are (a) whether the catheter is really the source of infection, and if it is, (b) does it require removal, or can the infection be cleared with antibiotic therapy? **Most nontunneled or implanted catheters** should be **removed**. For the more permanent catheters, the decision to remove the catheter depends on the patient's clinical state, identification of the organism, and the presence of complications such as endocarditis or septic venous thrombosis. Infected catheters may produce several manifestations: infections of the subcutaneous tunnel, infection at the exit site, or catheter-related bacteremia and sepsis. Generally, **erythema overlying the subcutaneous tract** of a tunneled catheter necessitates catheter removal. Leaving the catheter in place may result in severe cellulitis and soft-tissue necrosis. If there is only erythema at the exit site, it may be possible to salvage the line using antibiotics, usually vancomycin through the CVC.

Coagulase-negative *Staphylococci* such as *Staph. epidermidis* is the most common organism causing line infections.

In the absence of obvious tunnel or exit-site infection, authorities recommend obtaining two or more blood cultures to try to diagnose catheter-related bacteremia. Catheter-related infection is suspected when a patient has two or more positive blood cultures obtained from a peripheral vein, clinical manifestation of infection (e.g., fever, chills, and/or hypotension), and no apparent source for bloodstream infection except for the catheter. In some institutions, quantitative blood cultures are obtained, that is, counting colony-forming units (CFUs), with the idea that heavier colony counts will be obtained from blood drawn through an infected catheter than from blood obtained from a peripheral vein. If the catheter is removed, the tip of the catheter may be cut off and rolled across a culture plate, again using a quantitative culture method.

Staphylococcus aureus **and** ***coagulase-negative staphylococcus*** **are the most common causes of catheter-associated infections**. With ***coagulase-negative staphylococcus*** bacteremia, response to **antibiotic therapy without catheter removal** is possible up to 80% of the time; that is, one may seek to "sterilize" the CVC if it is deemed necessary. However, this is not usually advisable in critically ill or hemodynamically unstable patients in whom immediate catheter removal and rapid administration of antibiotics are essential. Bacteremia as a consequence of ***Staphylococcus aureus,*** **Gram-negative organisms, or fungemia caused by** ***Candida*** **species, respond poorly to antimicrobial therapy** alone, and **prompt removal of the catheter is recommended**.

Because of the serious complications associated with neutropenia, preventive measures are critical in cancer patients who are receiving chemotherapy. They should be **immunized against pneumococcus and influenza**, but administration of live-virus vaccines such as measles-mumps-rubella or varicella-zoster are contraindicated. **Granulocyte colony-stimulating factor** (G-CSF), which stimulates the bone marrow to produce neutrophils, is frequently used prophylactically in patients receiving chemotherapy to shorten the duration and depth of neutropenia, thereby reducing the risk of infection. It is also sometimes used once a neutropenic patient develops a fever, but at that point, its use is controversial. Prophylactic use of oral quinolones to prevent Gram-negative infection or antifungal agents to prevent *Candida* infection may reduce certain types of infection, but may select for resistant organisms, and is not routinely employed. In hospitalized patients with neutropenia, use of reverse isolation offers no benefit (the patient is most often infected with his or her own flora), and interferes with patient care.

Comprehension Questions

[27.1] Which of the following infectious agents is the most likely etiology associated with an infected central venous catheter?

A. *Staphylococcus aureus*
B. *Pseudomonas aeruginosa*

C. Coagulase-negative *Staphylococcus species*
D. *Klebsiella pneumoniae*
E. *Candida albicans*

[27.2] A 32-year-old man with acute myelogenous leukemia is undergoing chemotherapy. He was hospitalized 7 days ago for fever to 102°F with an absolute neutrophil count of 100 cells/mm^3, and has been placed on intravenous imipenem and vancomycin. He continues to have fever to 103°F without an obvious source. Which of the following is the best next step?

A. Lumbar puncture to assess cerebrospinal fluid
B. Continue present therapy
C. Stop all antibiotics because he likely has cancer-related fever
D. Add an aminoglycoside antibiotic
E. Add an antifungal agent

[27.3] A 68-year-old woman is diagnosed with acute leukemia and is undergoing induction of chemotherapy. Last cycle, she developed neutropenia with an absolute neutrophil count of 350 cells/mm^3, which has now resolved. Which of the following is appropriate therapy?

A. Immunization against varicella
B. Immunization against mumps
C. Use of recombinant erythropoietin before the next cycle of chemotherapy
D. Use of G-CSF after the next cycle of chemotherapy

Answers

[27.1] **C.** Coagulase-negative Staphylococci such as *Staphylococcus epidermidis*, is the most common etiology of catheter-related infections.

[27.2] **E.** Antifungal therapy should be added when the fever is persistent despite broad-spectrum antibacterial agents.

[27.3] **D.** Granulocyte colony-stimulating factor given after chemotherapy can decrease the duration and severity of neutropenia and the subsequent risk of sepsis. Live vaccines, such as varicella and mumps, are contraindicated. Erythropoietin is not indicated because the patient is not anemic.

CLINICAL PEARLS

❖ Fever in a neutropenic patient should be considered a medical emergency, and is associated with a high mortality rate.

❖ The usual sources of infection in neutropenic patients are Gram-positive skin flora or Gram-negative enteric flora, including *Pseudomonas*.

- Antifungal therapy should be started in neutropenic patients who have persistent fever despite broad-spectrum antibiotic therapy and who have no obvious source of infection.
- Vascular catheters with evidence of infection along a subcutaneous tract or purulent discharge at the exit site should be removed; replacement over a guidewire is insufficient.
- If a catheter is deemed necessary, but it is infected with coagulase-negative staphylococci, antibiotic treatment may sterilize the catheter, allowing it to remain in place. For *S. aureus,* Gram-negative rods, or fungal catheter infections, the catheter usually requires removal.

REFERENCES

2001 Guidelines for the management of intravascular catheter-related infections *CID* 2001;32:1249–1272.
2002 Guidelines for the use of antimicrobial agents in neutropenia patients with cancer. *CID* 2002;34:730–751.

CASE 28

A 25-year-old African American man is admitted to your service with the diagnosis of a sickle cell pain episode. He was admitted to the hospital six times last year with the same diagnosis, and he was last discharged 2 months ago. Again he presented to the emergency department complaining of abdominal and bilateral lower extremity pain, his usual sites of pain. When you go to examine him, you note he is febrile to 101°F, has a respiratory rate of 25 breaths per minute, a normal blood pressure, and slight tachycardia of 100 bpm. The lung examination reveals bronchial breath sounds and egophony in the right lung base. His oxygen saturation on 2 L/min nasal cannula is 92%. Besides the usual abdominal and leg pain, he is now complaining of chest pain, which is worse on inspiration. Although he is tender on palpation of his extremities, the remainder of his examination is normal. His laboratory exams reveal an elevated white blood cell and reticulocyte count, and a hemoglobin and hematocrit that are slightly lower than baseline. Sickle and target cells are seen on the peripheral smear.

- **What is the most likely diagnosis?**
- **What is your next step?**
- **What are the potential complications of this condition?**

ANSWERS TO CASE 28: Sickle Cell Crisis

Summary: A 25-year-old African American man with a history of numerous pain crises is admitted for abdominal and bilateral lower extremity pain. He is febrile to 101°F, has a respiratory rate of 25 breaths per minute, and slight tachycardia of 100 bpm. The lung examination reveals bronchial breath sounds and egophony in the right lung base. His oxygen saturation on 2 L/min nasal cannula is 92%. He is now complaining of chest pain, which is worse on inspiration. He has a leukocytosis, an elevated reticulocyte count, and a hemoglobin and hematocrit that are slightly lower than baseline. Sickle and target cells are seen on the peripheral smear.

- **Most likely diagnosis:** Acute chest syndrome.
- **Next step:** Chest radiograph and empiric antibiotic therapy.
- **Complications:** Respiratory failure, possible death.

Analysis

Objectives

1. Understand the pathophysiology of sickle cell anemia and acute painful episodes.
2. Learn the acute and chronic complications of sickle cell anemia.
3. Become familiar with treatment options available for the complications of sickle cell anemia.

APPROACH TO SICKLE CELL ANEMIA

Pathophysiology The molecular structure of a normal hemoglobin molecule consists of two alpha-globin chains and two beta-globin chains. Sickle cell anemia is an autosomal recessive disorder resulting from a substitution of valine for glutamine in the sixth amino acid position of the beta-globin chain. This substitution results in an alteration of the quaternary structure of the hemoglobin molecule. Individuals with only half of their beta-chains affected are heterozygous, a state referred to as sickle cell trait. When both beta chains are affected, the patient is homozygous and has sickle cell anemia. In patients with sickle cell disease the altered quaternary structure of the hemoglobin molecule causes polymerization of the molecules under conditions of deoxygenation. These rigid polymers distort the red blood cell into a sickle shape, which is characteristic of the disease. **Sickling** is promoted by **hypoxia**, **acidosis, dehydration, or variations in body temperature**.

Epidemiology Sickle cell anemia is the most common autosomal recessive disorder and the most common cause of hemolytic anemia in African Americans.

Approximately 8% of African Americans carry the gene (i.e., sickle cell trait), with 1 in 625 being affected by the disease.

Complications of Sickle Cell Disease *Acute painful episodes*, also known as pain crisis, are a consequence of microvascular occlusion of bones by sickled cells. The most common sites are the long bones of the arms, legs, vertebral column, and sternum. Acute painful episodes are precipitated by infection, cold exposure, dehydration, venous stasis, or acidosis. They usually last 2–7 days.

Infections are another complication. Patients with sickle cell disease are at a greater risk for infections, especially with encapsulated bacterial organisms. **Autoinfarction of the spleen** occurs during early childhood secondary to microvascular obstruction by sickled red blood cells. The spleen gradually regresses in size and by age 4 years is no longer palpable. As a consequence of infarction and fibrosis, the immunologic capacity of the spleen is diminished. Patients with sickle cell disease are at greater risk for pneumonia, sepsis, and meningitis by encapsulated organisms such as *Streptococcus pneumonia* and *Haemophilus influenza.* For the same reason, patients with sickle cell disease are at greater risk for osteomyelitis with *Salmonella* species.

Acute chest syndrome is a vasoocclusive crisis within the lungs and is associated with infection or pulmonary infarction. Patients with **acute chest syndrome** present with **hypoxia, dyspnea, fever, chest pain, and progressive pulmonary infiltrates** on radiography. These episodes may be precipitated by pneumonia causing sickling in the infected lung segments, or, in the absence of infection, intrapulmonary sickling can occur as a primary event. It is virtually impossible to clinically distinguish whether infection is present or not; thus, empiric antibiotic therapy is employed.

Aplastic crisis occurs secondary to viral suppression of red blood cell precursors, most often by parvovirus B19. It occurs because of the very short half-life of sickled red blood cells, and consequent need for brisk erythropoiesis. If red blood cell production is inhibited, even for a short time, profound anemia may result. The process is acute and usually reversible, with spontaneous recovery.

Other complications of sickle cell disease include hemorrhagic or ischemic stroke as a result of thrombosis, pigmented gallstones, papillary necrosis of the kidney, priapism, and congestive heart failure.

Treatment The mainstay of treatment for pain crisis is hydration and pain control with nonsteroidal antiinflammatory agents and narcotics. It is important to also provide adequate oxygenation to reduce sickling. One must search diligently for any underlying infection, and antibiotics are often used empirically when infection is suspected. **Acute chest syndrome** is treated with **oxygen, analgesia, and antibiotics**. Sometimes exchange transfusions are necessary. In general, blood transfusions may be required for aplastic crisis, for severe hypoxia in acute chest syndrome, or to decrease viscosity and cerebral thrombosis in patients with stroke. To protect against encapsulated organisms, all patients with sickle cell disease should receive **penicillin prophylaxis** and a **vaccination against pneumococcus**. Hydroxyurea is often used to reduce the occurrence of painful crisis by stimulating hemoglobin F production and thus decreasing hemoglobin S concentration.

Comprehension Questions

[28.1] Which of the following therapies would most likely decrease the number of sickle cell crises?

A. Hydroxyurea
B. Folate supplementation
C. Prophylactic penicillin
D. Pneumococcal vaccination

Match the finding in the first list with the syndrome it is commonly associated with in persons with sickle cell anemia in the questions 28.2–28.4.

A. Salmonella species
B. Streptococcus pneumonia
C. Parvovirus B19
D. Fat embolus
E. Hematuria

[28.2] Aplastic crisis

[28.3] Osteomyelitis

[28.4] Pneumonia

Answers

[28.1] **A.** Hydroxyurea has been found to decrease the incidence of sickle cell crises.

[28.2] **C.** Parvovirus B19 is associated with aplastic crisis, especially in individuals with sickle cell disease.

[28.3] **A.** Patients with sickle cell disease are at risk for *Salmonella* osteomyelitis.

[28.4] **B.** *Streptococcus pneumonial* is the most common causative agent for pneumonia.

CLINICAL PEARLS

❖ Treatment of an acute painful episode in sickle cell disease includes hydration, narcotic analgesia, adequate oxygenation, and search for underlying infection.

❖ Acute chest syndrome is characterized by chest pain, cough, dyspnea, fever, and radiographic pulmonary infiltrate, and can be caused by pneumonia, vaso-occlusion, or pulmonary embolism.

- ❖ Blood transfusion may be required for aplastic crisis, for severe hypoxemia in acute chest syndrome, or to decrease viscosity and cerebral thrombosis in patients with stroke.
- ❖ Hydroxyurea increases hemoglobin (Hb) F production (decreasing Hb S concentration) and thus reduces frequency of pain crises and other complications.

REFERENCES

Castro O, Brambilla DJ, Thorington B, et al. The acute chest syndrome in sickle cell disease: incidence and risk factors. The Cooperative Study of Sickle Cell Disease. Blood 1994;84:643–49.

Steinberg MH. Management of sickle cell disease. N Engl J Med 1999;340:1021–30.

CASE 29

A 20-year-old college student is your next patient. When you walk in the room, he's laying on the exam table, on his side, with his arm covering his eyes. The light in the room is off. You look down on his intake form, and see that the nurse recorded his temperature as 102.3°F, with a pulse of 110 bpm, and a blood pressure of 120/80 mmHg. When you gently ask how he's been feeling, he says that for the past 3 days he's had fever, body aches, and a progressively worsening headache. The light hurts his eyes and he is nauseated, but hasn't vomited. He's had some rhinorrhea, but no diarrhea, cough, or nasal congestion. He has no known ill contacts. On examination, there is no skin rash, but his pupils are difficult to assess because of photophobia. Ears and oropharynx are normal. His heart, lungs, and abdomen are normal. The neurologic exam is nonfocal, but flexion of his neck worsens his headache.

- **What condition are you concerned about?**
- **What diagnostic test would confirm the diagnosis?**

ANSWERS TO CASE 29: Bacterial Meningitis

Summary: A 20-year-old college student presents with a three-day history of fever, headache, myalgias, and nausea. He has no respiratory or gastrointestinal symptoms, but now has developed photophobia. He is febrile to 102.3° F, tachycardic, and normotensive. His physical examination is unremarkable with a nonfocal neurologic exam, but some neck stiffness. He has no skin rash.

- **Condition most likely concern:** Meningitis.
- **Diagnostic test to confirm diagnosis:** Lumbar puncture for evaluation of the cerebrospinal fluid, possibly preceded by a CT scan of the head.

Analysis

Objectives

1. Be familiar with the clinical presentations of viral and bacterial meningitis.
2. Know that lumbar puncture is the diagnostic test of choice for meningitis.
3. Be familiar with the treatment for meningitis.

Considerations

This 20-year-old college student has headache, nausea, photophobia, fever, and neck pain—all suggestive of meningitis. The most common causes are bacterial or viral. Of course, this could also be a flu-like syndrome; however, the history and exam are suggestive of meningitis. Studies show that in a patient without focal neurologic signs and a normal level of consciousness, CT scan may be unnecessary prior to performing a lumbar puncture. However, this is controversial. He has no rash, but if he had a reddish-purple skin rash, one would be suspicious of *Neisseria* meningitis, and appropriate antibiotics should be administered immediately. Nevertheless, in a 20-year-old, *N. meningitidis* is the most common cause of bacterial meningitis. Dosing of antibiotics in this case should not await the performance of any diagnostic test as the progression of the disease is rapid and mortality and morbidity is extremely high even when antibiotics are given in a timely manner.

APPROACH TO SUSPECTED MENINGITIS

Bacterial meningitis is the most common pus forming intracranial infection with an incidence of 2.5 per 10,000 persons. The microbiology of the disease has changed somewhat since the introduction of the *Haemophilus influenza* type B vaccine in the 1980s. Now ***Streptococcus pneumoniae* is the most common bacterial isolate**, with ***Neisseria meningitidis* a close second**. **Group B streptococcus** or *Streptococcus agalactiae* occurs in approximately 10% of cases, more frequently in neonates or in patients older than age 50 years or with chronic illnesses such as diabetes or liver disease.

Listeria monocytogenes also accounts for approximately 10% of cases and must be considered in pregnant women, the **elderly,** or patients with impaired cell-mediated immunity such as AIDS patients. *H. influenzae* is responsible for less than 10% of cases of meningitis. Resistance to penicillin and some cephalosporins is now of great concern in the treatment of *Streptococcus pneumoniae.*

Bacteria usually seed the meninges hematogenously after colonizing and invading the nasal or oropharyngeal mucosa. Occasionally, bacteria may directly invade the intracranial space from a site of abscess formation in the middle ear or sinuses. The gravity and rapidity of progression of disease depend upon both host defense and organism virulence characteristics. For example, patients with defects in the complement cascade are more susceptible to invasive meningococcal disease. Patients with cerebrospinal fluid (CSF) rhinorrhea caused by trauma or postsurgical changes may also be more susceptible to bacterial invasion. ***Staphylococcus aureus* and *S. epidermidis*** are common causes of meningitis in patients following **neurologic procedures** such as placement of **ventriculoperitoneal shunts**. The damage that occurs in meningitis is believed to be secondary to vigorous host inflammatory host response to components of the lysed bacteria, rather than the direct effects of the bacteria themselves.

Acute bacterial meningitis can progress over periods of hours to days. **Typical symptoms include fever, neck stiffness, and headache.** Patients may also complain of photophobia, nausea and vomiting, and more nonspecific constitutional symptoms. Approximately 75% of patients will experience some confusion or altered level of consciousness. Forty percent may experience seizures during the course of their illness.

Some physical exam findings may be useful in the evaluation of a patient with suspected meningitis. Classic findings include Kernig and Brudzinski signs. **Kernig sign** can be elicited with the patient on his/her back. The hip is flexed and the knees are flexed. The knee is then passively extended, and the test is positive if this maneuver elicits pain. **Brudzinski sign** is positive if the supine patient flexes the knees and hips when the neck is passively flexed. Neither sign is very sensitive for the presence of meningeal irritation. **Papilledema**, if present, would indicate **increased intracranial pressure**, and focal neurologic signs or altered level of consciousness or seizures may reflect ischemia of the cerebral vasculature or focal suppuration.

Differential Diagnosis

The differential diagnosis of bacterial meningitis is fairly limited, and can be narrowed depending upon the patient's age, as discussed above, exposure history, and the course of illness. Various viral infections may also cause meningitis. These include **enteroviruses**, which tend to be more common in the summer and fall, when patients may present with severe headache, accompanied by symptoms of gastroenteritis. The **CSF white blood cell count will be elevated,** with a **predominance of lymphocytes,** and usually **glucose and**

protein levels are normal (see Table 29–1). Either herpes simplex virus (HSV)-1 or -2 can cause herpes simplex meningitis. The CSF of these patients will also have a normal glucose, while protein and white blood cell count will be elevated with a predominance of lymphocytes. Typically, these patients have a high CSF red blood cell count, which is not seen in bacterial meningitis in the absence of a traumatic spinal tap. In a patient with HIV infection, fungal meningitis, specifically caused by *Cryptococcus,* should be considered. Tuberculous meningitis presents subacutely and is more common in older, debilitated patients, or in patients with HIV. Rickettsial disease, specifically Rocky Mountain spotted fever, may also present with meningitis. Intracranial empyema, or brain or epidural abscess, should be considered, especially if the patient has focal neurologic findings. The one nonsuppurative diagnosis in the differential is subarachnoid hemorrhage. These patients present with the sudden onset of the "worst headache of their lives," in the absence of other symptoms of infection. They may have photophobia, and the CSF will be grossly bloody; the supernatant will be xanthochromic, reflecting the breakdown of blood into bilirubin.

Blood cultures should be obtained in all patients with suspected meningitis. Critical to the diagnosis of meningitis is the lumbar puncture and evaluation of the cerebrospinal fluid. Table 29–1 lists typical findings in the CSF from various causes of meningitis.

The necessity of imaging of the head and brain prior to performing a lumbar puncture (LP) is controversial. Studies show that in the patient with suspected meningitis who does not have papilledema, focal neurologic signs, or altered level of consciousness, a LP may be safely performed without preceding imaging. However, in instances in which performance of the LP may be delayed, antibiotics should be administered after blood cultures while awaiting the radiologic studies. Ideally, the CSF should be examined within 30 minutes of antibiotics, but it has been shown that if the LP is performed within 2 hours of antibiotics, it will not significantly alter the CSF protein, glucose, white blood cell count, or Gram stain. If CSF is obtained, a culture and Gram stain should be sent, and if enough fluid is available, it should also be sent for cell count and glucose and protein levels. Latex agglutination tests for *S. pneumoniae* and *H. influenzae* can be useful in patients pretreated with antibiotics, and while not very sensitive, if positive they can rule in disease (high specificity). Polymerase chain reaction testing is available for some bacteria; however, it may be more useful in the diagnosis of herpes simplex, enteroviral, or tuberculous meningitis. In all, no more than 3.5–4 cc of CSF is necessary. The most critical issue in a patient with suspected bacterial meningitis, however, is the initiation of antibiotics. CSF examination and imaging studies can be deferred in this medical emergency.

During the course of treatment, most patients will undergo some cerebral imaging study. CT scans are most useful in the initial presentation to exclude intracranial mass or bleeding, or to evaluate for other signs of increased intracranial pressure. However, MRI is most helpful for demonstrating any

Table 29-1
CSF CHARACTERISTICS OF MENINGITIS

CAUSATIVE ORGANISM	OPENING PRESSURE	WHITE BLOOD CELL COUNT/TYPE	GLUCOSE	PROTEIN	RED BLOOD CELL COUNT	SPECIAL STAINS/TESTS
Bacteria	High	Elevated, predominantly neutrophilic	Low, <40 mg/dL	Elevated	None	Gram stain
Viral	Normal	Elevated, predominantly lymphocytic	Normal	Normal	none	Cell culture or PCR
Herpes simplex	Normal to high	As in other viral meningitis	Normal	Normal to high	High	PCR
Tuberculosis	Normal to high	Elevated, monocytes may be elevated	Very low	Very high	None	PCR, AFB smear (usually negative) and culture

Abbreviations: AFB = acid-fast bacillus; PCR = polymerase chain reaction.

Table 29-2
ETIOLOGIES OF BACTERIAL MENINGITIS BY AGE

AGE OF PATIENT	BACTERIA	EMPIRIC TREATMENT	COMMENTS
Neonate	1. Gram negative enteric bacteria (*Escherichia coli*) and group B streptococcus 2. Listeria monocytogenes	Ampicillin + cefotaxime	Vaginal organisms common
1–23 months	1. *Streptococcus pneumoniae* 2. *Neisseria meningitides* 3. *Haemophilus influenzae* type b (less since vaccine)	Cefotaxime (or ceftriaxone) + vancomycin	Previous to vaccine, *H. influenzae* caused 70% of meningitis in children
2–18 years	1. *N. meningitides* 2. *S pneumoniae* 3. *H. influenzae* type b (less common since vaccine)	Ampicillin + vancomycin ± ceftriaxone	
19–59 years	1. *S. pneumoniae* 2. *N. meningitides* 3. *H. influenzae* type b	Ampicillin + vancomycin ± ceftriaxone	
60+ years	1. *S. pneumoniae* 2. *Listeria monocytogenes* 3. Group B Streptococcus	Ampicillin + vancomycin + ceftriaxone (or cefotaxime)	*Listeria* more common

Source: Center for Disease Control, 2003.

focal ischemia or infarction caused by the disease. When HSV meningitis is suspected, MRI should demonstrate enhancement of the temporal lobes. In tuberculous meningitis, enhancement of the basal region may be seen. An EEG may be helpful in patients suspected of HSV meningitis. Within 2–15 days of the start of the illness, periodic sharp and slow wave complexes originating within the temporal lobes can be demonstrated at 2–3-second intervals. When skin lesions are present, biopsies may demonstrate *N. meningitidis* and can be helpful in the diagnosis.

Therapy

Treatment of meningitis is often empiric until specific culture data is available. Because of the growing incidence of resistant pneumococci as well as meningococci, the recommended empiric therapy in most areas is a **high-dose**

third-generation cephalosporin given concurrently with vancomycin. In other areas, if the disease presentation is typical for meningococcus (with the typical rash) or the organism is identified quickly on Gram stain of the CSF, therapy with high-dose penicillin can be started if the meningococcus in that area is known to be sensitive. **Ampicillin is added when there is a suspicion of Listeriosis. Acyclovir should be started for suspicion of HSV**, or four-drug anti-TB therapy if the presentation is suspicious for tuberculous meningitis. The administration of steroids is controversial. One study in adults demonstrated decreased mortality in patients with *S. pneumoniae* meningitis who were given glucocorticoids. However, other studies are more equivocal. There is also some evidence for benefit of steroids in severe tuberculous meningitis. Age may give a clue regarding etiology (see Table 29–2).

Prevention of meningitis can be achieved through the administration of **vaccines and chemoprophylaxis** of close contacts. **Specific vaccinations are available for *H. influenzae* type B and some strains of *S. pneumoniae*** and are now routinely administered to **children. Meningococcal vaccination** is recommended for those living in dormitory situations, such as college students and military recruits, but not for the general population. **Rifampin given twice a day for 2 days** or a single dose of ciprofloxacin is recommended for **household and close contacts** of an index case of **meningococcemia or meningococcal meningitis**.

Comprehension Questions

[29.1] An 18-year-old with a 1-week history of fever, headache, increasing confusion, and lethargy presents to the emergency department. His exam is normal and he has no focal neurologic signs. A CT of his head is negative. A lumbar puncture reveals a white blood cell count of 250/mm^3, with 78% lymphocytes, and 500 red blood cells (RBCs)/mm^3 in tube 1 and 630/mm^3 in tube 2. No organisms are seen on Gram stain. Which of the following is the best next step?

A. Intravenous ceftriaxone, acyclovir, and vancomycin
B. Intravenous fluconazole
C. Intravenous azithromycin
D. Careful observation with no antibiotics

[29.2] A 55-year-old with a long history of alcohol abuse presents with a 3-week history of progressive confusion and stupor. On examination he is afebrile, but has a new right sixth cranial nerve palsy and tremulousness of all four extremities. His CSF has 250 white blood cells (WBCs)/mm^3, with 68% lymphocytes. There are 300 RBCs/mm^3. Protein levels are high, and the CSF:serum glucose ratio is very low. He is started on ceftriaxone, vancomycin, and acyclovir. A purified protein derivative (PPD) placed on admission is positive, and bacterial cultures are negative at 48 hours. Which of the following would help to confirm the diagnosis?

A. Gram stain of throat scrapings
B. CT of the head with contrast
C. MRI of the head
D. Repeat LP after 48 hours of therapy
E. Herpes simplex virus PCR

[29.3] A 65-year-old man with colon cancer on chemotherapy presents with a fever and headache of 3 days duration. A lumbar puncture is performed, and Gram stain reveals Gram-positive rods. Which of the following therapies is most likely to treat the organism?

A. Vancomycin
B. Metronidazole
C. Ampicillin
D. Gentamicin
E. Ceftriaxone

Answers

[29.1] **A.** This young man most likely has a viral meningitis given the modest CSF pleocytosis count with predominant lymphocytes. Given the high RBC count, it may be HSV, so acyclovir should be instituted until more specific testing can be done. However, because bacterial meningitis cannot be excluded based on the CSF analysis alone, empiric antibacterials should be given until culture results are known, usually within 48 hours.

[29.2] **D.** Tuberculous meningitis is extremely difficult to diagnose and the index of suspicion should be high in susceptible individuals. Certain clinical findings, such as nerve palsies, and CSF findings, such as an extremely low glucose and high protein levels with a fairly low WBC count, are highly suggestive but not diagnostic. Mortality is high and related to the delay in instituting therapy. The only definitive test is acid-fast bacillus (AFB) culture, but it can take 6–8 weeks to grow. Polymerase chain reaction (PCR) test for *Mycobacterium tuberculosis* is diagnostic if positive; however, the sensitivity is low, so if the test is negative it does not rule out the disease. Findings such as a positive PPD, or CSF cell counts and protein levels that do not change with standard antimicrobial or antiviral therapies, can also suggest the diagnosis. Low CSF glucose is a hallmark of TB meningitis—-if the glucose goes down at 48 hours, it is highly suggestive of TB. CT scan and MRI may demonstrate basilar meningitis in TB, but the finding is not specific.

[29.3] **C.** *Listeria monocytogenes* is a Gram-positive rod that causes about 10% of all cases of meningitis. It is more common in the elderly and other patients with impaired cell-mediated immunity, such as patients on chemotherapy. It is also more common in neonates. It is not sensitive to cephalosporins, and specific therapy with ampicillin must be instituted if suspicion for this disease is high.

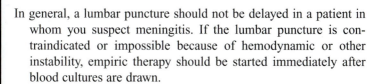

CLINICAL PEARLS

❖ In general, a lumbar puncture should not be delayed in a patient in whom you suspect meningitis. If the lumbar puncture is contraindicated or impossible because of hemodynamic or other instability, empiric therapy should be started immediately after blood cultures are drawn.

❖ The most common cause of bacterial meningitis in adults is *Streptococcus pneumoniae,* followed by *Neisseria meningitides. Listeria monocytogenes* meningitis occurs in neonates, immunocompromised or older patients.

❖ Patients who have had neurosurgical procedures, or skull trauma are at risk for Staphylococcal meningitis.

❖ Hemorrhagic CSF with evidence of temporal lobe involvement by imaging or EEG suggests HSV encephalitis; acyclovir is the treatment of choice.

❖ CASE 30

A 28-year-old man comes to the emergency room complaining of 6 days of fevers with shaking chills. Over the past 2 days, he has also developed a productive cough with greenish sputum, which is occasionally blood streaked. He reports no dyspnea, but sometimes experiences chest pain on deep inspiration. He does not have headache, abdominal pain, urinary symptoms, vomiting, or diarrhea. He has no significant past medical history. He does smoke cigarettes and marijuana regularly, drinks several beers daily, but he denies intravenous drug use.

On examination, his temperature is 102.5°F, with a heart rate of 109 bpm, blood pressure of 128/76 mmHg, and a respiratory rate of 23 breaths per minute. He is alert and talkative. He has no oral lesions and his funduscopic exam reveals no abnormalities. His jugular veins show prominent V waves, and his heart is tachycardic but regular with a harsh holosystolic murmur at the left lower sternal border that increases with inspiration. His chest exam reveals inspiratory rales bilaterally. On both of his forearms, he has linear streaks of induration, hyperpigmentation, with some small nodules overlying the superficial veins, but no erythema, warmth, or tenderness.

Laboratory examination is significant for an elevated white blood cell (WBC) count at 17,500/mm^3 with 84% polymorphonuclear cells, 7% band forms, and 9% lymphocytes, a hemoglobin concentration of 14 g/dL, a hematocrit of 42%, and a platelet count of 189,000/mm^3. Liver function tests and a urinalysis are normal. His chest radiograph shows multiple peripheral, ill-defined nodules, some with cavitation.

◆ **What is the most likely diagnosis?**

◆ **What is your next step?**

ANSWERS TO CASE 30: Endocarditis (Tricuspid)/Septic Pulmonary Emboli

Summary: A 28-year-old man complains of shaking chills and fever. He also has a productive cough, and denies intravenous drug use. He has a temperature of 102.5°F, a heart rate of 109 bpm, and a new holosystolic murmur at the left lower sternal border, which increases with inspiration. He has linear streaks of induration on both forearms, and a chest radiograph with multiple ill-defined nodules.

- **Most likely diagnosis:** Infective endocarditis involving the tricuspid valve, with probable septic pulmonary emboli.

- **Next step:** Obtain serial blood cultures and institute empiric broad-spectrum antibiotics.

Analysis

Objectives

1. Understand the differences in clinical presentation between acute and subacute, and left-sided versus right-sided endocarditis.
2. Learn the most common organisms that cause endocarditis, including "culture-negative" endocarditis.
3. Know the diagnostic and therapeutic approach to infective endocarditis, including the indications for valve replacement.
4. Understand the complications of endocarditis.

Considerations

Although this patient denied parenteral drug use, his track marks on the forearms are very suspicious for intravenous drug abuse. He has fever, a new heart murmur very typical of tricuspid regurgitation, and a chest radiograph suggestive of septic pulmonary emboli. Serial blood cultures, ideally obtained before antibiotics are started, are essential to establish the diagnosis of infective endocarditis. The rapidity with which one starts antibiotics depends on the clinical presentation of the patient: a septic, critically ill patient needs them immediately; a patient with a subacute presentation can wait many hours while cultures are obtained.

APPROACH TO SUSPECTED ENDOCARDITIS

Infectious endocarditis refers to a microbial process of the endocardium, usually involving the heart valves. The clinical presentation depends upon the valves involved (left-sided versus right-sided), as well as the virulence of the organism. Highly virulent species, such as *Staphylococcus aureus,* produce acute infection, and less virulent organisms, such as the viridans group of streptococci, tend to produce a more subacute illness, which may evolve over a period of weeks. **Fever is present in 95% of all cases**. For **acute endocarditis**, patients often present with high fever, acute valvular regurgitation, and embolic phenomena (e.g., to the extremities or to the brain, causing stroke.) **Subacute endocarditis** more often is associated with constitutional symptoms such as anorexia, weight loss, night sweats, and findings attributable to immune-complex deposition and septic vasculitis; these include petechiae, splenomegaly, glomerulonephritis, **Osler nodes (tender nodules on the finger or toe pads)**, **Janeway lesions (painless hemorrhagic macules** on the palms and soles), **Roth spots** (hemorrhagic retinal lesions with white centers), and **splinter hemorrhages**. These classic peripheral lesions, while frequently discussed, are actually seen in only 20–25% of cases.

Right-sided endocarditis usually involves the **tricuspid** valve, causing **pulmonary** emboli, rather involving the systemic circulation. Accordingly, patients develop pleuritic chest pain, purulent sputum or hemoptysis, and the radiographs may show multiple peripheral nodular lesions, often with cavitation. The murmur of tricuspid regurgitation may not be present, especially early in the illness.

In all cases of endocarditis, the critical finding is bacteremia, which is usually sustained. The initiating event is a transient bacteremia, which may be a result of mucosal injury, as in dental extraction, or a complication of the use of intravascular catheters. Bacteria are then able to seed valvular endothelium. Previously damaged, abnormal, or prosthetic valves form vegetations, which are composed of platelets and fibrin, and are relatively avascular sites where bacteria may grow protected from immune attack.

Serial blood cultures are the most important step in the diagnosis of endocarditis. Acutely ill patients should have **three blood cultures** obtained over a **2–3-hour** period prior to initiating antibiotics. In **subacute** disease, **three blood cultures over a 24-hour** period maximize the diagnostic yield. Of course, if patients are critically ill or hemodynamically unstable, no delay in initiating therapy is appropriate, and cultures are obtained on presentation, even while broad-spectrum antibiotics are administered. It is usually not difficult to isolate the infecting organism, because the hallmark of infective endocarditis is sustained bacteremia, and thus, all blood cultures are often positive for the micro organism. Table 30–1 lists typical organisms, frequency of infection, and associated conditions.

Culture-negative endocarditis, an uncommon situation in which routine cultures fail to grow, is most likely a result of prior **antibiotic** treatment, **fungal** infection (fungi other than candida species often require special culture media), or **fastidious** organisms. These organism can include *Abiotrophia spp., Bartonella spp., Coxiella burnetii, Legionella spp., Chlamydia,* and the **HACEK organisms** *(Haemophilus aphrophilus/paraphrophilus, Actinobacillus actinomycetemcomitans, Cardiobacterium hominis, Eikenella corrodens, Kingella kingae).* The clinical features, blood cultures, and echocardiography are used to diagnose cases of endocarditis using clinical

Table 30-1
CLINICAL MANIFESTATIONS OF ENDOCARDITIS

ORGANISM	FREQUENCY	ASSOCIATED CONDITIONS
Staphylococcus aureus	30–40% of native valve infection	Intravascular catheter, Intravenous drug users (Tricuspid valve endocarditis)
Coagulase-negative staphylococci	30–35% of early prosthetic valve infection	Neonates, Prosthetic valves
Viridans Streptococci	40–60% of native valve infection	Oral flora, after dental surgery
Enterococci	15%, usually in older patients	Previous genitourinary tract disease or instrumentation
Streptococcus bovis	5–10%	Elderly patients, often with underlying GI mucosal lesion; e.g., adenoma or malignancy
Candida species	5–10%	Intravascular catheters, IV drug use

criteria. Endocarditis is said to definitely be present if the patient satisfies two major criteria, or one major and three minor criteria, or five minor criteria (see Table 30–2).

One life-threatening complication of endocarditis is **congestive heart failure**, usually as a consequence of **infection-induced valvular damage**. Other cardiac complications are intracardiac abscesses, and conduction disturbances caused by septal involvement by infection. Systemic arterial embolization may lead to splenic or renal infarction or abscesses. Vegetations may embolize to the coronary circulation, causing a myocardial infarction, or to the brain causing a cerebral infarction. A **stroke syndrome** in a **febrile** patient should always suggest the possibility of **endocarditis**. Infection of the vasa vasorum may weaken the wall of major arteries and produce mycotic aneurysms, which can occur anywhere, but are most common in the cerebral circulation, sinuses of Valsalva, or abdominal aorta. These aneurysms may leak or rupture, producing sudden fatal intracranial or other hemorrhage.

Antibiotic treatment is usually begun in the hospital, but because of the prolonged nature of therapy, is often completed as an outpatient when the patient is clinically stable. **Treatment generally lasts 4–6 weeks.** If the organism is susceptible, such as **most streptococcus species, penicillin G** is the agent of choice. For ***S. aureus*, nafcillin** is the drug of choice, often used in combination with **gentamicin** initially for synergy, to help resolve bacteremia. Therapy for intravenous drug users should be directed against *S. aureus*. **Vancomycin**

Table 30-2
DIAGNOSTIC CRITERIA FOR ENDOCARDITIS

Major criteria

1. Isolation of typical organisms (viridans streptococci, *Staphylococcus aureus*, enterococci, *Streptococcus bovis*, or one of the HACEK organisms) from two separate blood cultures, or persistently positive blood cultures with other organisms
2. Evidence of endocardial involvement: either echocardiographic evidence of endocarditis, e.g., oscillating intracardiac mass, or new valvular regurgitation

Minor criteria

1. Predisposing valvular lesion or intravenous drug use
2. Fever of >38.0°C. (100.4°F)
3. Vascular phenomena: arterial or septic pulmonary emboli, mycotic aneurysm, Janeway lesions
4. Immunologic phenomena: glomerulonephritis, Osler nodes, Roth spots, positive rheumatoid factor
5. Positive blood cultures not meeting major criteria

Table 30-3
INDICATIONS FOR SURGICAL MANAGEMENT OF ENDOCARDITIS

Intractable congestive heart failure
More than one serious systemic embolic episode
Uncontrolled infection, e.g., positive cultures after 7 days of therapy
No effective antimicrobial therapy (e.g., fungal endocarditis)
Most cases of prosthetic valve endocarditis
Local suppurative complications such as a myocardial abscess

is used when **methicillin-resistant *S. aureus* or coagulase-negative staphylococci** are present. **Ceftriaxone is the usual therapy for the HACEK** group of organisms. Devising a rationale therapy for culture-negative endocarditis may be challenging, and depends on the clinical situation. Table 30–3 summarizes the commonly recognized indications for surgical intervention, that is, valve excision and replacement.

Comprehension Questions

[30.1] A 68-year-old man is hospitalized with *Streptococcus bovis* endocarditis of the mitral valve, and recovers completely with appropriate therapy. What is the most important next step?

A. Good dental hygiene and proper denture fitting to prevent reinfection of damaged heart valves from oral flora.

B. Repeat echocardiography in 6 weeks to ensure the vegetations have resolved.
C. Colonoscopy to look for mucosal lesions.
D. Mitral valve replacement to prevent systemic emboli such as cerebral infarction.

[30.2] A 24-year-old intravenous drug user is admitted with 4 weeks of fever. He has three blood cultures positive with *Candida* species and suddenly develops a cold blue toe. What is the appropriate next step?

A. Repeat echocardiography to see if the large aortic vegetation previously seen has now embolized.
B. Cardiovascular surgery consultation for aortic valve replacement.
C. Aortic angiography to evaluate for a mycotic aneurysm, which may be embolizing.
D. Switch from fluconazole to amphotericin B.

[30.3] Which of the following patients needs antimicrobial prophylaxis before dental surgery?

A. Atrial septal defect
B. Mitral valve prolapse without mitral regurgitation
C. Previous coronary artery bypass graft
D. Previous infective endocarditis

Answers

[30.1] **C.** Colonoscopy is necessary because a significant number of patients with *S. bovis* endocarditis have a colonic cancer or premalignant polyp, which led to the seeding of the valve by gastrointestinal flora. Heart valves damaged by endocarditis are more susceptible to infection, so good dental hygiene is important, but in this case, the organism came from the intestinal tract, not the mouth, and the possibility of malignancy is most important to address. Serial echocardiography would not add to the patient's care after successful therapy, because vegetations become organized and persist for months or years without late embolization. Prophylactic valve replacement would not be indicated, because the prosthetic valve is even more susceptible to reinfection than the damaged native valve, and would actually increase the risk of cerebral infarction or other systemic emboli as a consequence of thrombus formation, even if adequately anticoagulated.

[30.2] **B.** Fungal endocarditis, which occurs in intravenous drug users or immunosuppressed persons with indwelling catheters, frequently gives rise to large friable vegetations with a high risk of embolization (often to the lower extremities), and is very difficult to cure with antifungal medications. Valve replacement is usually necessary. Repeat echocardiography would not add to the patient's care, because the clinical diagnosis of peripheral embolization is almost certain, and it would not change the management. Medical therapy with any antifungal agent is unlikely to cure this infection. Mycotic aneurysms may occur in any artery as a consequence of endocarditis, and can cause late embolic complications, but in this case, the source is probably the heart.

[30.3] **D.** Prior endocarditis damages valvular surfaces, and these patients are at increased risk for reinfection during a transient bacteremia, such as may occur during dental procedures or some other GI or genitourinary tract procedures. All of the other conditions mentioned have a negligible risk of endocarditis, the same as the general population, and antibiotic prophylaxis is not recommended by the American Heart Association.

CLINICAL PEARLS

❖ The diagnosis of infective endocarditis is established by using clinical criteria, the most important of which are sustained bacteremia and evidence of endocardial involvement, usually by echocardiography.

❖ Right-sided endocarditis may be difficult to diagnose because it lacks the systemic emboli seem in left-sided endocarditis, and the new murmur of tricuspid regurgitation is often not heard.

❖ Left-sided native valve endocarditis is usually caused by viridans streptococci, *Staphylococcus aureus,* and *Enterococcus.* The large majority of right-sided endocarditis is caused by *S. aureus.*

❖ Valve replacement is usually necessary for persistent infection, recurrent embolization, or when medical therapy is ineffective, for example, in cases of large vegetations as seen in fungal endocarditis.

❖ Culture negative endocarditis is usually caused by prior administration of antibiotics prior to obtaining blood cultures, or infection with fungi, or fastidious organisms such as the HACEK group.

REFERENCES

Bayer A, Scheld WM. Endocarditis and Intravascular Infections. In: Mandell GL, Dolin R, Bennett JE, (eds.) Mandell, Douglas, and Bennett's Principles & Practice of Infectious Diseases, 5th ed. New york: Churchill-Livingstone.2000:857–884, 917–823.

Dajani AS, Taubert KA, Wilson W, et al. Prevention of Bacterial Endocarditis. Recommendations by the American Heart Association. *JAMA* 1997;277(22);1794–1801.

Mylonakis E, Calderwood SB, et al. Infective endocarditis in adults. *N Engl J Med* 2001;345(18):1318–30.

CASE 31

A 62-year-old man is brought to the clinic for a 3-month history of unintentional weight loss (12 lb). His appetite has diminished, but he reports no vomiting or diarrhea. He does report some depressive symptoms since the death of his wife a year ago, at which time he moved from Hong Kong to the United States to live with his daughter. He denies a smoking history. He complains of a 3-month history of productive cough with greenish sputum. He has not felt feverish. He takes no medications regularly, except a vitamin for "energy." On examination, his temperature is 99.4°F and his respiratory rate is 16 breaths per minute. His neck has a normal thyroid gland and no cervical or supraclavicular lymphadenopathy. His chest has few scattered rales in the left mid-lung fields and a faint expiratory wheeze on the right. His heart is regular with no gallops or murmurs. His abdominal exam is benign, his rectal exam shows no masses, and his stool is negative for occult blood. His chest x-ray is shown in Figure 31–1.

- **What is the most likely diagnosis?**
- **What is your next step?**

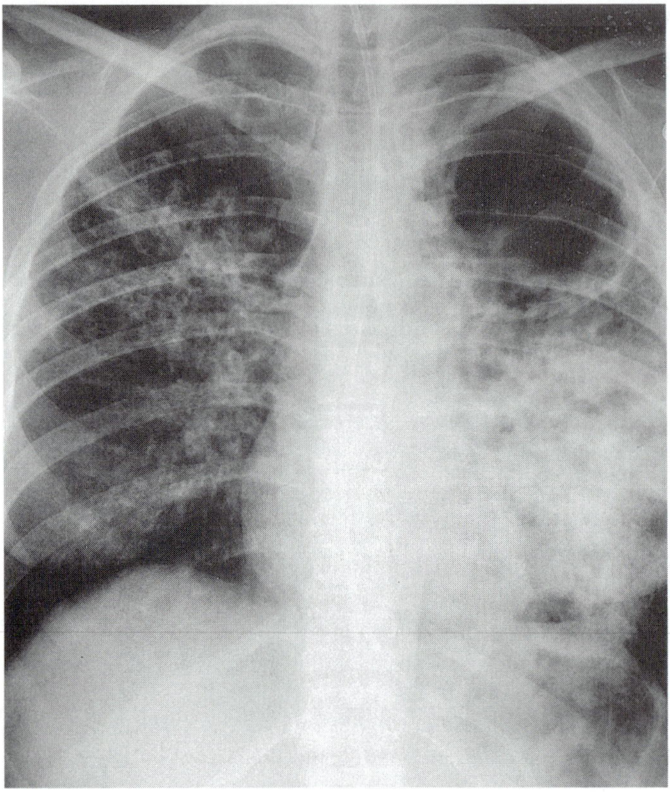

Figure 31–1. Chest x-ray. **(Reproduced with permission from Fishman AP. Fishman's Pulmonary Diseases & Disorders 3rd ed. New York: McGraw-Hill. 1998:2487.)**

ANSWERS to CASE 31: Tuberculosis (Pulmonary), Cavitary Lung Lesions

Summary: A 62-year-old man from Hong Kong has a 12-lb unintentional weight loss. His appetite has diminished, but he denies abdominal pain, vomiting, or diarrhea. He does report some depressive symptoms since the death of his wife a year ago. He denies tobacco use or fever. On examination, his temperature is 99.4°F and his respiratory rate is 16 breaths per minute. He has no cervical or supraclavicular lymphadenopathy. His chest has a few scattered rales in the left mid-lung fields and a faint expiratory wheeze on the right. His chest x-ray shows a cavitary lesion (left lower lobe).

- **Most likely diagnosis:** Pulmonary tuberculosis.
- **Next step:** Refer him to the hospital for admission so that serial sputum samples can be collected for identification of the organism, and for culture and sensitivities to guide antimicrobial therapy.

Analysis

Objectives

1. Know the natural history and the clinical and radiographic manifestations of primary and reactivation pulmonary tuberculosis, and of latent tuberculosis infection.
2. Understand the methods of diagnosis of tuberculosis.
3. Learn treatment strategies for tuberculosis.
4. Know the common extrapulmonary sites of tuberculosis, including pleurisy, lymphadenitis, miliary, meningeal, genitourinary, skeletal, and adrenal TB.

Considerations

This elderly Asian gentleman has symptoms suggestive of tuberculosis, such as weight loss, and productive cough. A chest radiograph is essential in helping to establish the diagnosis. His chest film is highly suggestive of tuberculosis, but many other diseases may cause cavitary lung lesions, including other infections, and malignancies. If the sputum samples do not reveal acid-fast organisms, then further testing, such as bronchoscopy, may be needed to rule out malignancy.

APPROACH TO SUSPECTED TUBERCULOSIS

Definitions

Latent tuberculosis: Asymptomatic infection of *Mycobacterium tuberculosis.*

Primary tuberculosis: The development of clinical illness immediately after infection with *Mycobacterium tuberculosis.*

Reactivation tuberculosis: Illness that occurs when latent tuberculosis becomes active and infectious after a period of dormancy, such as years after the initial infection.

Clinical Approach

Pulmonary Tuberculosis Tuberculosis is a bacterial infection caused by the acid-fast bacillus (AFB) *Mycobacterium tuberculosis,* and is usually transmitted through airborne spread of droplets from infected patients with pulmonary tuberculosis. The vast majority of cases occur in developing countries, but there was a resurgence in the United States during the mid-1980s as a consequence of various factors, including HIV infection. Untreated disease can have a 1-year mortality of 33% and a 5-year mortality rate as high as 50%.

Often seen in children, **primary pulmonary tuberculosis usually affects the middle and lower lung zones**. Lesions form in the periphery with hilar and paratracheal lymphadenopathy. Granulomatous lesions are caused by the inflammatory response of lymphocytes and macrophages. The center of the lesion may become necrotic (caseous necrosis) and liquefied, forming a cavity. Healed lesions are called **Ghon lesions**. Most patients exposed to *M. tuberculosis* do not manifest clinical symptoms, but may have a latent infection; years later, frequently during times of stress or immunosuppression, tuberculosis may reactivate, becoming symptomatic. **Reactivation tuberculosis** usually involves the **apical and posterior segments of the upper lobes** or the superior segments of the lower lobes of the lungs. The course may be rapid (weeks to months), chronic and slowly progressive ("consumption"), or spontaneously remit.

Signs and symptoms are nonspecific and subacute, including **fever, night sweats, malaise, weight loss, and anorexia**. The **cough is usually productive** of purulent sputum and sometimes **streaked with blood**. A lesion may erode into a vessel, causing massive hemoptysis. **Rasmussen aneurysm** is the rupture of a dilated vessel in a cavity. Physical findings can include fever, wasting, rales and rhonchi (if there is a partial bronchial obstruction), pallor, or finger clubbing from hypoxia. Some possible laboratory abnormalities are leukocytosis, anemia, and hyponatremia secondary to the syndrome of inappropriate secretion of antidiuretic hormone **(SIADH)**.

Extrapulmonary Tuberculosis The sites, in order of decreasing frequency of occurrence, are the **lymph nodes, pleura, genitourinary tract, bones and joints, meninges, and peritoneum**. Tuberculosis lymphadenitis is common in HIV-infected patients, children, and nonwhite women, and is generally **painless adenopathy**. Pleural disease can have an exudative effusion but may require pleural biopsy for diagnosis. Tuberculosis meningitis usually has cerebrospinal fluid with high protein, a lymphocyte predominance (or neutrophils in early infection), and low glucose level. **Adjunctive glucocorticoids** may improve the treatment response in TB meningitis. Genitourinary tuberculosis can be asymptomatic or have local symptoms such as dysuria, hematuria, and urinary frequency, and is characterized by the finding of leukocytes in the urine but negative bacterial cultures—"**sterile pyuria**." Skeletal tuberculosis affects weight-bearing joints, while **Pott disease involves the spine**. **Miliary tuberculosis** occurs by **hematogenous dissemination** with 1–2-mm granulomas that resemble millet seeds (hence the name). Adrenal tuberculosis can present as adrenal insufficiency.

Diagnosis The diagnosis of tuberculosis is made by combining the history and clinical picture with AFB stains or culture of a specimen (smear or tissue biopsy). When **pulmonary TB** is suspected, **three samples of early morning sputum** should be obtained while the patient is in isolation. Biopsy material should not be put in formaldehyde. Cultures may take from 4–8 weeks on ordinary solid media or 2–3 weeks on liquid media. Tuberculosis cases should be reported to the local public health department. Purified protein derivative (PPD) skin testing is useful for screening for latent infection, but has a limited role in diagnosing active infection, because there is often a false negative in this setting. A positive **PPD** is defined by induration after 48–72 hours that is **5 mm or greater in patients with HIV**, **close contacts** of patients with

TB, or patients with **chest x-ray findings consistent with TB**. People with other risk factors, such as health care workers or patients who are immunocompromised for reasons other than HIV, are considered to have a latent infection if the PPD is **10 mm** or more. Everyone else should have less than **15 mm of induration**.

Treatment The probable resistance pattern of the tuberculosis organism, based on the country of origin may help to guide the treatment. For individuals from areas with low drug-resistance, therapy generally starts with a **2-month course of isoniazid (INH), rifampin, and pyrazinamide. Multiple drugs are used to avoid resistance**. Directly observed treatment (watching patients take the medication) should be instituted in all patients in this phase. Subsequently, the patient should receive a 4-month course of INH and rifampin. Pyridoxine is frequently added to the regimen. Drug resistance or intolerable side effects may require alternate therapy, such as with amikacin, ethambutol, or streptomycin. Toxicity for which patients must be monitored includes **hepatitis**, hyperuricemia, and thrombocytopenia. Treatment failure is defined by positive cultures after 3 months or positive AFB stains after 5 months, and should be treated by adding two more drugs. **Latent TB infection** should be treated with INH for 9 months with the goal of preventing reactivation tuberculosis later in life.

Comprehension Questions

[31.1] A 42-year-old woman is being treated with corticosteroids for a exacerbation of immune thrombocytopenia purpura. After 2 days of intravenous steroid therapy, she develops a cough, fever, and night sweats. Which of the following is the most likely location of the tuberculosis?

A. Inferior aspect of the lung
B. Pleura of the lung
C. Apical aspect of the lung
D. Middle lobe of the lung

[31.2] A 24-year-old man has been treated with isoniazid, rifampin, and pyrazinamide for active pulmonary tuberculosis. After 3 months, he states that he is having numbness of his feet, but no back pain. He denies taking other medications. The most appropriate next step is:

A. CT scan of the lumbar spine
B. Initiate pyridoxine
C. Continue the tuberculosis agents and monitor for further neurological problems
D. Initiate a workup for tuberculosis adenopathy compression on the femoral nerve

[31.3] A 25-year-old woman is seen in the clinic because her father, who recently immigrated from South America, was diagnosed with and has been treated for tuberculosis. She denies a cough and her chest radiograph is normal. A PPD test shows 10 mm of induration. Her only medication is an oral contraceptive. Which of the following is the best next step?

A. Oral isoniazid and barrier contraception
B. Combination therapy including isoniazid, rifampin, and pyrazinamide
C. Observation
D. Induce three sputums

[31.4] Which of the following tests is the most important to follow for a patient receiving isoniazid and rifampin for tuberculosis treatment?

A. Renal function tests
B. Liver function tests
C. Slit-lamp examinations
D. Amylase and lipase tests

Answers

[31.1] **C.** Reactivation tuberculosis (triggered by steroids) usually involves the apical aspects of the lungs.

[31.2] **B.** Pyridoxine (vitamin B_6) is important in preventing the peripheral neuropathy that can complicate isoniazid therapy. If the numbness were caused by Pott disease, he should have back pain and other neurologic findings, such as lower-extremity weakness.

[31.3] **A.** Because this woman is a household contact of a patient with active TB, she is among the highest risk group: her skin test would be interpreted as positive if >5 mm. She has latent TB infection, and should be offered treatment to prevent reactivation TB later in life. Oral contraceptives may reduce drug levels, so barrier contraception might be a better option for her.

[31.4] **B.** Drug-induced hepatitis is a common complication of isoniazid and rifampin and requires periodic surveillance. Alcohol use, prior liver disease, and increased age are risk factors.

CLINICAL PEARLS

- Reactivation pulmonary tuberculosis most commonly presents radiographically with infiltrates or nodules in the apical and posterior segments of the upper lobes.
- Tuberculin skin testing is not a diagnostic test, but a useful screening test for potential contacts of infected persons; the response cutoff for a positive test depends on the patient's level of risk.

- ❖ Patients with a positive tuberculin skin test and no clinical or radiographic evidence of active disease are said to have *latent tuberculosis infection,* and can be treated with isoniazid to reduce their lifetime risk of developing reactivation TB.
- ❖ Individuals with active tuberculosis should be initiated on multiple agents such as isoniazid, rifampin, and pyrazinamide.
- ❖ Pyridoxine (vitamin B_6) is usually added to antituberculosis medications to prevent peripheral neuropathy.

REFERENCES

Horsburgh CR Jr, Feldman S, Ridzon R. Practice guidelines for the treatment of tuberculosis. Clin Infect Dis 2000;31(3):633–39.

Raviglione MC, O'Brian R. Tuberculosis. In: Braunwald E, Fauci AS, Kasper KL, et al., eds. Harrison's principles of internal medicine, 15th ed. New York: McGraw-Hill, 2001:1024–35.

CASE 32

A 42-year-old man complains of 2 days of worsening chest pain and dyspnea. Six weeks ago, he was diagnosed with stage II non-Hodgkin lymphoma with lymphadenopathy of the mediastinum and supraclavicular areas, and has been treated with radiation therapy. His most recent treatment was 1 week ago. He has no other medical or surgical history and takes no medications. His chest pain is constant and unrelated to activity. He becomes short of breath with minimal exertion. He is afebrile, his heart rate is 115 bpm with a thready pulse, his respiratory rate is 22 breaths per minute, and his blood pressure is 108/86 mmHg. The systolic blood pressure is noted to drop to 92 mmHg on inspiration. He appears uncomfortable and is diaphoretic. His jugular veins are distended to the angle of the jaw, and his chest is clear to auscultation. He is tachycardic, his heart sounds are faint, and no extra sounds are appreciated. The chest x-ray is shown in Figure 32–1.

- **What is the most likely diagnosis?**
- **What is your next step in therapy?**

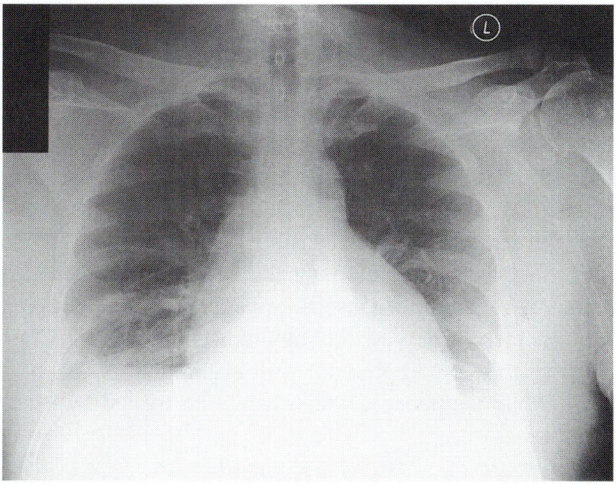

Figure 32–1. Chest x-ray. (Courtesy of Dr Jorge Albin).

ANSWERS TO CASE 32: Pericardial Effusion/Tamponade Caused by Malignancy

Summary: A man with a thoracic malignancy and history of radiotherapy to the chest now presents with chest pain, dyspnea, cardiac enlargement on chest x-ray (which could represent cardiomegaly or pericardial effusion), jugular venous distension, distant cardiac sounds, and pulsus paradoxus.

- **Most likely diagnosis:** Pericardial effusion causing cardiac tamponade.
- **Next step:** Urgent pericardiocentesis or surgical pericardial window.

Analysis

Objectives

1. Recognize pericardial tamponade; know how to check for pulsus paradoxus.
2. Know the features of cardiac tamponade, constrictive pericarditis, and restrictive cardiomyopathy, and how to distinguish among them.
3. Understand the treatment of each of these conditions.
4. Know the potential cardiac complications of thoracic malignancies and of radiation therapy.

Considerations

The patient described in the scenario, with his thoracic malignancy and history of radiation therapy, is at risk for diseases of the pericardium and of the myocardium. The jugular venous distension, distant heart sounds, and pulsus paradoxus are all suggestive of cardiac tamponade. All of these conditions can impede the diastolic filling of the heart, and lead to cardiovascular collapse. The major diagnostic considerations in this case, each with a very different treatment, are pericardial effusion causing cardiac tamponade, constrictive pericarditis, and restrictive cardiomyopathy. Urgent differentiation among these conditions is required, because the treatment is very different and the consequences of these diseases can be immediately fatal. Clinically, the patient's fall in systolic blood pressure with inspiration, pulsus paradoxus, is suggestive of cardiac tamponade, which would be treated by evacuating the pericardial fluid.

APPROACH TO SUSPECTED CARDIAC TAMPONADE

Cardiac tamponade refers to increased pressure within the pericardial space caused by an accumulating effusion, which compresses the heart and impedes diastolic filling. Because the heart can only pump out during systole what it receives during diastole, severe restrictions of diastolic filling leads to a marked decrease in cardiac output, which can cause cardiovascular collapse and death. If pericardial fluid accumulates slowly, the sac may dilate and hold up to 2000 mL (producing amazing cardiomegaly on chest x-ray) before causing diastolic impairment. If it accumulates rapidly, as in a hemopericardium caused by trauma or surgery, as little as 200 mL can produce tamponade. The classic description of **Beck triad (hypotension, elevated jugular venous pressure, and small quiet heart)**, is a description of **acute tamponade** with rapid accumulation of fluid, as in cardiac trauma or ventricular rupture. If the fluid accumulates slowly, the clinical picture may look more like congestive heart failure, with cardiomegaly on chest x-ray (although there should be no pulmonary edema), dyspnea, elevated jugular pressure, hepatomegaly, and peripheral edema. A high index of suspicion is required, and cardiac tamponade should be considered in any patient with hypotension and elevated jugular venous pressure.

The **most important physical sign** to look for **in cardiac tamponade** is the **pulsus paradoxus**. This refers to a **drop in systolic blood pressure during inspiration** of more than 10 mmHg. Although called "paradoxical," this drop in systolic blood pressure is actually not contrary to the normal physiologic variation with respiration; it is an exaggeration of the normal small drop in systolic pressure during inspiration. While not a specific sign of tamponade (e.g., it is often seen in patients with disturbed intrathoracic pressures during respiration, such as those with obstructive lung disease), the paradoxical pulse is fairly sensitive for hemodynamically significant tamponade in almost all cases. To test for this, one must use a manual blood pressure cuff, which is inflated above systolic pressure, and deflated very slowly until the first Korotkoff sound is heard during expiration, and then, finally, during both phases of respiration. The difference between these two pressure readings is the pulsus paradoxus. When the pulsus paradoxus is severe, it may be detected by palpation, as a diminution or disappearance of peripheral pulses during inspiration.

Constrictive pericarditis is a complication of previous pericarditis, either acute or chronic fibrinous pericarditis. The inflammation and resultant granulation tissue forms a **thickened fibrotic adherent sac**, which gradually contracts, encasing the heart, and **impairing diastolic filling**. In the past, tuberculosis was the most common cause of this problem, but this is now rare in the United States. Currently, this is **most commonly caused by radiation therapy**, **cardiac surgery**, or by any cause of acute pericarditis, such as **viral infection or uremia, or malignancy**. The pathophysiology of constrictive pericarditis is similar to cardiac tamponade, in that restricted ability of the ventricles to fill during diastole because of the thickened noncompliant pericardium.

Because the process is **chronic**, patients with **constrictive pericarditis** generally do not present with acute hemodynamic collapse, but rather with **chronic and slowly progressive weakness and fatigue and exertional dyspnea.** Patients commonly have what appears to be right-sided heart failure, that is, chronic lower-extremity edema, hepatomegaly, and ascites. Like patients with tamponade, they have elevated jugular venous pressures, but **pulsus paradoxus is usually absent**. Examination of neck veins does show an increase in jugular venous pressure during inspiration, termed **Kussmaul sign.** This is easy to see because it is the opposite of the normal fall in pressure as one inspires. Normally, the negative intrathoracic pressure generated by inspiration sucks blood into the heart, but because of the severe diastolic restriction, the blood cannot enter the right atrium or ventricle, so it fills the jugular vein. There is another physical finding characteristic of constrictive pericarditis, which is a **pericardial knock**, which is a high-pitched early diastolic sound occurring just after aortic valve closure. Chest radiography frequently shows cardiomegaly and a calcified pericardium.

Restrictive cardiomyopathy, like the previous diagnoses, is primarily a problem of impaired diastolic filling, usually with preserved systolic function. This is a relatively uncommon problem in the Western world. The **most common causes are amyloidosis**, an infiltrative disease of the elderly, in which an abnormal fibrillar amyloid protein is deposited in heart muscle, or fibrosis of the myocardium following radiation therapy or open heart surgery. In **Africa**, restrictive cardiomyopathy is much more common, because of a process called **endomyocardial fibrosis**, characterized by fibrosis of the endocardium along with fever and marked eosinophilia.

Clinically, it may be very difficutlt to distinguish restrictive cardiomyopathy from constrictive pericarditis, and various echocardiographic criteria have been proposed to try to distinguish between them. In addition, MRI can be very useful to visualize or exclude the presence of the thickened pericardium typical of constrictive pericarditis. Nevertheless, it may be necessary to obtain an **endomyocardial biopsy** to make the diagnosis. Differentiation between the two is essential because constrictive pericarditis is a potentially curable disease, whereas there is very little effective therapy for either the underlying conditions or the cardiac failure of restrictive cardiomyopathy. Table 32–1 compares features of these three entities.

Treatment

Treatment of cardiac tamponade consists of relief of the pericardial pressure, either by echocardiographically guided pericardiocentesis, or a surgical pericardial window. Resection of the pericardium is the definitive treatment for constrictive pericarditis. There is no effective treatment for restrictive cardiomyopathy.

Comprehension Questions

[32.1] A 35-year-old woman is noted to have a positive Kussmaul sign. Which of the following conditions is she most likely to have?

A. Constrictive pericarditis
B. Cardiac tamponade
C. Dilated cardiomyopathy
D. Diabetic ketoacidosis

[32.2] Which of the following is the most sensitive finding in patients with cardiac tamponade?

A. Disappearance of radial pulse during inspiration
B. Drop in systolic blood pressure of greater than 10 mmHg during inspiration
C. Rise in heart rate in greater than 20 bpm during inspiration
D. Distant heart sounds

[32.3] While awaiting pericardiocentesis, immediate supportive care of a patient with cardiac tamponade should include which of the following?

A. Diuresis with furosemide
B. Intravenous fluids
C. Nitrates to lower venous congestion
D. Morphine to relieve dyspnea

[32.4] Which of the following is most likely to cause restrictive cardiomyopathy?

A. Endomyocardial fibrosis
B. Viral myocarditis
C. Beriberi
D. Thyrotoxicosis

Answers

[32.1] **A.** Kussmaul sign, an increase in neck veins with inspiration, is seen with constrictive pericarditis.

[32.2] **B.** Pulsus paradoxus is a sensitive sign, although nonspecific for cardiac tamponade.

[32.3] **B.** Patients with cardiac tamponade are preload dependent, and diuresis may cause them to become hypotensive.

[32.4] **A.** Endomyocardial fibrosis is an etiology of restrictive cardiomyopathy, common in developing countries, that is associated with eosinophilia.

Table 32-1

FEATURES OF CARDIAC TAMPONADE, ACUTE PERICARDITIS, AND CONSTRICTIVE PERICARDITIS

DISEASE	PATHOPHYSIOLOGY	CLINICAL FEATURES	EKG FINDINGS
Cardiac tamponade	Increased pressure in pericardial space due to effusion, impeding diastolic filling	Pulsus paradoxicus, hypotension, elevated jugular venous distension, small quiet heart	Low voltages diffusely electrical alterans
Constrictive pericarditis	Inflammation and granulation tissue forms a thickened fibrotic adherent sac, commonly caused by radiation, viral infection, uremia	Absent pulsus paradoxicus, Kussmaul's sign, pericardial knock. Chronic and slow progressive weakness and exertional dyspnea	Low voltage
Acute pericarditis	Acute inflammation of the parietal pericardium and superficial myocardium	Chest pain, fever, pericardial rub	ST segment elevation, low voltage diffusely
Restrictive cardio-myopathy \	Myocardial fibrosis, hypertrophy, or infiltration leading to impaired diastolic filling	No pulsus paradoxus or Kussmaul sign. Progressive exertional dyspnea and dependent edema	

Harrison's 15th ed., 2001: McGraw-Hill

CLINICAL PEARLS

- Elevated jugular venous pressure and pulsus paradoxus are features of cardiac tamponade.
- Kussmaul sign and right-sided heart failure are features of constrictive cardiomyopathy, but pulsus paradoxus is not.
- Cardiac tamponade requires urgent treatment by pericardiocentesis, or a pericardial window.
- Constrictive pericarditis may show calcifications of the pericardium on chest x-ray or thickened pericardium on echocardiography. Definitive therapy is resection of the pericardium.
- Restrictive cardiomyopathy is most often caused by amyloidosis or radiation therapy. There is no effective therapy.

REFERENCE

Wynne J, Braunwald E. The Cardiomyopathies and Myocarditides. In: Braunwald E, Fauci AS, Kasper, KL, et al., (eds.). Harrison's principles of internal medicine, 15th ed. New York: McGraw-Hill, 2001:1359-1365.

❖ CASE 33

A 23-year-old man is your next patient to see in clinic. Under chief complaint, the nurse has written, "Wants a general check-up." You enter the room, and greet a generally healthy appearing young, white man, who seems nervous. He finally admits that he's been worried about a lesion on his penis. He denies pain or dysuria. He's never had any sexually transmitted diseases, and has an otherwise unremarkable past medical history. He is afebrile, and his exam is notable for a shallow, mildly tender to palpation, clean ulcer without exudates or erythema on the glans penis. There are some small, tender, inguinal lymph nodes bilaterally.

◆ **What is the most likely diagnosis?**

◆ **What is the likely treatment?**

ANSWERS TO CASE 33: Syphilis

Summary: A 23-year-old healthy man reluctantly requests evaluation of a nontender lesion on his penis. He's never had any sexually transmitted diseases and has an otherwise unremarkable past medical history. He is afebrile, and his exam is notable for a shallow, mildly tender to palpation, clean ulcer without exudates or erythema on the glans penis. There are some small, tender, inguinal lymph nodes bilaterally.

- **Most likely diagnosis:** Chancre of primary syphilis.
- **Likely treatment:** A single intramuscular injection of benzathine penicillin G.

Analysis

Objectives

1. Understand the pathogenesis and natural history of *Treponema pallidum* infection.
2. Know the differential diagnosis of genital ulceration and sexually transmitted diseases.
3. Learn the treatment of syphilis.

Considerations

This 23-year-old male reluctantly reveals his concern about a nontender ulcer of the penis. Although he has no history of sexually transmitted disease, the most common cause of a painless ulcer of the genital area in a young, immunocompetent person is syphilis. Sexually transmitted diseases often travel together so he should be evaluated for other STDs such as chlamydia or HIV. Also, other causes of genital ulcers should be considered, including chancroid and herpes virus (both usually painful), and a superficially infected skin lesion. Compliance with therapy and followup is crucial because syphilitic infections can progress to a chronic form that can lead to aneurysmal dilation of the aorta, as well as to permanent neurologic changes. He could also continue to spread the disease to others, and if he infects women of childbearing age, these women, if infected during pregnancy, could pass the infection to their newborns.

APPROACH TO SUSPECTED SYPHILIS

Definitions

Primary syphilis: Initial lesion of *T. pallidum* infection, usually in the form of the nontender ulcer, the chancre.

Secondary syphilis: Disseminated infection manifesting in a pruritic, maculopapular diffuse rash that classically involves the palms and soles, or the flat moist lesion of **condyloma lata**.

Clinical Approach

Syphilis is classically called the "great imitator" for its protean manifestations. After a decline in cases over the prior decades, the incidence of syphilis has been increasing since the 1980s. The public health consequences can be grave, so recognizing and correctly treating this disease is of great importance. There are an estimated 70,000 new cases of syphilis every year in the United States. Most occur in young adults in their twenties, and most cases are concentrated in the southern states. The number of cases reached its lowest point in the 1980s; however, the number of cases has increased since then, especially in heterosexuals, young women, and neonates. Some researchers believe this may be a result of cocaine use, sex for drugs trade, and perhaps the increased incidence of HIV infections.

Syphilis is caused by a spirochete, *Treponema pallidum*. The organism penetrates abraded skin or mucous membranes and then disseminates through the lymphatics and bloodstream to involve almost every organ. Within 1 week to 3 months of inoculation, a chancre will usually form at the site of entrance. Multiple ulcers may form, as in HIV-infected patients, but some patients may not notice the ulceration at all. The **chancre** of syphilis is typically **nonerythematous, with rolled borders and a clean base**. It is usually **painless,** although it may be tender if touched. Other diseases that may cause ulcerations include **chancroid**; however the ulcer in this disease is usually **painful, exudative, with ragged borders and a necrotic base**, and bleeds easily. The lymph nodes can also suppurate in chancroid, unlike in syphilis. The ulcers in **herpes simplex infections are typically painful, grouped vesicles on an erythematous base** that eventually ulcerate.

If untreated, syphilis progresses to a **second stage**, in which the disease disseminates widely, and the patient may present with a **pruritic, maculopapular diffuse rash that classically involves the palms and soles**. Patients may have these lesions orally as well, which are called "mucous patches," and they may suffer constitutional symptoms such as fever, myalgias, and headache. Other typical skin findings include **condyloma lata**, a gray papillomatous lesion found in intertriginous areas, and patchy hair loss.

If still left untreated, the patient will then pass into a quiescent, or latent, stage. Although relapses of symptoms of secondary syphilis can occur during this time, they become less frequent over years. Approximately 30% of patients will go on to develop **late-stage syphilis**. The symptoms of this stage result from the destruction of tissue caused by the chronic infection. The immune reaction to the organism causes a proliferative, obliterative endarteritis. In some organs, such as the skin, liver, and bone, these lesions are organized into **granulomas** with an amorphous or coagulated center called **gummas**. These lesions, in themselves, are benign; however, they can cause organ dysfunction through destruction of normal tissue. In the aorta, the obliterative endarteritis involves the vasa vasorum, which leads to necrosis of the media of the arterial wall. The resulting weakness of the wall leads to the formation of **saccular aneurysmal dilations of the aorta.**

Neurosyphilis is another form of tertiary disease, which may occur after secondary disease or from the latent stage. The organism disseminates to the central nervous system as well, causing symptoms of **meningitis, vertigo, or tinnitus**. In the CNS, this vasculitis leads to ischemia, stroke, and progressive neurologic deficits from the loss of nerve cells. Patients exhibit changes in personality, as well as specific neurologic findings as a result of demyelination of the posterior column and dorsal root ganglia (see Table 33–1).

The diagnosis of syphilis is always made fairly indirectly, as the organism has not yet been cultured. Nonspecific serologic tests, such as the RPR (rapid plasma reagin) and VDRL (Venereal Disease Research Laboratory) tests, which are actually tests for antibodies against lipid antigens that occur as part of the host reaction to *T. pallidum*, are fairly sensitive for the detection of disease. However, especially at low titers, they may be nonspecific and may result in false-positive tests. Therefore, **confirmatory testing** in the form of specific antibody testing for *T. pallidum*, such as the **FTA-Abs (fluorescent treponemal antibody absorption) or MHA-TP (microhemagglutination assay for *Treponema pallidum*) test,** is the next step to perform. **Darkfield microscopy**, in which scrapings from an ulcer are placed under a phase contrast lens to actually identify the organisms, is the classic method of diagnosis, but is rarely performed today. Biopsy of lesions such as those seen in secondary syphilis with special stains can also identify the organisms. To diagnose CNS disease, a positive cerebrospinal fluid (CSF) VDRL or RPR in

Table 33-1
SYMPTOMS AND SIGNS FOUND IN NEUROSYPHILIS

Changes in personality: lability, carelessness in appearance
Delusions, illusions, hallucinations
Deterioration of judgment, insight, and memory
Slurred speech
Small irregular pupils without reaction to light (Argyll-Robinson pupil)
"Gun barrel site"—loss of peripheral vision with destruction of the optic nerve
Hyperactive reflexes
Loss of facial expression (involvement of cranial nerves 7 and 8)
Posterior column involvement
Wide-based gait
Foot slap
Paresthesias
Bladder/bowel incontinence
Loss of position and vibratory sensation
Impotence

the setting of increased CSF leukocytosis and protein counts, sometimes with low glucose levels, is suggestive of CNS involvement. However, false-negative tests for VDRL in CSF are common, and the diagnosis is often made on clinical grounds.

Penicillin is the treatment of choice for syphilis. The most effective treatment and regimen, however, are truly unknown, because no therapeutic trials have been performed. However, current recommendations are to treat syphilis based on the stage of presentation (Table 33–2). Individuals with early disease, that is, with primary or secondary syphilis, or those with early latent syphilis (infection of less than 1 year), may be treated with a single intramuscular injection of benzathine penicillin G, a long-lasting intramuscular (IM) injection. For patients with late disease, that is, latent syphilis of an unknown duration (presumed to be >1 year), or with cardiovascular manifestations, or with gummas, treatment is given as three weekly IM injections of benzathine penicillin G. Neurosyphilis is notoriously difficult to treat. Those with CNS disease or patients concurrently infected with HIV and syphilis should receive high doses of intravenous penicillin G for 10–14 days, or longer. Pregnant women can receive either regimen, and all patients should be followed closely to ensure that their titer falls over the year after treatment. Pregnant women who are allergic to penicillin should be desensitized, and then receive penicillin because this is the only treatment known to prevent congenital infection.

T. pallidum infection usually leads to a **positive specific serologic test** (FTA-Abs or MHA-TP) for **life**, whereas an adequately treated infection will lead to a fall in RPR serology. A **normal response** is considered a **fourfold**

Table 33-2
TREATMENT OF SYPHILIS BASED ON STAGE

STAGE	CLINICAL MANIFESTATIONS	TREATMENT
Primary disease	Chancre	Single dose of intramuscular penicillin
Secondary disease, early latent (<1 year—no symptoms)	Maculopapular rash involving palms and soles, condyloma lata	Single dose of intramuscular penicillin
Late latent disease (>1 year—no symptoms)		Intramuscular penicillin at 1-week intervals for total of three doses
Tertiary syphilis, neurosyphilis	See Table 33-1	Intravenous pencillin for 10-14 days

drop in titers within 3 months, and a **negative or near-negative titer after 1 year**. A suboptimal response may mean inadequate treatment or undiagnosed tertiary disease. In any patient diagnosed with a sexually transmitted disease, the possibility that they may have other sexually transmitted diseases should be considered. Gonorrheal and chlamydial infections can be asymptomatic, especially in women. HIV is often asymptomatic early in the course of infection, and screening should be recommended to those persons who have histories of high risk behaviors or who have evidence of other sexually transmitted diseases. Hepatitis B and C are also, although less often, transmitted by sexual contact.

Comprehension Questions

[33.1] A 25-year-old man presents to your office complaining of left knee and right great toe pain, which started 1 week ago and have not responded to over-the-counter pain relievers. He also has felt feverish, achy, dysuria, and has developed an eye infection. About a month ago he was seen at an outside clinic and treated for syphilis. On examination, he is afebrile and both eyes are injected and very sensitive to light. His left knee and the metatarsophalangeal (MTP) joint of his right great toe are swollen and tender. What is your diagnosis?

A. Gouty arthritis
B. Reactive arthritis (Reiter syndrome)
C. Infectious arthritis
D. Rheumatoid arthritis
E. Syphilis

[33.2] As part of normal screening during pregnancy, a 28-year-old G2 P1 has a positive RPR with a titer of 1:64, and an MHA-TP that is also positive. She is allergic to penicillin, which causes shortness of breath and "swelling of her tongue." What treatment do you offer?

A. Erythromycin estolate
B. Doxycycline
C. Tetracycline
D. Penicillin after desensitization
E. Vancomycin
F. Wait until delivery of the baby before treatment

[33.3] A 23-year-old man is found to have late latent syphilis as part of a workup following his diagnosis with HIV. He is asymptomatic with a CD4 count of 350 and doesn't remember having lesions or rashes in the past. Prior to starting therapy with penicillin for the syphilis, he should:

A. Undergo a lumbar puncture to exclude neurosyphilis.
B. Have a skin biopsy to confirm the diagnosis of syphilis.
C. Have an MRI of his brain and an EEG.

D. Undergo skin testing to exclude penicillin allergy.
E. Have adjustment in his HIV medications to optimize his CD4 count prior to treatment for syphilis.

[33.4] A 28-year-old woman is noted to have a nontender ulcer of the vulva. A herpes culture is taken of the ulcer scraping which is negative, and the RPR titer is negative. Which of the following is your next step?

A. Empiric treatment for penicillin
B. Empiric treatment with acyclovir
C. Empiric treatment with azithromycin
D. Darkfield microscopy
E. Careful observation

Answers

[33.1] **B.** The triad of uveitis or conjunctivitis, urethritis, and arthritis are characteristic of reactive arthritis or Reiter syndrome. This poorly understood disease is thought to be caused by immune cross-reaction between antigens in infectious organisms and the host connective tissue. Commonly involved organisms include *Chlamydia trachomatis*, which this patient may have contracted when he contracted syphilis, but which may not have been treated. The arthritis typically involves large joints and is both progressive and additive. The uveitis can be difficult to treat; however, the dysuria of the urethritis can be transient. Patients with Reiter syndrome are often HLA-B27-positive.

[33.2] **D.** This patient should be desensitized and treated with penicillin, especially as she is pregnant and may pass the disease to her child. Following treatment, her titers should be closely followed and show at least a fourfold decrease. Treatment of the child after delivery with IV penicillin should be considered.

[33.3] **A.** This young man needs to have a spinal tap to look for signs of inflammation or infection, and to have CSF sent for either a VDRL or RPR. Approximately 40% of patients without immunodeficiency develop meningeal infection during the disseminated stage of syphilis, and in those with HIV, the risk of developing late stage or neurosyphilis may be higher. Because the therapy would change, neurosyphilis should be ruled out.

[33.4] **D.** About one-third of patients who have the primary lesion of the chancre will have negative serology and need either darkfield microscopy or biopsy with special stains to identify the spirochetes. The organism is too thin to be visualized by conventional light microscopy. Empiric treatment with penicillin is reasonable if darkfield microscopy is not available.

CLINICAL PEARLS

- ❖ Syphilitic chancres are generally clean, painless, ulcerative lesions and can be located anywhere on the body where inoculation occurred.
- ❖ The rash of secondary syphilis typically involves the palms and soles.
- ❖ The RPR and VDRL tests are nonspecific and may be falsely positive in several normal conditions (pregnancy) and disease states (systemic lupus erythematosus). Specific treponemal antibody tests, such as the MHA-TP and the FTA-Abs should be performed for confirmation, but once positive, they usually stay positive for life.
- ❖ A declining RPR titer can be followed to test the efficacy of therapy.
- ❖ CNS involvement can only be excluded through testing of the cerebrospinal fluid.
- ❖ Treatment of syphilis is based on stage: early syphilis can be treated with a single intramuscular injection of penicillin; late syphilis can be treated with three weekly injections; and neurosyphilis can be treated with intravenous penicillin for 10–14 days.

REFERENCE:

Tramont EC. Treponema pallidum (Syphilis). In: Mandell GL Dolin R, Bennett JE (eds.). Mandell, Douglas, and Bennett's principles of infectious diseases, 5th ed. New York: Churchill-Livingstone, 2000:2474-2490.

❖ CASE 34

A 58-year-old man from Venezuela comes to see you because of shortness of breath. He has had mild dyspnea on exertion for a few years, but more recently, he has noted worsening shortness of breath with minimal exercise and the onset of dyspnea at rest. He has difficulty reclining, and as a result, he spends the night sitting up in a chair trying to sleep. He reports a cough with production of yellowish-brown sputum every morning throughout the year. He denies chest pain, fever, chills, or lower extremity edema. He has smoked about two packs of cigarettes a day since age 15 years. He does not drink alcohol. A few months ago, the patient went to an urgent care clinic for evaluation of his symptoms, and he received a prescription for some inhalers, the names of which he doesn't remember; he was also told to find a primary care physician for further evaluation. On physical examination, his blood pressure is 142/90 mmHg, his heart rate is 96 bpm, his respiration rate is 22 breaths per minute, and temperature is 97.6°F. He is sitting in a chair, leaning forward. He appears uncomfortable with labored respirations and cyanotic lips. His neck was without lymphadenopathy, carotid bruit, or jugular venous distention. The chest examination reveals that the lower anterolateral costal margins move inward on inspiration and that wheezes and rhonchi are present bilaterally, but no crackles are noted. The anteroposterior diameter of the chest wall appears increased. Cardiovascular exam shows distant heart sounds but with a regular rate and rhythm. His extremities show no cyanosis, edema, or clubbing.

- **What is the most likely diagnosis?**
- **What is the next best diagnostic test?**
- **What is the best initial treatment?**

ANSWERS TO CASE 34: Chronic Obstructive Pulmonary Disease (COPD)

Summary: A 58-year-old Venezuelan smoker has noted worsening shortness of breath with minimal exercise and the onset of dyspnea at rest and difficulty reclining. He reports a productive cough with yellowish-brown sputum every morning throughout the year. He denies chest pain, fever, chills, or lower extremity edema. A few months ago, he was prescribed an inhaler. On physical examination, his blood pressure is 142/90 mmHg, his heart rate is 96 bpm, his respiration rate is 22 breaths per minute, and his temperature is 97.6°F. He is sitting in a chair leaning forward, and appears uncomfortable with labored respirations and cyanotic lips. The chest examination reveals lower chest retractions, and bilateral wheezes and rhonchi. The anteroposterior diameter of the chest wall appears increased. The cardiovascular exam shows distant heart sounds but with a regular rate and rhythm.

- **Most likely diagnosis:** Chronic obstructive pulmonary disease with a serious acute exacerbation.
- **Next diagnostic step:** Arterial blood gas to assess his oxygenation and acid–base status.
- **Best initial treatment:** Oxygen by nasal canula, followed closely by bronchodilators, and steroids for inflammatory component.

Analysis

Objectives

1. Know the definition and etiologies of chronic bronchitis, chronic obstructive pulmonary disease, and emphysema.
2. Be able to interpret arterial blood gases in a patient with chronic obstructive pulmonary disease.
3. Know about the treatment of acute exacerbations including the indications for intubation and mechanical ventilation.
4. Be familiar with the flow volume loops for obstructive lung disease.

Considerations

This 58-year-old long-time smoker complains of a 1-year history of worsening dyspnea and a productive cough. He is in respiratory distress with labored respirations, cyanosis, "barrel chest," wheezing, and distant heart sounds, all suggesting lung disease. The main issue is his respiratory status. Rapid clinical assessment is critical in case this patient is headed toward respiratory failure, necessitating intubation and mechanical ventilation. An arterial blood gas will quickly give information regarding the oxygenation status, and also the ventilatory efficiency via the PCO_2 (carbon dioxide pressure) level.

APPROACH TO CHRONIC OBSTRUCTIVE PULMONARY DISEASE

Definitions

Chronic bronchitis: Clinical diagnosis characterized by excessive secretion of bronchial mucus and productive cough for 3 months or more in at least two consecutive years in the absence of any other disease that might account for this symptom.

Chronic obstructive pulmonary disease (COPD): Disease state characterized by the presence of airflow obstruction caused by chronic bronchitis or emphysema. The airflow obstruction is usually progressive, may be accompanied by airway hyperreactivity, and may be partially reversible.

Emphysema: Pathologic diagnosis that denotes abnormal, permanent enlargement of air spaces distal to the terminal bronchiole, with destruction of their walls and without obvious fibrosis.

Clinical Approach

The most common etiology for COPD disease is inhalation injury, specifically cigarette smoking. Another important cause is **alpha$_1$-antitrypsin deficiency**, which is hereditary. The disease may become evident by the age of 40 years and often occurs without cough or smoking history. Therapy by replacement of alpha$_1$-antitrypsin enzyme is available. Characteristically, patients with COPD present with progressively worsening dyspnea (first on exertion, then with activity, then at rest). Patient may vary in appearance from a "blue bloater" (chronic bronchitis, overweight, edematous, cyanotic) to a "pink puffer" (emphysema, thin, ruddy cheeks).

Arterial blood gases are often normal in the early phase of the disease; however, in advanced cases, there is evidence of hypoxemia and hypercapnia. Usually, they are in a state of chronic respiratory acidosis as a consequence of CO_2 retention. **Spirometry is the most basic, inexpensive, and widely valuable pulmonary function test**. It helps to identify the type of lung disease, obstructive versus restrictive, along with potential reversibility, and gas exchanging capability of the lungs (DL_{CO}). **Flow volume loops** help to identify the type of lung disease (see Figure 34–1); restrictive lung diseases tend to have lower lung volumes, whereas obstructive diseases have larger lung volumes. Specific parameters help to classify the type and degree of lung dysfunction (see Table 34–1).

Management of severe COPD exacerbations focuses simultaneously on relieving airway obstruction and correcting life-threatening abnormalities of gas exchange. Bronchodilators (beta-agonist and anticholinergic agents) are administered via handheld nebulizers; high-dose systemic glucocorticoids accelerate the rate of improvement in lung function among these patients; antibiotics should be given if there is suspicion of a respiratory infection.

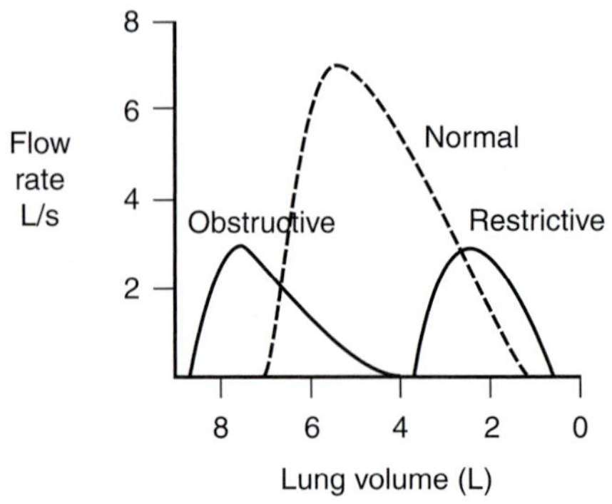

Figure 34–1. Expiratory flow volume loops of normal, obstructive, and restrictive lung disease.

Table 34-1
CHARACTERISTICS OF OBSTRUCTIVE VERSUS RESTRICTIVE LUNG DISEASE

	OBSTRUCTIVE LUNG DISEASE	RESTRICTIVE LUNG DISEASE	
Pulmonary Function Tests	Decreased FEV_1: FVC ratio; TLC usually normal or increased	Decreased lung volumes: decreased VC and TLC	
Example of Diseases	**BABE** **B**ronchiectasis (i.e., cystic fibrosis) **A**sthma **B**ronchitis (chronic) **E**mphysema	Extrapulmonary: poor breathing mechanics; **PMS** **P**oliomyelitis **M**yasthenia Gravis **S**coliosis	Pulmonary: poor lung expansion; **PAPI** **P**neumonia **A**RDS **P**ulumonary edema **I**nterstitial fibrosis

*Abbreviations: ARDS = acute respiratory distress syndrome; FEV_1 = forced expiratory volume in 1 second; FVC = functional vital capacity; TLC = total lung capacity; VC = vital capacity

Controlled oxygen administration with nasal oxygen at low flows or oxygen with Venturi masks will correct hypoxemia without causing severe hypercapnia. Caution must be exercised in those patients with chronic respiratory insufficiency whose respiratory drive is dependent on "relative hypoxemia"; these individuals may become apneic if excessive oxygen is administered.

Positive-pressure mask ventilation offers an alternative to intubation and mechanical ventilation in the treatment of cooperative patients with an acute exacerbation of COPD and severe hypercapnia. Signs of **acute respiratory failure** include **tachypnea** (respiratory rate >40 breaths per minute), **inability to speak** because of dyspnea, **accessory muscle use with fatigue** despite maximal therapy, **confusion, restlessness, agitation, lethargy, a rising PCO_2 level**, and extreme **hypoxemia**. Acute respiratory failure is generally treated with mechanical intubation. Endotracheal or nasotracheal intubation with ventilatory support helps to correct the gas-exchange disorders. Complications of mechanical intubation include difficulty in extubation, ventilator-associated pneumonia, pneumothorax, and acute respiratory distress syndrome. Long-term complications of COPD from hypoxemia can cause pulmonary hypertension, secondary erythrocytosis, exercise limitation, and impaired mental functioning. These patients must be encouraged to quit smoking and undergo evaluation for oxygen therapy. They are susceptible to lung infections, and should receive pneumococcal immunization and annual influenza vaccination.

Comprehension Questions

[34.1] Which of the following can be useful in the diagnosis of occult pulmonary hemorrhage?

A. Forced expiratory volume in 1 second (FEV_1)
B. Forced vital capacity (FVC)
C. Total lung capacity (TLC)
D. Diffusing capacity of lung for carbon monoxide (DL_{CO})
E. Functional residual capacity

[34.2] Which of the following is a 50-year-old man with severe kyphoscoliosis most likely to have?

A. Enlarged overall lung volume
B. Alveolar hyperventilation
C. Left rather than right ventricular failure
D. Increased lung compliance
E. Recurrent pulmonary infections

[34.3] Which of the following is the best measure of airflow obstruction?

A. Diffusing capacity of lung for carbon monoxide (DL_{CO})
B. Residual volume (RV)
C. Forced expiratory volume in 1 second (FEV_1)
D. Forced expiratory volume in 1 second/forced vital capacity ratio (FEV_1/FVC)
E. Forced vital capacity (FVC)

[34.4] Which of the following best characterize restrictive ventilatory defects?

A. Low lung volumes
B. A decrease in the forced expiratory volume in 1second /forced vital capacity (FEV_1/FVC) ratio

C. An increased vital capacity (VC)
D. A decreased diffusing capacity of lung for carbon monoxide (DL_{CO})
E. An increased airway resistance (R_{AW})

Answers

[34.1] **D.** The diffusing capacity for carbon monoxide attempts to measure the surface area of alveolar capillary membrane by determining the amount of hemoglobin in the thorax using the avid hemoglobin that binds carbon monoxide. Because hemoglobin that binds carbon monoxide can be intravascular or extravascular, as in the case of pulmonary hemorrhage, the diffusing capacity can quantitate the degree of pulmonary hemorrhage. This may be useful in certain disorders such as Goodpasture syndrome, in which new hemorrhage can be relatively occult.

[34.2] **E.** Bony deformities of the chest can lead to respiratory failure with elevated PCO_2 levels, as well as with recurrent pulmonary infection. The pattern on pulmonary function testing is usually that of a restrictive pattern, or decreased lung volumes and compliance.

[34.3] **D.** A decrease in the forced expiratory volume in 1 second/forced vital capacity ratio is the hallmark of airflow obstruction. The FEV_1 is decreased in obstructive, as well as in restrictive, lung disease. The diffusing capacity and the residual volume do not identify airway obstruction. The DL_{CO} indicates the adequacy of the alveolar-capillary membrane; the RV is the volume of air remaining in the lungs after a maximal expiratory effort.

[34.4] **A.** Restrictive disorders are characterized by low lung volumes. Diffusing capacity may or may not be decreased in pulmonary fibrosis, a type of restrictive disease. Vital capacity and airway resistance are decreased in restrictive lung disorders.

CLINICAL PEARLS

❖ Patients with obstructive lung disease have trouble blowing air out, whereas patients with restrictive lung disease have trouble getting air in.

❖ For simple acid–base disorders, think the following: If pH and PCO_2 move in the same direction, think metabolic acidosis/alkalosis. If pH and PCO_2 move in opposite directions, think respiratory acidosis/alkalosis.

❖ The mainstay for treatment of COPD exacerbations includes bronchodilators, oxygen, and glucocorticoids.

- ❖ Controlled supplemental oxygen along with positive-pressure ventilation may easily prevent intubation.
- ❖ Home oxygen therapy to treat chronic hypoxemia is the only way to improve survival among persons with COPD.

REFERENCE

Hong EG, Ingram RH. Chronic Bronchitis, Emphysema, and Airways Obstruction. In: Braunwald E, Fauci AS, Kasper KL, et al., eds. Harrison's principles of internal medicine, 15th ed. New York: McGraw-Hill, 2001.

❖ CASE 35

A 47-year-old man presents to your office with the complaint of cough. The cough began about 2 months prior to this appointment, and it has become more annoying to the patient. It is non-productive, and worse at night. He recently re-started an exercise program after about two years of a more sedentary lifestyle, and says he's having a much harder time with the exertion; he just runs out of breath earlier than he used to and coughs a great deal. He has not had any blood tinged sputum or weight loss. He denies nasal congestion and headaches. He does not smoke, though he does have hypertension, which has been well controlled for years with hydrochlorothiazide. His examination is notable for a blood pressure of 134/78 mmHg, and lungs that are clear to auscultation bilaterally, except for an occasional expiratory wheeze on forced expiration. A chest radiograph is read as normal.

- **What is the most likely diagnosis?**
- **How would you confirm the diagnosis?**

ANSWERS TO CASE 35: Chronic Cough/Asthma

Summary: A 47-year-old nonsmoking man complains of a 2-month history of a nonproductive cough that is worse at night. He becomes dyspneic more easily and denies any blood-tinged sputum, weight loss, nasal congestion, or headaches. He is hypertensive and has been taking hydrochlorothiazide for years. He is normotensive and his lungs are clear to auscultation bilaterally, except for an occasional expiratory wheeze on forced expiration. A chest radiograph is read as normal.

- **Most likely diagnosis:** Reactive airway disease (asthma).
- **Confirmation of diagnosis:** Pulmonary function tests, with methacholine challenge if indicated.

Analysis

Objectives

1. Know the differential diagnosis of chronic cough in adult patients.
2. Understand the stepwise approach to finding the cause of cough in these patients.
3. Learn how to diagnose and treat reactive airway disease (asthma).

Considerations

This is a 47-year-old male who presents with a chronic cough of more than 2 weeks duration. With the history of exercise intolerance, worsening cough at night, and the occasional wheezes on examination, asthma is the most likely diagnosis in this patient. His age is atypical for the presentation; thus, the chest radiograph is important to evaluate for more serious processes such as tumor, infection, or a parenchymal abnormality; this is especially true of smokers but also in nonsmokers. Because the chest radiograph is normal, many of the less-common causes of chronic cough are unlikely. If the patient has a history of exposure to environmental irritants or is taking a medication associated with cough, the offending agent should be removed. Medications should be investigated, but this patient is taking hydrochlorothiazide; for example, angiotensin-converting enzyme (ACE) inhibitors can induce cough, which can start anywhere from 3 weeks to 1 year after initiation of the drug. If the cough does not resolve, consider empiric treatment for postnasal drip or gastroesophageal reflux disease (GERD), as both these conditions can be silent; patients often have multiple causes for chronic cough.

APPROACH TO CHRONIC COUGH

Definitions

Acute cough: Condition for less than 3 weeks, most commonly caused by acute upper respiratory infection, but may also be caused by congestive heart failure, pneumonia, and pulmonary embolism.

Asthma: Chronic inflammatory condition of the airways associated with widespread bronchospasm that is reversible.

Chronic cough: Condition for longer than 3 weeks, which in a smoker may be suspicious for chronic obstructive pulmonary disease (COPD) or bronchogenic carcinoma, and in a nonsmoker with a normal chest radiograph and not taking an ACE inhibitor, may be postnasal drip, GERD, or asthma.

Clinical Approach

Chronic cough represents a common complaint and a large portion of health care dollars. Ironically, the complications from the cough, including subjective perceptions of exhaustion and self-consciousness, along with symptoms of hoarseness, musculoskeletal pain, sweating, and urinary incontinence, usually drive the patient to the doctor's office. Physiologically, the cough serves two main functions: (a) to protect the lungs against aspiration and (b) to clear secretions or other material into more proximal airways to be expectorated from the tracheobronchial tree. Patients with hemoptysis, immunocompromised states, comorbidities such as chronic obstructive pulmonary disease or cystic fibrosis, current or previous infections such as tuberculosis or HIV, and significant symptoms such as weight loss, night sweats, and chills, are beyond the scope of this discussion.

The evaluation of chronic cough begins with a detailed history and physical, including smoking habits, complete medication list, environmental and occupational exposures, and any history of asthma or obstructive lung disease. Specific questions regarding the precipitating factors, duration, character, and development of the cough should also be elicited. Although the physical exam or nature of the cough rarely identifies the cause, meticulous review of the ears, nose, throat, and lungs may suggest a particular diagnosis. For example, a cobblestone appearance of the oropharynx (representing lymphoid hyperplasia) or boggy erythematous nasal mucosa can be consistent with postnasal drip. **End-expiratory wheezing suggests active bronchospasm**, whereas **localized wheezing may be consistent with a foreign body or a bronchogenic tumor.**

In more than 90% of cases, a negative chest radiograph in an immunocompetent nonsmoker guides the physician to one of three diagnoses: **postnasal drip, asthma, or GERD**. In the outpatient setting, the mainstay of diagnosis relates to the response with empiric therapy, and multiple etiologies are addressed in terms of treatment. Often, a definitive diagnosis for chronic cough depends on observing a successful response to therapy. The American College of Chest Physicians developed a stepwise approach to diagnosing and treating chronic cough (see Figure 35–1). Referral to a pulmonologist is recommended when the diagnostic and empiric therapy options are exhausted. If suspicion for carcinoma is high, a high-resolution CT scan of the thorax or bronchoscopy should be actively pursued. A diagnosis of psychogenic cough should be one of exclusion.

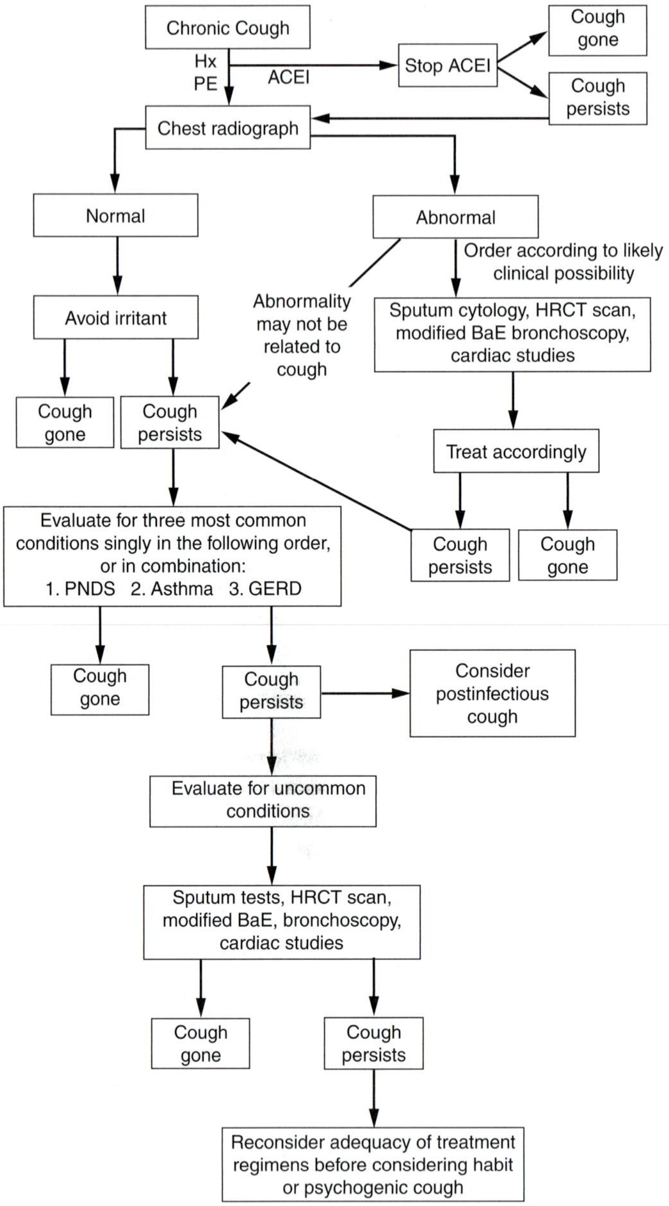

Figure 35–1. Algorithm for the diagnosis and treatment of chronic cough. ACEI = angiotensin-converting enzyme inhibitor; BaE = barium esophagography; GERD = gastroesophageal reflux disease; HRCT = high-resolution computed tomography; Hx = history; PE = physical exam; PNDS = postnasal drip syndrome. **(Reproduced with permission from Irwin RS, Boulet L-P, Cloutier MM, et al. Managing cough as a defense mechanism and as a symptom: a consensus panel report of the American College of Chest Physicians. Chest 1998;114(Suppl):133S–181S.)**

Postnasal Drip Postnasal drip syndrome may be attributed to sinusitis and the following types of rhinitis, alone or in combination: nonallergic, allergic, postinfectious, vasomotor, drug-induced, and environmental-irritant–induced. Because the symptoms may be nonexistent or nonspecific (such as frequent throat clearing, nasal discharge, or sensation of liquid in the throat), no definitive diagnostic criteria exists for postnasal drip, and response to therapy confirms the diagnosis. Initial treatment for a nonallergic etiology usually includes combination treatment with a first-generation antihistamine and a decongestant for 3 weeks. For allergic rhinitis, a newer-generation antihistamine, along with a nasal corticosteroid, should be used. If the patient's symptoms do not improve, sinus radiographs may be ordered. Opacification, air–fluid levels, or mucosal thickening could suggest sinusitis, which should be treated with antibiotics.

Asthma Although wheezing is considered a classic sign of reactive airway disease, cough is often the only symptom. Cough-variant asthma usually presents with a dry cough that occurs throughout the day and night that is worsened by airway inflammation from viral infections of the upper respiratory tract, allergies, cold air, or exercise. Although the history may be suggestive of asthma, the diagnosis should be confirmed with pulmonary function tests. The pulmonary function test typically demonstrates reversible air obstruction with a histamine or methacholine challenge. A negative methacholine test usually excludes asthma as a cause of the cough. The astute clinician will recognize that other conditions can also contribute to the asthma. Management of asthma should be aimed at controlling airway inflammation. Initial empiric treatment usually includes inhaled or oral corticosteroids and a short-acting bronchodilator for intermittent bronchospasm. Modification of therapy is based on frequency and severity of symptoms (see Table 35–1).

Gastroesophageal Reflux GERD often can be silent, and it may be the primary or coexisting cause of the cough, often as a result of aspiration and vagal stimulation. The initial treatment includes lifestyle modification along with medical therapy. Recommendations include a high-protein, low-fat diet, antireflux diet for 3–4 weeks; elevation of the head of the bed; consumption of the last meal of the day at least 3 hours before bedtime; avoidance of caffeine, alcohol, peppermint, and chocolate; smoking cessation; and weight reduction. If the cough does not resolve with lifestyle changes, daily treatment with an H_2-receptor antagonist (cimetidine, famotidine, nizatidine, or ranitidine) or a proton pump inhibitor (omeprazole) should be initiated. If acid suppression does not cause symptoms to resolve, one can use a gastric motility stimulant such as metoclopramide. To maximize the therapeutic response, these medications may be used in combination.

Patients who remain symptomatic after maximal medical treatment often benefit from 24-hour esophageal pH monitoring to confirm the diagnosis. An esophagogastroduodenoscopy showing esophagitis or an upper gastrointestinal radiographic series demonstrating reflux further supports the diagnosis. Of note, gastrointestinal symptoms may resolve prior to the resolution of the cough, and full resolution may require 2–3 months of intensive medical therapy.

Table 35-1
GUIDELINES FOR THE DIAGNOSIS AND MANAGEMENT OF ASTHMA

CLASSIFICATION	STEP	DAYS WITH SYMPTOMS	NIGHTS WITH SYMPTOMS	DAILY MEDICATION	QUICK RELIEF MEDICATION
Severe persistent	4	Continual	Frequent	High-dose inhaled steroids and long-acting inhaled β_2-agonist; if needed, add oral steroids	Short acting inhaled β_2-agonist, as needed; oral steroids may be required
Moderate persistent	3	Daily	>1/week	Low-to-medium–dose inhaled steroids and long-acting β_2-agonist (preferred) or medium-dose inhaled steroids or low-to-medium–dose inhaled steroids and either leukotriene modifier or theophylline	Short-acting inhaled β_2-agonist, as needed; oral steroids may be required
Mild persistent	2	>2/week, but <1 time/day	>2/month	Low-dose inhaled steroids (preferred) or cromolyn, leukotriene modifier, or nedocromil, or sustained-release theophylline to serum concentration of 5–15 μg/mL	Short acting inhaled β_2-agonist, as needed; oral steroids may be required
Mild intermittent	1	<2/week	<2/month	No daily medications	Short-acting inhaled β_2-agonist, as needed; oral steroids may be required

Comprehension Questions

[35.1] Patient with known asthma on inhaled corticosteroid and intermittent (short-acting) β_2-agonist presents with complaints of nocturnal awakenings secondary to cough and occasional wheezing. This occurs three to four times a week. Pulmonary function tests in the past have shown mild obstructive lung disease. What is the best next step?

A. Oral steroids
B. Leukotriene inhibitors
C. Long acting β_2 agonists
D. Theophylline
E. Antireflux therapy

[35.2] Which of the following is most accurate?

A. Cough caused by captopril will usually resolve with switching to enalapril
B. Initial treatment of a chronic cough should include codeine or a similar opiate derivative to suppress the cough
C. Cough caused by reflux can be effectively ruled out by a negative history of heartburn or dyspepsia
D. More than one condition is often responsible for causing a chronic cough in a given patient

[35.3] A 22-year-old African American woman presents with fatigue, arthralgias, and a nagging dry cough for the past 6 weeks, but no shortness of breath. On physical exam, her lungs are clear to auscultation, and she has bilateral pretibial tender erythematous raised nodules. What is your best next step?

A. Chest radiograph
B. High-resolution CT
C. Empiric treatment for postnasal drip
D. Antinuclear antibody
E. Initiation of antituberculosis therapy

[35.4] An obese 50-year-old man with history of asthma returns with complaints of occasional dyspepsia and cough. He wakes up in the morning with a sour taste in his mouth. His current medications include inhaled corticosteroid and a short-acting β_2-agonist. What should be your next step?

A. 24-Hour esophageal pH monitoring
B. Chest radiograph
C. Initiation of omeprazole
D. Short course of oral corticosteroids
E. Initiation of allergy desensitization

Answers

[35.1] **C.** Long-acting β_2-agonists are helpful in this situation. The asthma would be classified as moderate persistent, and the recommended treatment is long-acting β_2-agonists such as salmeterol, which are particularly helpful with nocturnal symptoms.

[35.2] **D.** Often more than one condition is responsible for causing a chronic cough in a given patient. Cough from angiotensin inhibitor are class dependent, and change to another class of antihypertensives is more appropriate. The etiology of chronic cough should be addressed prior to suppression of the cough, for treatment of the underlying condition is the most effective approach. GERD may present with the sole manifestation of cough, or it may present "silently."

[35.3] **A.** Chest radiography is the next step. The patient likely has sarcoidosis given the new cough, myalgias, and description of erythema nodosum. The initial, most cost-effective study is a chest radiograph. Hilar lymphadenopathy with or without interstitial infiltrates would solidify a diagnosis of sarcoidosis. A high-resolution CT may be ordered if the patient has interstitial lung disease, but it is not the first study of choice. Postnasal drip does not explain the patient's other symptoms. An antinuclear antibody would not necessarily identify the cause of the cough or provide a diagnosis.

[35.4] **C.** Initiation of omeprazole, a proton pump inhibitor. Dyspepsia and the sour taste suggest GERD. Other recommendations include dietary modifications and weight reduction. Twenty-four–hour esophageal pH monitoring is only indicated if the medications did not help. Oral corticosteroids could be a consideration if the clinical scenario was more consistent with asthma exacerbation.

CLINICAL PEARLS

- ❖ A normal chest radiograph excludes most, **but not all**, of the serious and uncommon causes of chronic cough.
- ❖ The three most common causes of chronic cough in immunocompetent nonsmokers who are not taking ACE inhibitors are postnasal drip, asthma, and GERD.
- ❖ Cough caused by ACE inhibitors can occur in patients who have been stable on their medication for some time.
- ❖ The treatment of asthma is a stepwise process based on frequency of symptoms and response to prescribed medications.

- ❖ Asthma can be the cause of cough in a patient with normal exam and pulmonary function tests. If suspicion is high, a methacholine challenge, if positive, has a high predictive value.
- ❖ Definitive diagnosis of the etiology of chronic cough is not always necessary for successful treatment.

REFERENCES

Irwin RS, Boulet L-P, Cloutier MM, et al. Managing cough as a defense mechanism and as a symptom: a consensus panel report of the American College of Chest Physicians. Chest 1998;114(Suppl):133S–181S.

Irwin RS, Madison JM. The diagnosis and treatment of cough. N Engl J Med 2000;343(23):1715–1721.

Williams SG, Schmidt DK, Redd SC, Storms W. National Asthma Education and Prevention Program. Key clinical activities for quality asthma care. Recommendations of the National Asthma Education and Prevention Program. MMWR Recomm Rep 2003;52(RR-6):1–8.

CASE 36

A 63-year-old African American woman is brought to the emergency room for upper arm pain and swelling following a fall at home. The family has noted that for about the past 2 months, the patient has become progressively fatigued, absent-minded, and has developed loss of appetite and weight loss. She has been getting up to urinate several times a night and complains of thirst; however, a test for diabetes in her doctor's office was negative. This morning, she lost her balance because of feeling "lightheaded" and fell, landing on her left arm. The examination is notable for an elderly, thin woman in mild distress as a result of pain. Her blood pressure is 110/70 mmHg, her heart rate is 80 bpm, and she is afebrile. Her thyroid gland is normal to palpation. Her mucus membranes are somewhat dry and sticky. Her heart and lung examinations are normal, and the carotid auscultation reveals no bruits. The examination of her extremities is significant only for deformity of the left mid-humerus with swelling. The left radial pulse is 2+ and symmetric. The radiologist calls you to confirm the fracture of the mid-left humerus, but also states that there is the suggestion of some lytic lesions of the proximal humerus, and suggests a skull film. The serum creatinine level is 2.1 mg/dL, normal electrolytes and glucose, but her serum calcium is 13 mg/dL.

- **What is the most likely diagnosis?**
- **What is the most likely underlying etiology in this patient?**
- **What is your next therapeutic step?**

ANSWERS TO CASE 36: Hypercalcemia/Multiple Myeloma

Summary: A 63-year-old African American woman is evaluated for a humeral fracture sustained during a fall because of lightheadedness. She has a 2-month history of fatigue, absent-mindedness, loss of appetite and weight, and nocturia. Her vital signs are normal. Her thyroid gland is normal to palpation. Her mucus membranes are somewhat dry and sticky. She has a deformity of the left mid-humerus with swelling, but with normal distal pulses. In addition to the fracture seen on x-ray, she also has lytic lesions of the proximal humerus. She has renal insufficiency and hypercalcemia.

- **Most likely diagnosis:** Hypercalcemia with pathologic fracture of the left humerus.
- **Most likely underlying etiology:** Multiple myeloma.
- **Next therapeutic step:** Initial therapy of the hypercalcemia with IV fluids could be started in the emergency department.

Analysis

Objectives

1. Know the clinical presentation and differential diagnosis of hypercalcemia.
2. Know the treatment for symptomatic hypercalcemia.

Considerations

The patient presents with acute confusion, fatigue, and lethargy, all symptoms of hypercalcemia, consistent with the calcium level of 13 mg/dL. The first step in therapy should be intravenous hydration. An electrocardiograph is important because hypercalcemia may lead to cardiac arrhythmias. A focused diagnostic strategy should focus on the possibility of hyperparathyroidism, and malignancy, including multiple myeloma. Given the rapidity of onset of symptoms, weight loss, age, and presence of lytic bone lesions, the first concern should be for malignancy, such as multiple myeloma, breast or lung cancer. Other causes for hypercalcemia to consider include granulomatous disease, hyperparathyroidism, vitamin toxicity, drugs, and some hereditary causes of hypercalcemia. A skull x-ray would be helpful if it shows lytic bone lesions. Both serum and urine electrophoresis would help to identify the presence of a monoclonal gammopathy. A serum parathyroid hormone (PTH) and parathyroid hormone-related protein (PTHrP) if normal, would exclude other causes of hypercalcemia (see Figure 36–1 for diagnostic algorithm and Table 36–1 for causes). Treatment then can be aimed at etiology (see Table 36–2).

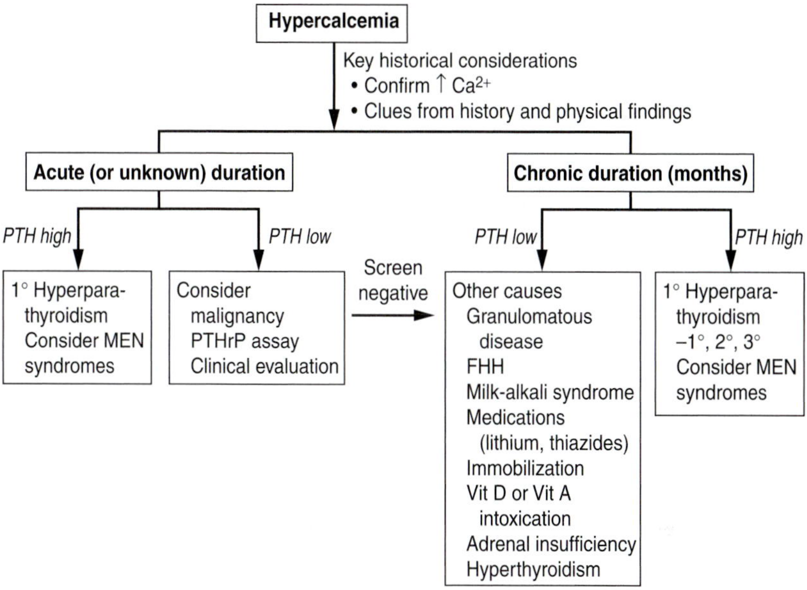

Figure 36–1. Algorithm for evaluation of patients with hypercalcemia. PTHrP = Parathyroid Hormone related protein; PTH = Parathyroid Hormone; FHH = Familial Hypercalciuric hypercalemia. **(Reproduced with permission from Potts JT. Diseases of the Parathyroid Gland and Other Hyper- and Hypocalcemia Disorders. In: Braunwald E, Fauci AS, Kasper KL, et al., eds. Harrison's principles of internal medicine, 15th ed. New York: McGraw-Hill, 2001:2205-2226.**

APPROACH TO HYPERCALCEMIA

Definitions

Corrected calcium level: Add 0.8 mg/dL to the serum total calcium for every 1 g/dL of albumin level below 4 g/dL. Example: if the serum calcium level = 9.0 mg/dL and the albumin level is 2.0 g/dL, the corrected calcium level = 10.6 mg/dL.

Hypercalcemia: Elevated serum calcium levels after correction for albumin concentration (normal range about 8.8–10.4 mg/dL).

Clinical Approach

Hypercalcemia **The most common causes of hypercalcemia include malignancies or hyperparathyroidism**. Other causes include granulomatous disorders such as sarcoid and tuberculosis; less commonly, hypercalcemia may be the presentation of intoxication with vitamins A, D, or calcium-containing antacids, or occur as a side effect of drug therapies such as lithium or thiazide diuretics. Genetic conditions such as familial hypocalciuric hypercalcemia and

Table 36-1
CAUSES OF HYPERCALCEMIA

DISEASE PROCESS	MECHANISM	CLINICAL PRESENTATION	DIAGNOSTIC CRITERIA	TREATMENT
Primary hyperparathyroidism	Elevated parathyroid hormone leading to increased turnover of bone	Solitary adenoma or part of multiple endocrine neoplasia (MEN); nephrolithiasis, peptic ulcers and mental changes (bones, groans, etc.)	Hypercalcemia, hypophosphatemia, elevated PTH	Medical therapy for mild symptoms; surgery for symptoms or hypercalciuria, renal insufficiency, or osteoporosis
Lithium therapy	Stimulation of PTH	Same as with primary hyperparathyroidism	Same as with primary hyperparathyroidism	Discontinue lithium if symptoms
Malignancy-related hypercalcemia	Local destruction of bone (multiple myeloma or leukemia or lymphoma) or humoral release of PTH-rH (solid tumors such as breast, renal, or lung cancer)	Symptoms of hypercalcemia, and of the particular cancer	Imaging of bones (either plain film or CT), PTH-rP levels, bone marrow biopsy	Treatment of the tumor and control of cancer, biphosphonates

Sarcoidosis (and other granulomatous disorders)	Excess $1,25(OH)_2D$ synthesized in macrophages and lymphocytes	Usually few symptoms	Low PTH levels and elevated $1,25(OH)_2D$ levels	Avoidance of sunlight, decrease vitamin D and calcium intake; if needed glucocorticoids
Excessive vitamin D intake	Increased calcium intestinal absorption, and if severe, bone resorption	Symptoms of hypercalcemia	Low PTH levels and markedly elevated levels of 25(OH)D, and normal $1,25(OH)_2$ D levels	Glucocorticoids and, if needed, intensive hypercalcemia management
Renal insufficiency	Secondary hyperparathyroidism as a result of partial resistance to PTH effects	Bone pain, pruritus, ectopic calcification, osteomalacia	Elevated renal function tests	Limit dietary phosphate intravenous calcitriol

Table 36-2
TREATMENT FOR HYPERCALCEMIA

TREATMENT	ONSET	ADVERSE EFFECTS
Hydration	Acute (effect seen in hours)	Volume overload, electrolyte disturbances
Bisphosphonates	Subacute (1–2 days)	Hypophosphatemia, hypomagnesemia, hypocalcemia, fever
Calcitonin	Acute (hours)	Efficacy short-lived (tachyphylaxis)
Phosphate (oral or IV)	Subacute to acute	Renal insufficiency, hypocalcemia
Glucocorticoids (effective in cancer-induced hypercalcemia)	Lengthy (days)	Hyperglycemia, osteoporosis, immune suppression
Dialysis (renal insufficiency)	Acute (hours)	Volume shifts, electrolyte disorders, complicated procedure

hyperparathyroidism as part of a multiple endocrine neoplasia syndrome are less common causes.

The differential diagnosis can be narrowed based on the chronicity of the patient's presentation and the presence or absence of other symptoms and signs. **Primary hyperparathyroidism**, usually caused by a **solitary parathyroid adenoma**, is the most likely cause when hypercalcemia is discovered in an otherwise **asymptomatic** patient on routine laboratory screening. Most patients have no symptoms with mild hypercalcemia below 12 g/dL, except perhaps some polyuria and dehydration. With levels above 13 mg/dL, patients begin developing increasingly severe symptoms, including CNS symptoms (lethargy, stupor, coma, mental status changes, psychosis), gastrointestinal symptoms (anorexia, nausea, constipation, peptic ulcer disease), kidney problems (polyuria, nephrolithiasis), and musculoskeletal complaints (arthralgias, myalgias, weakness). The **symptoms of hyperparathyroidism** can be remembered as **stones** (kidney), **moans** (abdominal pain), **groans** (myalgias), **bones** (bone pain), and **psychiatric overtones.** Diagnosis can be established by finding hypercalcemia, hypophosphatemia, with inappropriately elevated PTH levels. Symptomatic patients can be treated with parathyroidectomy.

However, a patient presenting with **symptomatic hypercalcemia** is more likely to have a **malignancy**. Multiple myeloma, lymphoma, and leukemia can all present with hypercalcemia, as can solid tumors such as breast, lung, and kidney cancers. Some of these cancers cause elevated calcium levels by **stimulat-**

ing osteoclast activity through direct bone marrow invasion (multiple myeloma, leukemia, and breast cancer). Others produce **excess 1,25 vitamin D** (lymphomas), while others secrete a **parathyroid hormone-related protein** that binds the PTH receptor (kidney and lung). Cancer-related hypercalcemia can be differentiated from primary hyperparathyroidism by a suppressed PTH level.

Electrolytes, to assess acid–base status, and renal function are important tests to consider. A normal complete blood count (CBC) and peripheral smear would make leukemia a less-likely cause. Levels of parathyroid hormone and specific assays for parathyroid hormone-related protein are generally measured. If multiple myeloma is suspected, serum and urine electrophoresis for monoclonal antibody spikes should be examined. Radiographs showing lytic or blastic lesions may be helpful; finally, a bone marrow biopsy may be considered.

Multiple Myeloma Multiple myeloma is a neoplastic proliferation of plasma cells that usually produce monoclonal IgA or IgG antibodies. Patients typically present with **lytic bone lesions**, **hypercalcemia**, **renal insufficiency**, **anemia**, and an elevated globulin fraction on serum chemistries, which if separated by electrophoresis, shows a **monoclonal proliferation** (M-spike). The **diagnosis** of multiple myeloma requires laboratory and clinical criteria: a **monoclonal antibody spike** in the serum or light chains in the urine, and **more than 10% atypical plasma cells in the bone marrow and lytic bone lesions**.

Patients with increased IgA or IgG antibodies without the signs or symptoms of multiple myeloma have what is termed a monoclonal gammopathy of undetermined significance. Long-term studies demonstrate that approximately 16% of these patients will go on to develop multiple myeloma. It is impossible to predict which patients will progress. Risk factors include older age, male gender, black race, and a positive family history of multiple myeloma.

Therapy for multiple myeloma includes a **combination of chemotherapy** with melphalan and prednisone. Other chemotherapeutic regimens are used but have not been shown to increase survival. Some patients may be candidates for autologous bone marrow transplant.

Comprehension Questions

[36.1] On routine blood work done for a life insurance application, a 53-year-old woman was found to have a calcium level of 12 mg/dL (normal = 8.8–10.4 mg/dL) and a phosphate level of 2 mg/dL (normal = 3.0–4.5 mg/dL). She is not anemic and has no symptoms. Her past medical history is significant for osteoporosis, discovered on a dual-energy x-ray absorptiometry (DEXA) scan done at the time of her menopause 1 year ago. What is the most likely cause of her hypercalcemia?

A. Multiple myeloma
B. Parathyroid adenoma

C. Familial hypocalciuric hypercalcemia
D. Lymphoma
E. Breast Cancer

[36.2] A 62-year-old woman is noted to have multiple myeloma and an elevated calcium level. Which of the following therapies is useful for treating the hypercalcemia?

A. Bisphosphonates
B. Erythropoietin
C. Melphalan
D. Interferon alpha
E. Parathyroid hormone replacement

[36.3] A 22-year-old African-American woman presents with worsening cough and shortness of breath over 6 weeks, which did not improve with a course of antibiotics or antitussives. Her serum calcium level is found to be 11.5 mg/dL, and a chest x-ray reveals bilateral hilar lymphadenopathy. Which of the following is the most likely diagnosis?

A. Sarcoidosis
B. Mycoplasma pneumonia
C. Leukemia
D. Diabetes mellitus
E. Pulmonary embolism

[36.4] A 66-year-old man with known metastatic squamous cell carcinoma of the esophagus is brought to the emergency department for increasing lethargy and confusion. He is clinically dehydrated, his serum calcium level is 14 mg/dL, and his creatinine is 2.5 mg/dL, when 1 month ago it was 0.9 mg/dL. Which therapy for his hypercalcemia should be instituted first?

A. Intravenous bisphosphonate
B. Intravenous furosemide
C. Glucocorticoids
D. Intravenous normal saline
E. Chemotherapy for squamous cell carcinoma

Answers

[36.1] **B.** An asymptomatic, most likely chronically elevated calcium level is most likely caused by primary hyperparathyroidism caused by a parathyroid adenoma. The chronicity of this patient's hypercalcemia can be guessed at because she has osteoporosis and is only 1-year postmenopausal.

[36.2] **A.** Bisphosphonates are helpful in controlling hypercalcemia through inhibiting osteoclastic bone reabsorption. Erythropoietin is useful in treating the anemia associated with multiple myeloma, and melphalan, in combination with prednisone, is useful in treatment of the disease itself.

[36.3] **A.** Both sarcoidosis and lymphoma can present with cough, dyspnea, and hilar adenopathy on chest x-ray. In approximately 10% of cases, sarcoidosis can cause elevated calcium levels through the production of 1,25 vitamin D that occurs in the macrophages of the granulomas. This can also be seen in granulomas caused by tuberculosis and in lymphoma. Leukemia usually does not present in this manner, although it can cause hypercalcemia through invasion of the bone itself.

[36.4] **D.** Although all of the other therapies listed may be helpful in the treatment of hypercalcemia, given the clinical findings of dehydration and elevated creatinine with a history of previously normal renal function, volume expansion with normal saline would correct the dehydration and presumed prerenal azotemia, allowing the kidneys to more efficiently excrete calcium. Other therapies could be added if the response to normal saline alone is insufficient.

CLINICAL PEARLS

- Hypercalcemia that is acutely symptomatic is most likely caused by cancer. Asymptomatic hypercalcemia is most likely caused by primary hyperparathyroidism.
- In primary hyperparathyroidism, the serum parathyroid hormone (PTH) and calcium levels are elevated, and the phosphate levels are decreased. In malignancy-related hypercalcemia, calcium is high and PTH levels are suppressed.
- Symptoms of hyperparathyroidism can be remembered as stones, moans, groans, bones, and psychiatric overtones.
- Asymptomatic monoclonal gammopathy and multiple myeloma are most likely on opposite ends of a spectrum of neoplastic disease of plasmacytes.
- The classic triad of multiple myeloma consists of: a monoclonal antibody spike in the serum or light chains in the urine, 10% plasma cells in the bone marrow, and lytic bone lesions.

REFERENCES

Bataille R, Harousseau J. Multiple myeloma. N Engl J Med 1997;336(23):1657–64.

Longo DL. Plasma Cell Disorders. In: Braunwald E, Fauci AS, Kasper KL, et al, (eds). Harrison's principles of internal medicine, 15th Edition. New York: McGraw-Hill. 2001:727-733.

Deftos LJ. Hypercalcemia in malignant and inflammatory diseases. Endocrinol Metab Clin North Am 2002;31(1):141-158.

CASE 37

A 48-year-old woman calls 911 and is brought to the emergency room complaining of a sudden onset of dyspnea. She reports she was standing in the kitchen making dinner, when she suddenly felt as if she could not get enough air, her heart started racing, and she became light-headed and felt as if she would faint. She denied chest pain or cough. Her past medical history is only significant for gallstones, for which she underwent a cholecystectomy 2 weeks previously, which was complicated by a wound infection, requiring her to stay in the hospital for 8 days. She takes no medications regularly, only acetaminophen as needed for pain at her abdominal incision site.

On examination, she is tachypneic with a respiratory rate of 28 breaths per minute, her oxygen saturations are 84% on room air, and her heart rate is 124 bpm with a blood pressure of 118/89 mmHg. She appears uncomfortable, diaphoretic, and frightened. Her oral mucosa is slightly cyanotic, her jugular venous pressure is elevated, and her chest is clear to auscultation. Her heart is tachycardic but regular with a loud second sound in the pulmonic area, but no gallop or murmur. Her abdominal exam is benign, with a clean incision site without signs of infection. Her right leg is moderately swollen from mid-thigh to her feet, and her thigh and calf are mildly tender to palpation. Laboratory studies including cardiac enzymes are normal, her EKG reveals only sinus tachycardia, and her chest x-ray is interpreted as normal.

- **What is the most likely diagnosis?**

- **What is the most appropriate diagnostic step?**

ANSWERS TO CASE 37: Pulmonary Embolism

Summary: A 48-year-old woman is brought to the hospital for a very acute onset of dyspnea and is found to be tachypneic, tachycardic, and hypoxemic. On physical examination, she has elevated jugular venous pressure and a loud pulmonic closure sound, perhaps signifying acutely elevated pulmonary pressures. All of this, especially the finding of hypoxemia despite a clear chest radiograph, strongly suggests a pulmonary embolism, most likely caused by a lower-extremity deep venous thrombosis, a late complication of her recent hospitalization and relative immobilization.

- **Most likely diagnosis:** Pulmonary embolism.
- **Most appropriate diagnostic step:** Ventilation–perfusion lung scan or CT angiography, depending on availability in the hospital.

Analysis

Objectives

1. Understand the factors that predispose patients to develop thromboembolic disease.
2. Recognize the clinical presentation of pulmonary embolism.
3. Know the strategies to diagnose pulmonary embolism.
4. Understand the goals and methods of treatment of thromboembolism.

Considerations

Pulmonary embolism is a difficult diagnosis to establish because of the nonspecificity of presenting signs and symptoms, and the probabilistic nature of the most common noninvasive diagnostic tests. In patients with suspected pulmonary embolism, initial treatment is supportive to maintain adequate oxygenation and hemodynamic, and efforts are undertaken to try to diagnose the pulmonary embolism or other cause of the patient's symptoms. Often, a series of diagnostic tests is necessary to try to arrive at the likely diagnosis. Specific treatment of pulmonary embolism may include thrombolysis or surgical embolectomy for unstable patients, or initiation of anticoagulation as a long-term measure to prevent recurrence.

APPROACH TO SUSPECTED PULMONARY EMBOLISM

Definition

Deep venous thrombosis: Blood clot in the deep venous system that usually affects the lower extremities or pelvic veins.

Clinical Approach

Etiology and Risk Factors The successful treatment and management of pulmonary embolism requires a combination of clinical suspicion and the appropriate use of diagnostic tools. Pulmonary emboli (PE) usually arise from deep venous thrombi (DVT) and occasionally from less-common sources, including air, fat, tumor, bone marrow, talc, amniotic fluid, arthroplasty cement, and sepsis. More than 100 years ago, Rudolf **Virchow postulated three factors** that predispose to venous thrombus: **local trauma to vessel wall, a state of hypercoagulability, and venous stasis**. Genetic predisposition to hypercoagulability accounts for approximately 20% of PEs. **The most common inherited condition is the factor V Leiden mutation** expressed as resistance to the anticoagulant protein C; Table 37–1 lists other conditions. Malignancies can complicate or occasionally be diagnosed by venous thrombosis. These neoplastic cells are thought to generate thrombin or to synthesize various procoagulants. Even surgery has been found to significantly increase the risk of PE as late as 1 month postoperation.

Pathophysiology When venous thrombi dislodge from their site of formation, they may embolize to the pulmonary arteries causing pulmonary embolism. The **deep proximal lower extremity veins** are the **most common site of clot formation resulting in PE**, although thromboses in pelvic, calf, and upper extremity veins may also embolize. The obstruction to the pulmonary artery causes platelets to release vasoactive agents such as serotonin, thereby elevating pulmonary vascular resistance. The resulting increase in alveolar dead space and subsequent redistribution of blood flow creates areas of ventilation to perfusion mismatch (V/Q mismatch) and impairs gas exchange. Reflex bronchoconstriction causes increasing airway resistance. This cascade can result in pulmonary edema, hemorrhage, or loss of surfactant further decreasing lung compliance. As pulmonary vascular resistance increases, right-heart wall tension rises, resulting in dilation and dysfunction that may ultimately impair left heart function. **Progressive heart failure is the usual cause of death from pulmonary embolism.**

Table 37-1
CAUSES OF HYPERCOAGULABLE STATES

Heritable conditions
Factor V Leiden mutation
Hyperhomocysteinemia
Prothrombin gene mutation
Protein C and S deficiency
Antiphospholipid antibodies (or lupus anticoagulant)
Antithrombin III deficiency
Nonheritable conditions
Pregnancy
Oral contraceptive use
Hormone replacement therapy
Malignancy
Surgery

Clinical and Nonimaging Evaluation Pulmonary embolism can often mimic other cardiopulmonary diseases, making the diagnosis challenging. Acute onset of dyspnea is the most common symptom of PE, while tachypnea is the most frequently observed sign. Severe dyspnea accompanied by syncope, hypotension, or cyanosis may indicate massive PE, while pleuritic pain, cough, or hemoptysis may suggest a smaller more peripheral embolus causing infarction of lung tissue. Classic findings on physical exam, include tachycardia, low-grade fever, and signs of right ventricular dysfunction, including bulging neck veins, a left parasternal lift, an accentuated pulmonic component of the second heart sound, and a systolic murmur that increases with inspiration. Findings suggestive of DVT include pain, swelling, and erythema to the lower extremity, particularly the back of the leg below the knee. Some people will complain of calf tenderness.

Nonimaging diagnostic tools include laboratory tests and EKG. The serum D-dimer enzyme-linked immunoabsorbent assay (ELISA) is elevated (>500 ng/mL) in 90% of patients with PE, reflecting the breakdown of fibrin and thrombolysis. While the D-dimer ELISA has a high negative predictive value (thus is useful in excluding PE), it lacks specificity. Elevations may be seen in myocardial infarction, pneumonia, heart failure, cancer, or sepsis. While traditional teaching once stressed the importance of arterial blood gases (ABGs), more recent data indicates that ABGs may lack diagnostic utility. Abnormalities in the EKG may be useful in the evaluation of PE; the most frequent finding is T-wave inversions in the anterior leads (especially V1-V4). Other common findings include sinus tachycardia, new-onset atrial fibrillation, and an S wave in lead I, a Q wave in lead III, and an inverted T wave in lead III, (S1 Q3 T3).

Imaging Modalities Radiological studies have become critical in the diagnosis of pulmonary embolism and deep venous thrombosis. A plain film of the chest is often the first study ordered in a symptomatic patient with new-onset dyspnea. Although physicians are often taught that a normal chest x-ray is the most common finding in PE, nonspecific abnormalities such as atelectasis or parenchymal defects are actually more common; nevertheless, a normal chest radiograph does not exclude a PE. Other findings, such as an elevated hemidiaphragm, small pleural effusions, or cardiomegaly, may lead the physician to an alternative diagnosis, but often two separate diseases occur simultaneously. Nonspecific abnormalities, such as atelectasis or minimal parenchymal defects, are common in PE; nevertheless, a normal chest radiograph is entirely consistent with pulmonary embolism. In general, **acute onset** of **hypoxemia in a patient with a normal chest x-ray should be interpreted as PE until otherwise proven!** Classic abnormalities associated with PE include Westermark sign (a nonspecific prominence of the central pulmonary artery with decreased pulmonary vascularity), Hampton hump (a peripheral wedge-shaped density above the diaphragm), and Palla sign (enlargement of the right descending pulmonary artery). The chest radiograph is probably more important in identifying significant lung parenchymal disease (pneumonia, pulmonary edema) and cardiac disease (cardiomyopathy), as the cause of the respiratory symptoms.

Perfusion lung scanning (V/Q scan) remains the principal screening test for ruling out PE in patients without underlying cardiopulmonary disease. Generally, a normal V/Q scan effectively rules out PE; however the clinical suspicion must be combined with the imaging result. Low-, intermediate-, and high-probability scans detect 98% of PEs. The positive predictive value (PPV) of a high-probability scan is 87%, and when combined with high clinical suspicion, the PPV rises to 96%. The negative predictive value (NPV) of a low-probability scan is 86%, and when combined with low clinical suspicion, the NPV increases to 96%. For a normal/near normal scan, the NPV is also 96%. However, as many as 40% of patients with a high clinical suspicion of PE but a low-probability scan are actually found to have PE on further evaluation.

Preexisting cardiopulmonary disease significantly decreases the utility of the V/Q scan, such that 60% of patients with chronic obstructive pulmonary disease (COPD) have indeterminate scans. A nondiagnostic V/Q scan is often followed by venous ultrasonography of the lower extremities. The confirmation of DVT in a symptomatic patient is adequate to diagnose PE. Approximately 80–90% of clinically suspected PEs are thought to originate from deep vein thrombosis. However, about one-third of patients with a pulmonary embolism have no evidence of DVT on ultrasonography, possibly because the clot has already embolized to the lung or lies in the pelvic veins where ultrasonography is inadequate. In patients with clinically suspected PE, **pulmonary angiography is the gold standard** for making a definitive diagnosis after thorough evaluation with other imaging modalities remains unclear. The 95% specificity and sensitivity make this study ideal for detecting small emboli (1–2 mm); however, significant disadvantages include the invasiveness and lack of general availability. An alternative to the conventional lung scanning and pulmonary angiography is the spiral chest computed tomography. This approach best identifies PE in the proximal pulmonary vasculature (but is less sensitive for peripheral defects) and is less invasive than standard angiography. However, if CT findings are normal and the index of suspicion remains high, pulmonary angiography should be performed (see Figure 37-1 for algorithm).

Treatment Treatment options may be categorized in terms of primary and secondary therapy based on different management goals. **Primary therapy** consists of clot dissolution or **thrombolysis or removal of clot by surgical embolectomy,** and is usually reserved for patients with a **high risk of adverse outcomes if the clot remains,** that is, those with **right-heart failure or hypotension.**

When **right-heart function remains normal**, patients typically **have good outcomes with anticoagulation as secondary therapy**. Anticoagulation with heparin and Coumadin or placement of an inferior vena caval filter serves to

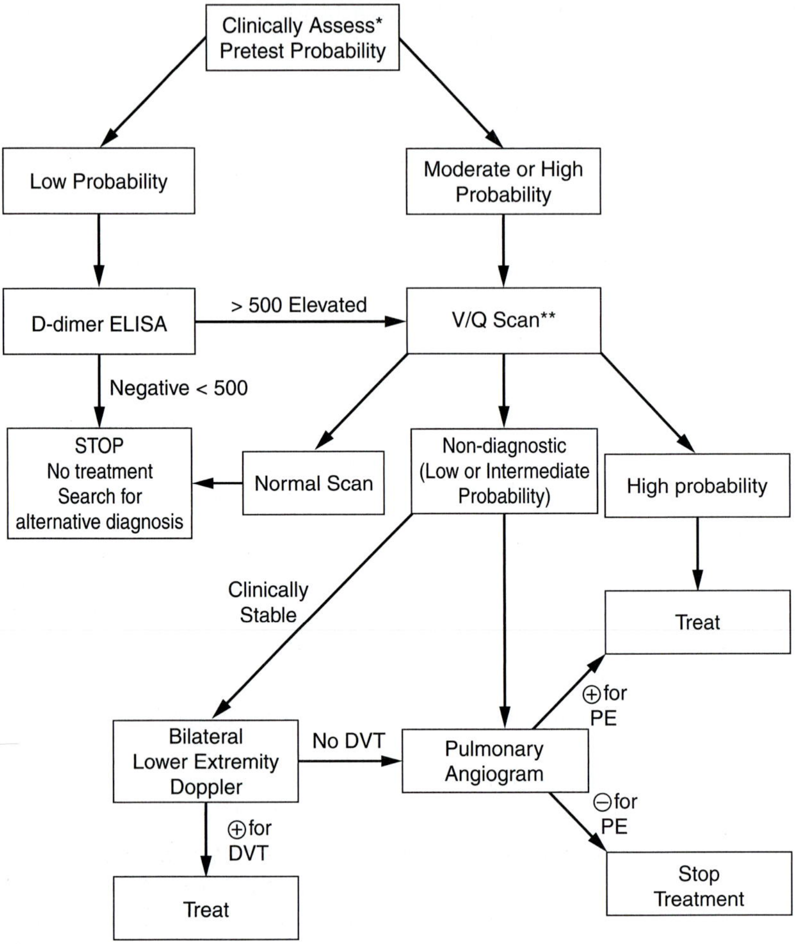

* Clinical clues:

1. Sudden onset of dyspnea or worsening of chronic dyspnea
2. Pleuritic chest pain or pleural rub
3. Hypoxemia ($SaO_2 < 92\%$)
4. Hemoptysis
5. Recent surgery or immobilization
6. Prior Hx of DVT or PE

** CT Angiography can be considered

Figure 37–1. Diagnostic Algorithm for Suspected Pulmonary Embolism..

prevent recurrent PE rather than removing existing clots. Guidelines for the prevention of recurrent PE include the following:

1. Treat DVT or PE with heparin for at least 5 days while overlapping with oral anticoagulation until the international normalized ratio (INR) has been therapeutic for 2 consecutive days.
2. Continue oral anticoagulation for at least 3 months with target INR of 2.5.
3. Patients with reversible or time-transient risk factors can be treated for 3–6 months. Patients with the first episode of DVT should be treated for at least 6 months. Patients with recurrent venous thrombosis or continuing risk factors, such as cancer or antiphospholipid antibody syndrome, should be treated indefinitely.
4. Inferior vena caval filter placement is recommended when there is contraindication to or failure of anticoagulation.

Comprehension Questions

[37.1] A 35-year-old woman complains of calf tenderness and acute dyspnea. The arterial blood gas reveals a PO_2 (pressure of oxygen) of 76 mmHg. Which of the following is the most common physical examination finding of pulmonary embolism?

A. Wheezing
B. Increased pulmonary component of the second heart sound
C. Tachypnea
D. Calf swelling
E. Pulmonary rales

[37.2] A 39-year-old man is noted to have a deep venous thrombosis without any known risk factors. He notes that his brother also developed a pulmonary embolism at age 45 years, and his mother developed a "clot in the leg" when she was in her thirties. Which of the following is the most likely inherited disorder in this patient?

A. Protein S deficiency
B. Antithrombin III deficiency
C. Factor V Leiden mutation
D. Antiphospholipid antibody syndrome
E. Familial malignancy syndrome

[37.3] A 54-year-old woman is noted to have a cervical cancer and presents with significant vaginal bleeding with a hemoglobin level of 7 g/dL. Her left leg is swollen, which on Doppler investigation reveals a deep venous thrombosis. Which of the following is the best treatment for the thrombus?

A. Intravenous unfractionated heparin
B. Fractionated subcutaneous heparin

C. Subcutaneous unfractionated heparin
D. Oral Coumadin
E. Vena cava filter

Answers

[37.1] **C.** Tachypnea is the most common physical sign associated with pulmonary embolus.

[37.2] **C.** Factor V Leiden mutation is the most common hereditary thrombophilia.

[37.3] **E.** Cervical cancer with significant vaginal bleeding is a relative contraindication for anticoagulation. Thus, a vena cava filter is the most appropriate choice in this patient.

REFERENCES

Goldhaber SZ. Pulmonary Thromboembolism. In: Braunwald E, Fauci As, Kasper KL, et al, (eds). Harrison's Principles of Internal Medicine, 15th ed. New York: McGraw-Hill. 2002:1509-1513. .

Goldhaber S. Pulmonary embolism. N Engl J Med 1998;339:93–101.

Tabas J. Radiological imaging in acute pulmonary embolism. Resident Staff Physician 2002;(48(7):12–18.

CASE 38

A 68-year-old woman is brought to the emergency room after coughing up a cupful of red blood. For the previous 3–4 months, she has had a chronic nonproductive cough, but no fevers. More recently, she has noticed some blood-streaked sputum. On review of her symptoms, she reports increased fatigue, decreased appetite, and a 25-lb weight loss in the past 3 months. She denies chest pain, fever, chills, or night sweats. The patient has smoked one pack of cigarettes per day for the past 35 years. She drinks two martinis every day and has not had any significant mental illness. She worked in a library in the New England area for 35 years. She does not take any medication except for one aspirin per day.

This is a thin woman who is mildly anxious, alert, and oriented. Her blood pressure is 150/90 mmHg, her heart rate is 88 bpm, her respiratory rate is 16 breaths per minute, and her temperature is 99.2°F. Her neck examination reveals no lymphadenopathy, thyromegaly, or carotid bruit. The chest has scattered rhonchi bilaterally, but there are no wheezes or crackles. The cardiovascular examination reveals a regular rate and rhythm, without rubs, gallops, or murmurs. The abdomen is benign with no hepatosplenomegaly. Examination of her extremities reveals 1+ ankle edema and no cyanosis; there is finger clubbing. The neurological examination is normal.

- **What is your next step?**

- **What is the most likely diagnosis?**

ANSWERS TO CASE 38: Hemoptysis, Lung Cancer

Summary: A 68-year-old female smoker has coughed up a cupful of red blood. For the previous 3–4 months, she has had a chronic nonproductive cough, and more recently, some blood-streaked sputum. She reports increase fatigability, reduced appetite, and a 25-lb weight loss in the past 3 months. She denies chest pain, fever, chills, or night sweats. On examination, her chest reveals scattered rhonchi bilaterally without wheezes or crackles. She has clubbing of the fingers.

◆ **Next step:** Chest x-ray film, posterioanterior and lateral.

◆ **Most likely diagnosis:** Lung cancer.

Analysis

Objectives

1. Know the differential diagnosis of hemoptysis.
2. Be familiar with the risk factors for and the clinical presentation of lung cancer (including superior vena cava [SVC] syndrome and Horner syndrome).
3. Know the workup of the solitary pulmonary nodule.
4. Be familiar with the general principles of treatment of lung cancer.

Considerations

This is a 68-year-old woman with a past medical history significant for tobacco use for more than 25 years who presents to the emergency room with hemoptysis, cough, reduced appetite, and weight loss. The most likely diagnosis in this case is lung cancer. On physical exam, there was clubbing. Finger clubbing is defined as an enlargement of the terminal digital phalanges with the loss of the nail bed angle. Clubbing of the fingers is seen in a variety of conditions, including congenital heart disease and a number of pulmonary diseases. Clubbing can also be congenital and unassociated with any disease. In pulmonary disease, clubbing of fingers is most commonly seen in patients with lung cancer or with chronic septic conditions, such as bronchiectasis or lung abscess. Finger clubbing is not commonly seen in patients with chronic obstructive lung disease or chronic TB, and if it appears in patients with these conditions, it should lead to suspicion of development of a tumor. Our patient's finger clubbing is, therefore, another element on physical examination that reinforces the suspicion of lung cancer.

APPROACH TO HEMOPTYSIS

Definitions

Horner syndrome: Symptoms are ptosis, loss of pupillary dilation (miosis), and loss of sweating on the same side of the face (anhydrosis) caused by compression of the superior cervical ganglion.

Superior vena cava syndrome (SVCS): Obstruction of venous drainage leads to dilation of collateral veins of the upper part of the chest and neck, edema of the face, neck and upper part of the torso, shortness of breath, and CNS symptoms, such as confusion, headache, and visual problems.

Clinical Approach

Hemoptysis is defined as a coughing up blood as a result of bleeding from the respiratory tract. It is an alarming symptom, both because it may be a manifestation of a serious underlying diagnosis such as malignancy, and because massive amounts of hemoptysis can fill up alveolar air spaces and cause asphyxiation. Hemoptysis, particularly if in large quantity or recurrent, is a potentially fatal event requiring an immediate search for the cause and precise location of the bleeding. A reasonable definition of massive hemoptysis is ≥600 mL of blood in 24 hours. Hemoptysis must be differentiated from hematemesis and from blood dripping into the bronchial passages from the nose, mouth, and nasopharynx. **Currently, the most common causes of hemoptysis in the United States are bronchitis and lung cancer.** Historically, the most common causes have been tuberculosis, lung abscess, and bronchiectasis. History is an important diagnostic step: blood-streaked purulent sputum suggests bronchitis; **chronic copious sputum production suggests bronchiectasis. Hemoptysis with an acute onset of pleuritic chest pain and dyspnea** suggests a **pulmonary embolism**. Every patient with hemoptysis should undergo a chest x-ray to look for a mass lesion, evidence of bronchiectasis, or parenchymal disease. If the chest radiograph reveals a pulmonary mass, the patient should undergo fiberoptic bronchoscopy to localize the site of bleeding, and to visualize and attempt to biopsy any endobronchial lesion. Patients with massive hemoptysis require measures to maintain their airway and to prevent spilling blood into unaffected areas of the lungs. They should be kept at rest with suppression of cough. If the bleeding is localized to one lung, the affected side should be placed in a dependent position so bleeding does not flow into the contralateral side. They may also require endotracheal intubation, and rigid bronchoscopy for better airway control and suction capacity.

Clinical Presentation of Lung Cancer The manifestation (symptoms and signs of lung cancer) depends on the tumor's location and the type of spread. Some patients may be completely asymptomatic. In these cases, a lung nodule is usually found on routine chest x-ray. Most primary lung tumors are endobronchial. Therefore, patients typically present with cough with or without hemoptysis. In patients with chronic bronchitis, increases in intensity and intractability of the existing cough may suggest the presence of malignancy. Sputum production is usually not excessive, but occasionally it may be watery and profuse, as in alveolar cell carcinoma, and is often blood-streaked. Chest pain is also a possible symptom of lung cancer and suggests the neoplastic invasion of the chest wall. Symptoms of weight loss, malaise, and fatigue usually develop later in the disease course. **Malignant serosanguineous pleural effusion is common and often large and recurrent**. Patients may present with a complaint of chest pain and an increasing shortness of breath. **Horner syndrome is caused by the invasion of the cervicothoracic sympathetic nerves and occurs with apical tumors (Pancoast tumor)**. Phrenic nerve invasion may cause diaphragmatic paralysis. Superior vena cava obstruction is produced by direct extension of the tumor or by compression from the neighboring lymph nodes. Superior vena cava syndrome has a dramatic clinical presentation and requires urgent care. Small cell lung cancer and squamous cell lung cancer frequently cause SVCS.

Lung cancer may also be accompanied by numerous extrapulmonary paraneoplastic manifestations. All levels of the nervous system may be affected, leading to encephalopathy, subacute cerebellar degeneration, Eaton-Lambert syndrome, and peripheral neuropathy. Small cell carcinoma may secrete adrenocorticotropic hormone (ACTH), resulting in Cushing syndrome, or antidiuretic hormone (ADH) with water retention and hyponatremia. Squamous cell tumors may secrete parathyroid hormone-like substances that produce hypercalcemia. Other endocrine syndromes associated with primary lung cancer include thyrotoxicosis, gynecomastia, and skin pigmentation. Several hematologic disorders, including thrombocytopenic purpura, leukemoid reaction, polycythemia, and myelophthisic anemia may also occur.

Once a patient presents with symptoms or radiographic findings suggestive of lung cancer, the next steps are

1. Tissue diagnosis to establish malignant diagnosis and histologic type.
2. Staging to determine resectability or curative potential.
3. Cancer treatment: surgery, radiotherapy, or chemotherapy.

Risk Factors of Lung Cancer Primary lung cancer is the leading cause of cancer deaths in both men and women. The incidence of lung cancer is increasing, mainly among women. Approximately 85% of lung cancers are linked to smoking. Cigarette smoking accounts for 90% of cases in men and approximately 70% of cases in women. A small proportion of lung cancers, 16% in men and 5% in women, are related to occupational agents, often overlapping with smoking, such as asbestos, radiation, and nickel chromate exposure. The exact role of air pollution is uncertain. Occasionally, lung cancers, especially adenocarcinoma and alveolar cell carcinoma, are associated with pulmonary scars. Damage to DNA, oncogene activation, and genetic factors are also thought to be of primary importance in the pathophysiology of lung cancer.

Histologically, primary lung cancer can be divided into three large categories: small cell lung cancer (SCLC), nonsmall cell lung cancer (NSCLC), and a group of miscellaneous types. Nonsmall cell lung cancer is farther divided into three types: squamous cell carcinoma, adenocarcinoma, and large cell carcinoma. Small cell lung cancer and nonsmall cell lung cancer constitute 95% of primary lung cancer. As compared with NSCLC, SCLC tends to metastasize much earlier and more widely, and is more likely to respond to chemotherapy. The relative frequency of the histologic type is 20–25% for SCLC and 70–75% for NSCLC. Squamous and small cell cancers are usually central lesions. Adenocarcinoma and large cell cancer are peripheral lesions. Adenocarcinoma metastasizes early, especially to the CNS, bones, and adrenal glands, and they usually present as solitary nodules. Adenocarcinoma has the least association with smoking and a stronger association with pulmonary scars. Squamous cancer does not usually metastasize early. It usually is a central/hilar lesion with local extension and may present with symptoms caused by bronchial obstruction, such as atelectasis and pneumonia; it may present on chest x-ray as a cavitary lesion. Squamous cell lung cancer is by far the most likely lung cancer to cavitate. Small cell cancer, previously called oat cell, is extremely aggressive. Eighty percent of patients have metastasis at the time of diagnosis, so its treatment is usually different from that of other lung cancers. Contrary to other lung cancers, cavitation never occurs in small cell cancer. Small cell lung cancer can cause syndrome of inappropriate antidiuretic hormone secretion (SIADH), ectopic ACTH production, and Eaton-Lambert syndrome. Large cell cancer is usually a peripheral lesion and tends to metastasize to the CNS and mediastinum, causing SVCS or hoarseness as a consequence of laryngeal nerve paralysis. If there is a history of asbestos exposure, squamous cancer, adenocarcinoma, and mesothelioma should all be considered. Table 38–1 lists lung cancer characteristics.

Solitary Pulmonary Nodule The solitary pulmonary nodule is defined as a nodule surrounded by normal parenchyma. Approximately 35% of solitary pulmonary nodules are malignant. Proper management of a solitary nodule in an individual patient depends on a variety of elements: age, risk factors, presence of calcifications and size of the nodule. The presence and type of calcification on a solitary pulmonary nodule can be helpful. "Popcorn," and "bull's-eye" calcifications suggest a benign process. In low-risk patients, age 35 years and younger and nonsmokers, a solitary calcified nodule can be followed every 3 months with chest x-rays and it is considered benign after 2 years if there is no growth. The risk of malignancy in such patients is less than 1%. High-risk patients require a more aggressive approach: a bronchoscopy with biopsy of the lesion is highly recommended to sort out benign from malignant lesions. The size of the nodule is another important factor, because the likelihood of malignancy increases with size. Lesions greater than 2.5cm in diameter are highly suspicious for malignancy.

General Principles of Treatment Treatment of lung cancer is performed with either curative or palliative intent.

The treatment of lung cancer consists of surgical resection, chemotherapy and/or radiation therapy in different combinations, depending on the tissue type and on extent of the disease.

Table 38-1
LUNG CANCER CHARACTERISTICS

	SMALL CELL	SQUAMOUS CELL	ADENOCARCINOMA	LARGE CELL
Location	Central	Central	Peripheral	Peripheral
Associated with smoking	Yes	Yes	No	Yes
Cavitation	Rare	Most likely		
Metastases	Early	Late	Early	Late
Extrapulmonary manifestations	SIADH, ectopic ACTH, Eaton-Lambert, Cushing, peripheral neuropathy	Hypercalcemia	Thrombophlebitis	SVC syndrome or hoarseness

Abbreviations: ACTH = adrenocorticotropic hormone; SIADH = syndrome of inappropriate antidiuretic hormone secretion; SVC = superior vena cava.

Small cell lung cancer is nearly always metastatic at time of diagnosis, and therefore, not eligible for surgical resection. It is staged as either limited disease, that is, disease confined to one hemithorax that can be treated within a radiotherapy port, or extensive disease, that is, contralateral lung involvement or distant metastases. All patients with untreated small cell lung cancer have a grim prognosis, with survival measured in weeks. With treatment, survival can be prolonged, and approximately 20–30% of patients with limited stage disease can be cured with radiotherapy and chemotherapy.

Once the diagnosis of nonsmall cell lung cancer is made, the next step is to stage the disease by the TNM (tumor, node, metastasis) system (size, local spread of tumor, node involvement, and metastatic spread) (see Table 38–2). Patients with NSCLC who are stage I or II, or some with IIIA, may be candidates for curative resection and radiotherapy. The next big decision is whether the patient can withstand an operation. Because most lung cancer occurs in older patients who have been smokers, they frequently have underlying cardiopulmonary disease and require preoperative evaluation,

Table 38-2
SUMMARY OF STAGING

Staging of lung cancer is based on the TNM system. T is for tumor size or extension to adjacent tissues; N is for nodal involvement; and M is for distant metastases.

Stage I: Tumor is without nodal involvement or distant metastasis.

IA: Tumor <3 cm without extension to adjacent tissues

IB: Tumor either (a) is >3 cm or (b) invades visceral pleura, causes atelectasis of less than entire lung, or extends at least 2 cm from carina.

Stage II: Tumor is without distant metastasis.

IIA: Tumor <3 cm with ipsilateral hilar and/or ipsilateral bronchial nodal involvement.

IIB: (a) Stage IB with involvement of ipsilateral hilar or bronchial nodes or (b) tumor invading chest wall, diaphragm, mediastinal pleura, pericardium, or (c) tumor with atelectasis of entire lung or extending within 2 cm of carina.

Stage III: Tumor is without distant metastasis.

IIIA: Tumor invading chest wall, diaphragm, mediastinal pleura, pericardium, or tumor with atelectasis of entire lung, or tumor extending within 2 cm of carina with ipsilateral hilar or bronchial nodal involvement, or (b) tumor with involvement of ipsilateral mediastinal and/or subcarinal nodes.

IIIB: Involvement of contralateral nodes or of scalene or supraclavicular nodes (either side), or (b) tumor invading mediastinum, heart or great vessels, trachea/esophagus, vertebral body or carina, or (c) tumor with malignant pleural or pericardial effusion, or (d) satellite tumor nodules within same lobe as primary tumor.

Stage IV: Distant metastasis (including tumor nodules in different lobe from primary tumor).

including pulmonary function testing, to predict whether they have sufficient pulmonary reserve to tolerate a lobectomy or pneumonectomy.

Comprehension Questions

[38.1] A 67-year-old long-time smoker with COPD presents with 3 days of headaches and plethoric swelling of his face and right arm. Which of the following is the most likely diagnosis?

A. Angioedema
B. Hypothyroidism
C. SVC syndrome
D. Trichinosis

[38.2] A 64-year-old woman comes to your office complaining of hoarse voice for 4 months. She has not had fever, sore throat, or a cough. On exam, she has expiratory wheezes in her left mid-lung fields. What is the best next step?

A. Prescribe antibiotics for bronchitis
B. Order a chest x-ray
C. Advise gargling with salt-water solution
D. Prescribe an albuterol inhaler

[38.3] A 33-year-old woman who is a nonsmoker had lost 30 lb of weight and had a cough. She is noted to have a lung mass on chest radiograph. Which of the following lung cancers is the most likely cell type?

A. Squamous cell
B. Adenocarcinoma
C. Small cell
D. Large cell

[38.4] A 52-year-old man presents with dyspnea and chest x-ray shows a hilar mass with ipsilateral pleural effusion. What is the best next step?

A. CT scan of the chest, head, and abdomen for cancer staging
B. Pulmonary function testing to evaluate pulmonary reserve to evaluate for pulmonectomy
C. Obtain a specific tissue diagnosis by biopsy of the hilar mass
D. Initiate palliative radiation because the patient is not a candidate for curative resection

Answers

[38.1] **C.** The patient has features of SVC syndrome, caused by compression of the superior vena cava, almost always by a thoracic malignancy. Urgent diagnosis and treatment is mandatory because of impaired cerebral venous drainage, and resultant increased intracranial pressure or possibly fatal intracranial venous thrombosis. Angioedema, hypothyroidism, and trichinosis may all cause facial swelling, but not the plethora or swelling of the arm.

[38.2] **B.** This patient has chronic hoarseness and unilateral wheezing. This suggests an intrathoracic mass causing bronchial obstruction and impairment of the recurrent laryngeal nerve, causing vocal cord paralysis, thus an imaging study of the chest is essential.

[38.3] **B.** Ninety percent of patients with lung cancer of *all* histologic types have a smoking history. The most common form of lung cancer that is found in nonsmokers, young patients, and in women is adenocarcinoma.

[38.4] **C.** Tissue diagnosis is essential to proper treatment of any malignancy, and should always be the first step. Once a specific tissue diagnosis is obtained, the cancer is staged for prognosis and to guide therapy; that is, Is there a possibility of curative resection? Questions for this patient include the tissue type, location of spread, and whether the pleural effusion is caused by malignancy.

CLINICAL PEARLS

- Almost all patients with hemoptysis require evaluation with bronchoscopy. Massive hemoptysis may result in death by asphyxiation.
- Lung cancer is the leading cause of cancer deaths in men and women.
- A solitary pulmonary nodule in a nonsmoker <35 years old can be followed radiographically. For other patients, a biopsy is necessary, either bronchoscopic, percutaneous, or surgical.
- The steps in management of a patient with suspected lung cancer include tissue diagnosis, staging, preoperative evaluation, and treatment with surgery, radiotherapy, or chemotherapy.
- Small cell lung cancer is usually metastatic at time of diagnosis, and not resectable. Nonsmall cell lung cancer is curable by resection if it is stage I or II disease, and some stage IIIA.

REFERENCES

Minna JD. Neoplasms of the Lung. In: Braunwald E, Fauci AS, Kasper KL, et al., (eds). Harrison's Principles of Internal Medicine, 15th ed. New York: McGraw-Hill. 2001:562-571.

CASE 39

A 44-year old man presents with the sudden onset of shaking chills, fever, and a productive cough. He was in his usual state of good health until 1 week ago, when he developed mild nasal congestion and achiness. He otherwise felt well until last night, when he became fatigued, feverish, and developed cough associated with right-side pleuritic chest pain. His past medical history is remarkable only for a 15 pack-year history of smoking. In your office, his vital signs are normal except for a temperature of 102°F. His oxygen saturation on room air is 100%. He is comfortable, except when he coughs. His exam is unremarkable except for bronchial breath sounds and end inspiratory crackles in the right lower lung field.

- **What is your diagnosis?**

- **What is your next step?**

ANSWERS TO CASE 39: Community-Acquired Pneumonia

Summary: A 44-year-old healthy man presents with the sudden onset of shaking chills, fever, and a productive cough. One week ago, he developed mild nasal congestion and achiness. Last night, he became fatigued, feverish, and developed cough associated with right-side pleuritic chest pain. He has a 15 pack-year smoking history. His vital signs are normal except for a temperature of 102°F. His oxygen saturation on room air is 100%. He is comfortable, except when he coughs. His exam is unremarkable except for bronchial breath sounds and end inspiratory crackles in the right lower lung field.

- **Most likely diagnosis:** Community-acquired pneumonia.
- **Next step:** Oral antibiotic therapy, pain relievers, antipyretics, and cough suppressants for relief of symptoms. Close outpatient followup (with followup in 1–2 weeks).

Analysis

Objectives

1. Know the causative organisms in community-acquired pneumonia and the appropriate therapeutic regimens.
2. Understand the clinical criteria indicating inpatient versus outpatient therapy.
3. Discuss the role of radiologic and laboratory evaluation in the diagnosis of pneumonia.
4. Understand the difference between aspiration pneumonitis and aspiration pneumonia.

Considerations

This previously healthy 44-year-old man has an acute onset of productive cough, fatigue, fever, and shaking chills. He is a smoker. The pulmonary examination suggests a focal consolidation of the lungs, which is consistent with a bacterial process, such as infection with *Streptococcus peneumoniae*.

APPROACH TO SUSPECTED PNEUMONIA

Pneumonia is an infection of the parenchyma of the lungs. Patients may present with any of a combination of cough, fever, pleuritic chest pain, sputum production, shortness of breath, hypoxia, or respiratory distress. Certain clinical presentations are associated with particular infectious agents. For example, the "typical" pneumonia is often described as having a sudden onset of fever, cough with productive sputum, is often associated with pleuritic chest pain, and may have **rust-colored sputum**. This is the classical description of pneumococcal pneumonia. The **"atypical" pneumonia** is characterized as having a **more insidious onset, with a dry cough**, prominent extrapulmonary symptoms such as **headache, myalgias, sore throat**, and a chest radiograph that appears much worse than the auscultatory findings. This type of presentation is usually attributed to *Mycoplasma pneumoniae*. Although there is some diagnostic value to these characterizations, it is very difficult to reliably distinguish between typical and atypical organisms based on clinical history and physical examination as the cause of a specific patient's pneumonia. Therefore, pneumonias are typically classified according to the immune status of the host, the radiographic findings, and the setting in which the infection was acquired, in an attempt to identify the likely causative organism and to guide initial empiric therapy.

Typical community-acquired pneumonia, as opposed to nosocomial or hospital-acquired pneumonia, is most commonly caused by streptococcus pneumonia, *Moraxella catarrhalis*, or *Haemophilus influenzae*. Viruses, such as influenza and adenovirus, can also cause pneumonia. Atypical pneumonia, which is characterized by a more insidious onset, a dry cough, muscle aches, headaches, and sore throat, is typically caused by *Mycoplasma pneumoniae*. However, other organisms such as *Legionella* (typically associated with preceding gastrointestinal symptoms), and *Chlamydia pneumoniae* should be considered. In a patient with specific risk factors *Chlamydia psittaci* (bird exposure), coccidiomycosis (travel to the American southwest), or histoplasmosis (endemic to the Mississippi Valley) may be the cause. In a patient with AIDS or immunosuppression, *Pneumocystis carinii* should be added to the differential diagnosis. Tuberculosis is a possibility in patients with a history suggestive of exposure or predisposition, such as AIDS, to this disease.

Those with hospital- or nursing home-acquired infection, termed nosocomial pneumonia, should have antibiotic coverage for Gram-negative organisms. An inability to perform basic hygiene leads to colonization of the oral cavity with enteric Gram-negative bacteria such as E. coli. In these cases, the patient's normal defenses against pulmonary infection are often compromised. A patient's level of consciousness may be depressed; he may be intubated or unable to cough efficiently, leading to an increased risk of pulmonary infection.

Once the clinical diagnosis of pneumonia has been made, the next step is to try to risk stratify the patients, to decide which patients can be treated safely as outpatients with oral antibiotics and which need hospitalization. In 1997, Fine and colleagues described a prediction rule that accurately identified those patients with community-acquired pneumonia who had a low risk of death or other adverse outcomes. The PORT study used some basic demographic, historical questions and physical exam findings to separate out those patients with higher risk of complications that may benefit from hospitalization, as opposed to those who could be discharged on oral antibiotics with close followup. Patients younger than age 50 years without these medical problems or physical exam findings are assigned to risk class I and have about a 0.1% risk of death and a 5.1% risk of hospitalization over the next 30 days. Patients who are hypoxemic, hemodynamically unstable, or who have multiple risk factors (see Table 39–1) have poor prognoses and usually require hospitalization. Patients in risk classes I to III can usually be safely treated as outpatients with

Table 39-1
RISK STRATIFICATION OF PNEUMONIA

History consistent with high risk
Age over 50 years
History of cancer
Congestive heart failure
Cerebrovascular disease
Renal or liver disease
Physical findings of high risk
Altered mental status
Tachycardia (≥125 beats per minute)
Tachypnea (>30 breaths per minute)
Hypotension (<90 mmHg systolic)
Temperature <35°C (95°F) >40°C (104°F)

oral antibiotics. Those in risk classes IV and V, or who are hypoxemic or hemodynamically unstable, require inpatient therapy.

While outpatients are usually diagnosed and empiric treatment is begun based on clinical findings, further diagnostic evaluation is important in hospitalized patients. Chest radiography is important to try to define the cause and extent of the pneumonia and to look for complications, such as parapneumonic effusion or lung abscess. Unless the patient cannot mount an immune response, as in severe neutropenia, or the process is very early, every patient with pneumonia will have a visible pulmonary infiltrate. The pattern of infiltration can yield diagnostic clues*. Diffuse interstitial infiltrates are common in *Pneumocystis carinii* pneumonia and viral processes. Conversely, pleural effusions are almost never seen in *Pneumocystis carinii* pneumonia. Bilateral apical infiltrate suggests tuberculosis. Appearance of **cavitation** suggests a necrotizing infection such as *Staphylococcus aureus*, tuberculosis, or Gram-negative organisms such as *Klebsiella pneumoniae*. Serial chest radiography on inpatients is usually unnecessary, because it takes many weeks for the infiltrate to resolve, and is typically done if the patient is not clinically improving, or has a pleural effusion, or has a necrotizing infection.

Microbiologic studies, such as sputum Gram stain and culture, and blood cultures are important to try to identify the specific etiologic agent causing the illness. However, use of sputum Gram stain and culture is limited by the frequent contamination by upper respiratory flora as the specimen is expectorated. However, if the sputum appears purulent, and it is minimally contaminated (>25 polymorphonuclear cells and <10 epithelial cells per low-powered field), the diagnostic yield is good. Additionally, blood cultures can be helpful, because 30–40% of patients with pneumococcal pneumonias are bacteremic.

*Infection with *Streptococcus pneumoniae* classically presents with a dense lobar infiltrate, often with an associated parapneumonic effusion.

Serologic studies can be performed to diagnose patients who are infected with organisms not easily cultured, for example, *Legionella*, *Mycoplasma*, or *Chlamydia pneumoniae*.

Finally, fiberoptic bronchoscopy with bronchoalveolar lavage is often done in seriously ill or immunocompromised patients, or in those patients who are not responding to therapy, to try to obtain a specimen from the lower respiratory tract for routine Gram stain and culture, as well as more sophisticated resting, such as direct fluorescent antibody testing for various organism, for example, *Legionella*.

Initially, empiric treatment is based upon the most common organisms given the clinical scenario. For outpatient therapy of **community-acquired pneumonia**, macrolide antibiotics such as **azithromycin**, or antipneumococcal **quinolones** such as gatifloxacin or levofloxacin, are good choices to treat Streptococcus pneumoniae, *Mycoplasma*, and other common organisms. **Hospitalized patients** with community-acquired pneumonia are usually treated with an **intravenous third-generation cephalosporin plus a macrolide** or with an antipneumococcal quinolone. For immunocompetent patients with hospital-acquired or ventilator-associated pneumonias, the causes include any of the organisms that can cause community-acquired pneumonia, *Pseudomonas aeruginosa,* or *Staphylococcus aureus*, as well as more Gram-negative enteric bacteria and oral anaerobes. Accordingly, the initial antibiotic coverage is broader and includes an antipseudomonal beta-lactam, such as piperacillin or cefepime, plus an aminoglycoside, and may include clindamycin.

For immunocompromised patients, such as AIDS patients, the spectrum of potential pathogens is much broader and includes *Pneumocystis carinii* pneumonia, unusual bacteria such as *Rohodococcus equi*, tuberculosis, as well as fungal organisms such as *Histoplasma* or *Cryptococcus*. It should be remembered, however, that even in AIDS patients, the most common cause of pneumonia is *S. pneumoniae*. If an AIDS patient presents with an acute onset of fever and a productive cough with purulent sputum, pneumococcal pneumonia is the most likely diagnosis.

Two other commonly confused pulmonary syndromes deserve mention at this point. **Aspiration pneumonitis** is a chemical injury to the lungs caused by aspiration of acidic gastric contents into the lungs. Because of the high acidity, gastric contents are normally sterile, so this is not an infectious process, but rather a chemical burn, which causes a severe inflammatory response, which is proportional to the volume of the aspirate and the degree of acidity. This inflammatory response can be profound, and produce respiratory distress and a pulmonary infiltrate which is apparent within four to six hours, and typically resolves within 48 hours. Aspiration of gastric contents is most likely to occur in patients with a depressed level of consciousness, such as those under anesthesia, or suffering from a drug overdose, or after a seizure.

Aspiration pneumonia, by contrast, is an infectious process caused by inhalation of oropharyngeal secretions that are colonized by bacterial pathogens. It should be noted that many healthy adults frequently aspirate small volumes of oropharyngeal secretions while sleeping (this is the primary way that bacteria gain entry to the lungs), but usually the material is cleared by coughing, ciliary transport, or normal immune defenses, so that no clinical infection results. However, any process that increases the volume or bacterial organism burden of the secretion, or impairs the normal defense mechanisms can produce clinically apparent pneumonia. This is most commonly seen in elderly patients with dysphagia, such as stroke victims, who may aspirate significant volumes of oral secretions, and those with poor dental care. The affected lobe of the lung depends upon the patient's position: in recumbent patients, the posterior segments of the upper lobes and apical segments of the lower lobes are most common. In contrast to aspiration pneumonitis, where aspiration of vomitus may be witnessed, the aspiration of oral secretions is typically silent, and should be suspected when any institutionalized patient with dysphagia presents respiratory symptoms and pulmonary infiltrate in a dependent segment of the lung.

Antibiotic therapy for aspiration pneumonia is similar to that of other pneumonias, that is, it should cover typical respiratory pathogens such as *S. pneumoniae* and *H. influenzae*, as well as Gram-negative organisms and oral anaerobes. Treatment for aspiration pneumonitis, because it is usually not infectious, is mainly supportive. Antibiotics are often added if secondary bacterial infection is suspected because of failure to improve within 48 hours, or if the gastric contents are suspected to be colonized because of acid suppression or because of bowel obstruction.

Comprehension Questions

[39.1] A 65-year-old cigarette smoker with a history of hypertension and mild congestive heart failure presents to the emergency room with worsening cough, fever, and dyspnea at rest. The illness began one week ago with fever, muscle aches, abdominal pain, and diarrhea, with the nonproductive cough developing later that week, and rapidly becoming worse. Therapy for which atypical organism must be considered in this case?

A. *Chlamydia pneumoniae*
B. *Mycoplasma pneumoniae*
C. *Legionella pneumophila*
D. Coccidiomycosis
E. *Aspergillus fumigatus*

[39.2] An 85-year-old nursing home resident has dementia, requiring that she have assistance in all activities of daily life. She has a 3-day history of fever and productive cough. Chest x-ray reveals a right middle lobe consolidation. Which of the following is the most likely description of the mechanism of infection?

A. Aspiration of oral flora
B. Aspiration of gastric contents

C. Inhalation of *M. tuberculosis* droplet nuclei.
D. Hypersensitivity pneumonitis

[39.3] A 56-year-old man is brought into the emergency room intoxicated with alcohol. He has repeated bouts of emesis and is found choking. Lung examination reveals some crackles in the right lung base. Which of the following is the most appropriate management?

A. Initiate azithromycin
B. Initiate corticosteroid therapy
C. Initiate haloperidol therapy
D. Observation

Answers

[39.1] **C.** *Legionella* typically presents with myalgias, abdominal pain, diarrhea, and a severe pneumonia.

[39.2] **A.** This nursing home resident likely has aspirated oral bacterial flora. There is no history of a choking episode or emesis.

[39.3] **D.** Antibiotic therapy is generally not indicated for aspiration pneumonitis.

CLINICAL PEARLS

❖ It is difficult to reliably distinguish clinically between typical and atypical causes of pneumonia. Therefore, diagnosis and empiric treatment of pneumonia is based upon the setting in which it was acquired (community acquired or nosocomial) and the immune status of the host.

❖ Clinical criteria, such as patient age >50 years, coexisting illnesses, tachycardia, and tachypnea, can be used to risk stratify patients with pneumonia to decide who can be treated as an outpatient and who requires hospitalization.

❖ Although initial antibiotic therapy is empiric, the etiologic agent can frequently be identified based on chest radiography, blood cultures, or sputum Gram stain and culture (if >25 polymorphonuclear cells and <10 epithelial cells per low-power field).

❖ Aspiration pneumonitis is a noninfectious chemical burn caused by inhalation of acidic gastric contents in patients with decreased level of consciousness, such as seizure or overdose.

❖ Aspiration pneumonia is pulmonary infection caused by aspiration of colonized oropharyngeal secretions and is seen in patients with impaired swallowing, such as stroke victims.

REFERENCES

Fine MJ, Auble TE, Yealy DM, et al. A prediction rule to identify low-risk patients with community-acquired pneumonia. *N Engl J Med* 1997;336(4):243–50.

Halm EA, Teirstein AS, et al. Management of community-acquired pneumonia. *N Engl J Med* 2002;347:2039–45.

Marik P. Aspiration pneumonitis and aspiration pneumonia. *N Engl J Med* 2001;344:665–71.

CASE 40

A 58-year-old woman comes to the office after a near-fainting spell she experienced 1 day ago. She was outside playing tennis and became lightheaded. She vomited and felt light-headed, and spent the rest of the day lying down with mild, diffuse, abdominal pain and nausea. She had no fever or diarrhea. She reports several months of worsening fatigue, mild, intermittent, generalized abdominal pain, and loss of appetite with a 10–15-lb unintentional weight loss. Her medical history is significant for breast cancer that was treated with mastectomy and radiation 3 years previously, and for which she was apparently cured. She takes no medications. On exam, her temperature is 99.8°F, her heart rate is 102 bpm, her blood pressure is 89/62 mmHg, and she has a normal respiratory rate. She does become lightheaded and her heart rate rises to 125 bpm upon standing. She is alert and well-tanned with hyperpigmented creases in her hands. Her chest is clear and her heart is tachycardic but regular. The breast exam reveals a 2 cm mass in her remaining breast, and some axillary lymphadenopathy. On abdominal exam, she has normal bowel sounds and mild diffuse tenderness without guarding. Her pulses are rapid and thready. She has no peripheral edema. Initial laboratory studies are significant for Na (121 mEq/L), K (5.8 mEq/L), HCO_3 (16 mEq/L), glucose (52 mg/dL), and creatinine (1.0 mg/dL).

- **What is the most likely diagnosis?**

- **What is your next step?**

ANSWERS TO CASE 40: Adrenal Insufficiency

Summary: A 58-year-old woman presents with orthostatic hypotension, intermittent chronic abdominal pain, and constitutional symptoms such as fatigue and unintentional weight loss. She also has hyponatremia, hyperkalemia, acidosis, and hypoglycemia. All of this patient's clinical features are consistent with acute adrenal insufficiency. Although the most common cause of adrenal insufficiency is idiopathic autoimmune destruction, in her case, it may be due to adrenal metastases from breast cancer.

- **Most likely diagnosis:** Primary adrenal insufficiency.
- **Next step:** After drawing a cortisol level, immediate administration of intravenous saline with glucose, and stress-dose corticosteroids.

Analysis

Objectives

1. Know the presentation of primary and secondary adrenal insufficiency and of adrenal crisis.
2. Know the most common causes of primary and secondary adrenal insufficiency.
3. Know the treatment for adrenal insufficiency.

Considerations

This patient has a low-grade fever, which may be a feature of adrenal insufficiency, or it may signify infection, which can precipitate an adrenal crisis, or may produce a similar clinical picture. It is important to diagnose and treat any underlying infection. Because of the adrenal insufficiency and the aldosterone deficiency, she has volume depletion and hypotension. Thus, intravenous replacement with normal saline is critical.

APPROACH TO SUSPECTED ADRENAL INSUFFICIENCY

Etiology

Primary adrenal insufficiency refers to adrenal failure to destruction or infiltration of the adrenal glands. The **most common cause in the United States is autoimmune destruction** of the **adrenal glands**. The most common cause worldwide is tuberculous adrenalitis. Other causes include chronic granulomatous infections (histoplasmosis, coccidiomycosis), bilateral adrenal hemorrhage (usually in the setting of sepsis with disseminated intravascular coagulation [DIC]), adrenal metastases (commonly from lung, breast, or stomach cancers), or X-linked adrenoleukodystrophy, a genetic disorder with adrenal and neurologic manifestations. Patients with AIDS often develop adrenal involvement as a result of infection with Cytomegalovirus (CMV) or *Mycobacterium avium-intracellulare.* In primary adrenal insufficiency, the glands themselves are destroyed, so the patient becomes deficient in cortisol and aldosterone. Primary adrenal insufficiency is a relatively uncommon disease in clinical practice. A high level of suspicion, particularly in those individuals who have suggestive signs or symptoms, or who are susceptible by virtue of associated autoimmune disorders or malignancies must be maintained. The nonspecific symptoms might be otherwise missed for many years until a stressful event leads to crisis and death.

Secondary adrenal insufficiency is adrenal failure caused by a lack of adrenocorticotropic hormone (ACTH) stimulation from the pituitary gland. It can be caused by an autoimmune, infiltrative, metastatic disease of the pituitary. The **most common reason, however, is chronic exogenous administration of corticosteroids**, which can suppress the entire hypothalamic–pituitary–adrenal axis. Because of the widespread use of corticosteroids, secondary adrenal insufficiency is relatively common. In secondary adrenal insufficiency, the rennin–angiotensin system is usually able to maintain near-normal levels of aldosterone, so the patient is only deficient in cortisol.

Clinical Features

The clinical presentation depends on the relative deficiency of glucocorticoids, mineralocorticoids, ACTH excess, and other associated disorders. **Acute adrenal insufficiency**, or Addisonian crisis, may presents with **weakness, nausea, vomiting and abdominal pain, fever, hypotension, and tachycardia**. Laboratory findings may **include hyponatremia, hyperkalemia, metabolic acidosis**, azotemia as a consequence of aldosterone deficiency, and hypoglycemia and eosinophilia as a consequence of cortisol deficiency. Patients with adrenal insufficiency may go into crisis when stressed by infection, trauma, or surgery. The clinical features may appear identical to septic shock; the only clues that the cause is adrenal disease may be the hypoglycemia (blood sugar is often elevated in sepsis), and profound hypotension, which may be refractory to administration of pressors, but is reversed almost immediately when steroids are given.

Chronic adrenal insufficiency has nonspecific clinical features such as **malaise, weight loss, chronic fatigue, and gastrointestinal symptoms such as anorexia, nausea, and vomiting.** A patient may have hypoglycemia and postural hypotension as a result of volume depletion. **Hyperpigmentation** is seen over time in primary adrenal insufficiency caused by elevated melanocyte-stimulating hormone production from the pituitary as a by-product of high ACTH levels. It is typically seen as generalized hyperpigmentation of skin and mucous membranes, and is increased in sun-exposed areas or over pressure areas, such as elbows and knees, and may be noted in skin folds. In secondary adrenal insufficiency, patients are deficient in cortisol because of a lack of ACTH from the pituitary, but aldosterone production is maintained by the renin–angiotensin system. Therefore, volume depletion and hyperkalemia are not present, and the patient will not manifest the typical hyperpigmentation.

Diagnosis Cortisol levels show a diurnal variation. Cortisol levels are high in the morning and low as the day progresses, and should be elevated in stressful situations such as acute medical illness, surgery, or trauma. A **morning plasma cortisol level** of ≤5 mcg/dL in an acutely ill patient is definitive evidence of adrenal insufficiency. Conversely, a random cortisol level of >20 mcg/dL is usually interpreted as evidence of intact adrenal function. **The ACTH stimulation test** is used to confirm primary adrenal insufficiency. Synthetic ACTH (cosyntropin) 250 mcg is administered intravenously, and serum cortisol levels are measured at baseline, then at 30- and 60-minute intervals. An increase in the cortisol level of 7 mcg/dL, or a maximal stimulated level over 18 mcg/dL is considered normal, and indicates intact adrenal function. If cosyntropin-stimulation testing indicates probable adrenal insufficiency, ACTH levels can then be measured to distinguish between primary (high ACTH) and secondary (low ACTH) adrenal failure.

The insulin-glucose tolerance test is the gold standard for testing the entire hypothalamic–pituitary axis. It is based on the principle that if a stressful situation is induced (in this case, hypoglycemia), the ACTH level should rise with a consequent increase in cortisol levels. CT scan and MRI are helpful in evaluating adrenal and pituitary disease after biochemical confirmation.

Treatment Treatment of Addisonian crisis includes **intravenous 5% glucose with normal saline** to correct volume depletion and hypoglycemia and administration of **corticosteroid therapy**. Hydrocortisone is usually given intravenously at doses of 100 mg every 6-8 hours, or it can be given as a bolus followed by a continuous infusion. At high doses, the hydrocortisone provides both glucocorticoid and mineralocorticoid activity. A cortisol level should be drawn before treatment to confirm the diagnosis. Causes of the acute crisis should be identified and treated; in particular, there should be a search for infection.

Long-term treatment of patients with primary adrenal insufficiency includes replacement doses of glucocorticoids (e.g., hydrocortisone 25–30 mg/d) and mineralocorticoids (e.g., fludrocortisone 0.1–0.2 mg/d). Patients with secondary adrenal insufficiency still produce aldosterone, as mentioned before, so only glucocorticoids need to be replaced. In both cases, to avoid long-term complications of glucocorticoid excess (diabetes, hypertension, obesity, osteoporosis, cataracts), patients should not be over treated. Stress doses of steroids should be given for intercurrent illnesses. Patients should wear a medical alert bracelet.

Comprehension Questions

[40.1] Which of the following is the most common cause of secondary adrenal insufficiency?

A. Autoimmune process
B. Surgical excision
C. Hemorrhagic shock
D. Exogenous corticosteroids
E. ACTH failure due to panhypopituitarism

[40.2] A 30-year-old woman takes prednisone 15 mg/d for systemic lupus erythematosus. She is admitted to the hospital for a cholecystectomy. Which of the following is the most important intervention for her?

A. Hydrocortisone intravenously before surgery and every 6 hours for 24 hours
B. Double the prednisone the night before and hold her steroids the day of the surgery
C. Use of cyclophosphamide in lieu of corticosteroids for 2 weeks following surgery to promote wound healing
D. Cancel the surgery and use lithotripsy to break up the stones

[40.3] A 30-year-old woman is noted to have adrenal insufficiency and a very distinct tan, although she hardly ventures outside. Which of the following is the most likely etiology?

A. Long-term steroid use
B. Sheehan syndrome (pituitary insufficiency)
C. Brain tumor
D. Autoimmune adrenal destruction

Answers

[40.1] **D.** Long-term steroid use, with secondary suppression of the pituitary secretion of ACTH is the most common cause of secondary adrenal insufficiency. Autoimmune adrenalitis is the most common cause of primary adrenal insufficiency.

[40.2] **A.** A stress dose of corticosteroids is important to prevent adrenal insufficiency before surgery.

[40.3] **D.** The hyperpigmentation occurs as a result of increased melanocyte-stimulating factor, a by-product of ACTH. Secondary causes of adrenal insufficiency result in low ACTH levels and do not cause the "tanned" appearance. Autoimmune adrenal destruction is the most common cause of primary adrenal insufficiency in the United States.

CLINICAL PEARLS

- ❖ Primary adrenal insufficiency presents with weakness, fatigue, abdominal pain with vomiting, hyperpigmentation, and hyponatremia with hypotension, which may be refractory to pressors.
- ❖ The treatment of adrenal crisis is immediate administration of Salt (saline), Sugar (glucose), and Steroids (hydrocortisone).
- ❖ The most common causes of primary adrenal insufficiency in the United States are autoimmune destruction, metastatic disease, and infectious causes (e.g., CMV in advanced AIDS). The most common cause worldwide is tuberculosis.
- ❖ Secondary adrenal insufficiency is the most common form of the illness, and is usually a result of suppression of the hypothalamic–pituitary axis by exogenous corticosteroids.

REFERENCE

Aron DC, Findling JW, Tyrrell B, et al. Glucocorticoids and adrenal androgens. In: Greenspan FS, Gardner DG, (eds.) Basic and clinical endocrinology, 6th ed. NewYork: Lange Medical Books/McGraw-Hill. 2001:334-377.

CASE 41

A 57-year-old man comes to the office complaining of malaise for several weeks. He says that he hasn't been feeling well for some time, with fatigue, depressed mood, loss of appetite, and a 20-lb unintentional weight loss. In addition, he has been bothered by generalized itching of his skin, and has tried moisturizing lotions and creams without improvement. He denies fevers, abdominal pain, nausea, vomiting, or diarrhea. He does think his stools have been lighter in color recently. He has no other medical history, and takes no medications except a multivitamin. He drinks alcohol occasionally, and smokes cigars.

On examination, he is afebrile, with a heart rate of 68 bpm and a blood pressure 128/74 mmHg. He has a flat affect and a somewhat disheveled appearance. He has noticeable icterus of his sclera and skin. His chest is clear and his heart is regular without murmurs. His abdomen is soft and nontender with active bowel sounds, a liver span of 10 cm, and no splenomegaly or masses. His skin has a few excoriations on his arms and back, but no rashes or telangiectasias.

Blood is obtained for laboratory analysis; the results are available the next day. His serum albumin is 3.1 g/dL, his alkaline phosphatase is 588 IU/L, with a total bilirubin of 8.5 mg/dL, a direct bilirubin of 6 mg/dL, and alanine aminotransferase (ALT) of 175 IU/L and aspartate aminotransferase (AST) of 140 IU/L. His hemoglobin is 13.5 g/dL. Prothrombin time (PT) is 15 seconds and partial thromboplastin time (PTT) is 32 seconds.

- **What is the most likely diagnosis?**

- **What is the next step?**

ANSWERS TO CASE 41: Painless Jaundice, Pancreatic Cancer

Summary: A 57-year-old man presents with pruritus, weight loss, and light-colored stools, and is found to be jaundiced with markedly elevated alkaline phosphatase and conjugated hyperbilirubinemia. All of this points towards cholestasis. The light-colored, or acholic, stools suggest the cholestasis is most likely caused by biliary obstruction. The absence of abdominal pain makes gallstone disease less likely.

◆ **Most likely diagnosis:** Biliary obstruction, most likely caused by malignancy.

◆ **Next step:** Imaging procedure of his biliary system, either ultrasonography or CT scan.

Analysis

Objectives

1. Know the causes and evaluation of a patient with unconjugated hyperbilirubinemia.
2. For a patient with conjugated hyperbilirubinemia, be able to distinguish between hepatocellular disease and biliary obstruction.
3. Understand the evaluation of a patient with cholestasis.
4. Know the treatment and complications of biliary obstruction.

Considerations

In patients with jaundice, one must try to distinguish between hepatic and biliary disease. In the patient with suspected biliary obstruction, without the pain typically associated with gallstones, one should be suspicious of malignancy or strictures. In the case presented, the clinical picture is worrisome for a malignant cause of biliary obstruction, such as pancreatic caner.

APPROACH TO PAINLESS JAUNDICE

Definitions

Cholestasis: Deficient bile flow that can result from intrahepatic disease or extrahepatic obstruction.

Conjugated bilirubin (direct-reacting bilirubin): Bilirubin that has entered the liver and been enzymatically bound to glucuronic acid forming bilirubin mono- or diglucuronide.

Jaundice or **icterus:** Yellowing of the skin or whites of the eyes, indicating hyperbilirubinemia

Unconjugated bilirubin (indirect-reacting bilirubin): Bilirubin that has not been enzymatically bound to glucuronic acid by the liver and is in the serum reversibly and noncovalently bound to albumin.

Clinical Approach

Jaundice, or icterus, is the visible manifestation of **hyperbilirubinemia**, and can usually be noticed by physical examination when the serum bilirubin exceeds 2.0–2.5 mg/dL. Traditional instruction regarding the jaundiced patient divides the mechanism of hyperbilirubinemia into prehepatic (excessive production of bilirubin), intrahepatic, or extrahepatic (as in biliary obstruction.) For most patients with jaundice, it is probably more clinically useful to think about hepatic or biliary diseases that cause conjugated hyperbilirubinemia, because that represents most clinically important causes of jaundice.

The term **unconjugated hyperbilirubinemia** is used when the conjugated (or direct-reacting fraction) does not exceed 15% of the total bilirubin. It is almost always caused by hemolysis, or Gilbert syndrome. In these conditions, the serum bilirubin is almost always <5 mg/dL, and there is usually no other clinical signs of liver disease. In addition, there should be no bilirubinuria (only conjugated bilirubin can be filtered and renally excreted). Hemolysis is usually clinically apparent, as in sickle cell disease or autoimmune hemolytic anemia. Gilbert syndrome is a benign condition caused by a deficiency of hepatic enzymatic conjugation of bilirubin, which results in intermittent unconjugated hyperbilirubinemia, often precipitated by such events as stress, fasting, and febrile illnesses. It is associated with no liver dysfunction and requires no therapy.

Conjugated hyperbilirubinemia almost always reflects either hepatocellular disease, or biliary obstruction. These two conditions can be differentiated by the pattern of elevation of the liver enzymes. Elevation of serum aspartate aminotransferase and alanine aminotransferase levels are characteristic of hepatocellular disease as a result of the inflammation/destruction of the hepatocytes and the release of these enzymes into the blood. The serum alkaline phosphatase level is elevated in cholestatic disease as a consequence of inflammation, destruction, or obstruction of the intrahepatic or extrahepatic bile ducts with relative sparing of the hepatocytes. The serum aspartate aminotransferase and alanine aminotransferase levels may be mildly elevated in cholestasis, but usually not to the levels seen in primary acute hepatocellular disease. Other tests such as serum albumin, or prothrombin time, generally reflect the capacity of hepatocytes to synthesize proteins such as clotting factors. When they are abnormal, they most often reflect hepatocellular disease. Table 41–1 summarizes the liver test patterns seen in various categories of hepatobiliary disorders.

The patient discussed in the above case has a pattern consistent with cholestasis, and the first diagnostic test in a patient with cholestasis is usually an ultrasound. It is noninvasive and is very sensitive for detecting stones in the gallbladder as well as intrahepatic or extrahepatic biliary dilatation. The **most common cause of biliary obstruction in the United States is gallstones**, which may become lodged in the common bile duct. However, obstructing stones causing jaundice are usually associated with epigastric or right upper quadrant colicky pain. Extrahepatic dilatation without evidence of stones war-

Table 41-1
LIVER TEST PATTERNS IN HEPATOBILIARY DISORDERS

TYPE OF DISORDER	BILIRUBIN	AMINOTRANSFERASES	ALKALINE PHOSPHATASE	ALBUMIN	PROTHROMBIN TIME
Hemolysis/Gilbert's syndrome	Normal to 5 mg/dl 85% due to indirect fractions No bilirubinuria	Normal	Normal	Normal	Normal
Acute hepatocellular necrosis (viral and drug hepatitis. hepatotoxins, acute heart failure)	Both fractions may be elevated. Peak usually follows aminotransferases Bilirubinuria	Elevated, often >500 IU/L ALT >AST	Normal to <3 times normal elevation	Normal	Usually normal >5× above control and not corrected by parenteral vitamin K, suggests poor prognosis
Chronic hepatocellular disorders	Both fractions may be elevated Bilirubinuria	Elevated, but usually <300 IU/L	Normal to <3 times normal elevation	Often decreased	Often prolonged. Fails to correct with parenteral vitamin K

Alcoholic hepatitis Cirrhosis	Both fractions may be elevated Bilirubinuria	AST:ALT >2 suggests alcoholic hepatitis or cirrhosis	Normal to <3 times normal elevation	Often decreased	Often prolonged. Fails to correct with parenteral vitamin K
Intra- and extra-hepatic cholestasis (Obstructive jaundice)	Both fractions may be elevated Bilirubinuria	Normal to moderate elevation Rarely >500 IU/L	Elevated, often >4 times normal elevation	Normal, unless chronic	Normal. If prolonged. will correct with parenteral vitamin K
Infiltrative diseases (tumor, granulomata): partial bile duct obstruction	Usually normal	Normal to slight elevation	Elevated, often > 4 times normal elevation Fractionate, or confirm liver origin with 5' nucleotidase or gamma glutamyl transpeptidase	Normal	Normal

(Reprinted, with permission, from Braunwald E, Fauci AS, Kasper KL, et al (eds). Harrison's Principles of Internal Medicine, 15th ed. New York, NY: McGraw-Hill, 2001.)

rants further study with CT or ERCP (endoscopic retrograde cholangiopancreatography) to detect stones and exclude malignant causes of common bile duct and pancreatic duct obstruction including cholangiocarcinoma, pancreatic cancer, and ampullary cancer (ampulla of Vater).

Other possible causes include strictures, which can result from prior biliary surgery, prior inflammatory conditions such as pancreatitis (rarely), inflammatory diseases of the biliary tree, or infection in the setting of AIDS. The two most important primary conditions are primary sclerosing cholangitis and primary biliary cirrhosis. Table 41–2 compares features of these two entities.

The complications of biliary obstruction include development of cholangitis as a result of ascending infection, or secondary hepatic cirrhosis, if the obstruction is chronic or recurrent. The patient in this scenario has painless jaundice, liver enzymes consistent with a cholestatic process, and light-colored stools, suggesting obstruction of bile flow into the intestine. Because he has no history of abdominal or biliary surgery that might have caused a stricture, malignancy is the most likely cause of his biliary obstruction. The most common malignancy to present in this way is pancreatic cancer. He should undergo an imaging procedure of his abdomen, which includes a right upper quadrant ultrasound to evaluate the biliary tree, as well as a CT scan or MRI to visualize the pancreas. Endoscopic ultrasound with fine needle aspirateion is highly accurate in establishing a tissue diagnosis.

Pancreatic cancer is the fifth leading cause of cancer death in the United States. Peak incidence is in the seventh decade of life, with two-thirds of cases occurring in persons older than 65 years of age. There is a slight male predominance and a higher incidence in the black population. The median survival is 9 months, with an overall 5-year survival rate of 3%. Clinically apparent metastatic disease is found in 80% of patients at the time of diagnosis. For patients without obvious metastases, the best hope for cure is surgical resection by pancreaticoduodenectomy (Whipple procedure), which in experienced hands has a perioperative mortality rate of <5%. Since there is a high rate of recurrence of cancer, even in disease that is considered to be resectable. Many treatment programs include neoadjuvant chemotherapy. Alternate palliative therapy includes pancreatic and common bile duct stenting to relieve the obstruction.

Table 41-2
COMPARISON OF PRIMARY SCLEROSING CHOLANGITIS AND PRIMARY BILIARY CIRRHOSIS

EPIDEMIOLOGY	DISEASE	LOCATION OF DISEASE	ASSOCIATED CONDITIONS	SEROLOGIC MARKERS	COMPLICATIONS
Younger males	Primary sclerosing cholangitis	Larger intra- and extrahepatic ducts	Ulcerative colitis	None	Stricture; infection (cholangitis); cholangiocarcinoma
Older females	Primary biliary cirrhosis	Smaller intra-hepatic bile ducts	Autoimmune diseases such as rheumatoid arthritis	Antimitochondrial antibody (AMA)	Cirrhosis

Comprehension Questions

Match the following diagnoses (A to F) with the most likely clinical situation [41.1 to 41.4]:

A. Hemolysis
B. Alcoholic hepatitis
C. Gilbert disease
D. Pancreatic cancer
E. Gallstones
F. Primary sclerosing cholangitis

[41.1] A 38-year-old man with a 12-pack of beer per day alcohol history presents with jaundice, ascites, and dark urine. His lab results are AST 350 U/mL, ALT 150 U/mL, alkaline phosphatase 120 U/mL, total bilirubin 25 mg/dL, direct bilirubin 12 mg/dL, and albumin 2.1 g/dL.

[41.2] A 40-year-old moderately obese woman presents with abdominal pain after eating and mild scleral icterus. Her lab results are AST 200 U/L, ALT 150 U/L, alkaline phosphatase 355 U/L, total bilirubin 3.5 mg/dL, direct bilirubin 1.8 mg/dL, and albumin 3.5 g/dL.

[41.3] A 25-year-old man presents with 3 days of scleral icterus but has been otherwise feeling well. His lab results are AST 45 U/L, ALT 48 U/L, alkaline phosphatase 100 U/L, total bilirubin 4.0 mg/dL, direct bilirubin 0.2 mg/dL, and albumin 3.5 g/dL. Complete blood count is normal.

[41.4] A 32-year-old man with a 5-year history of episodic bloody diarrhea and abdominal cramping pain presents with scleral icterus and fever. His lab results are AST 100 U/L, ALT 125 U/L, alkaline phosphatase 550 U/L, total bilirubin 5.5 mg/dL, direct bilirubin 3.0 mg/dL, and albumin 2.9 g/dL.

Answers

[41.1] **B.** The patient's labs show a conjugated hyperbilirubinemia with evidence of hepatocellular disease (hypoalbuminemia, ascites). The AST and ALT show the 2:1 ratio consistent with alcohol-related liver disease.

[41.2] **E.** The patient's labs show a conjugated hyperbilirubinemia consistent with an obstructive pattern. She has the risk factors for gallstones of being middle-age, female, and obese, and has symptoms of postprandial abdominal pain.

[41.3] **C.** The patient's labs show an unconjugated hyperbilirubinemia without other abnormality. He is otherwise healthy without symptoms of systemic disease or anemia. No treatment is necessary.

[41.4] **F.** The patient's labs show a conjugated hyperbilirubinemia with an obstructive pattern. The history is consistent with inflammatory bowel disease, which is associated with primary sclerosing cholangitis. The initial evaluation should include ultrasonography to rule out gallstones, and if negative, ERCP could confirm the diagnosis by demonstrating multiple strictures of the extrahepatic bile ducts. Treatment options include stenting of the larger bile duct strictures and immunosuppression to slow the progression of the disease.

CLINICAL PEARLS

- ❖ Unconjugated hyperbilirubinemia is usually caused by hemolysis or Gilbert syndrome.
- ❖ Conjugated hyperbilirubinemia is commonly caused by hepatocellular disease, with elevations of AST and ALT, or to biliary obstruction, with elevations of alkaline phosphatase.
- ❖ An imaging procedure such as ultrasonography is the initial study of choice in a patient with cholestasis to evaluate for intrahepatic or extrahepatic biliary obstruction.
- ❖ The most common causes of biliary obstruction are gallstones, which should be painful if obstructing, and strictures or neoplasms, which are often painless.
- ❖ The prognosis for pancreatic cancer is very poor; the best hope for cure is resection by a pancreaticoduodenectomy (Whipple procedure).

REFERENCES

Brower ST, Benson AB, Myerson RJ. Pancreatic, neuroendocrine GI, and adrenal cancers. In: Pazdur R, Coia LR, Hoskins WJ, Wagman LD, eds. Cancer management: a multidisciplinary approach, 6th ed. Melville, New York: PRR, 2002:249–61.

Pratt DS, Kaplan MM. Jaundice. In: Braunwald E, Fauci AS, Kasper KL, et al., eds. Harrison's principles of internal medicine, 15th ed. New York: McGraw-Hill, 2001:255–59; 1711–20.

CASE 42

While seeing patients in your preceptor's clinic, you have the opportunity to meet and examine one of her long-time patients, a 46-year-old woman who presents for her yearly physical exam. She has been fine, and has no complaints today. Her past medical history is notable only for borderline hypertension and moderate obesity. Last year her fasting lipid profile was acceptable for someone without known risk factors for coronary artery disease. Her mother and older brother have diabetes and hypertension. At prior visits, you see that your preceptor has counseled her on a low-calorie, low-fat diet and recommended that she start an exercise program. However, the patient says she has not made any of these recommended changes. With her full-time job and three children she finds it difficult to exercise, and admits that her family eats out frequently. Today her blood pressure is 140/92 mmHg. Her body mass index (BMI) is 27 kg/m^2. Her exam is notable for acanthosis nigricans at the neck, but is otherwise normal. A Papanicolaou (Pap) smear is performed, and a mammogram is offered. The patient has not eaten yet today, so on your preceptor's recommendation, a fasting plasma glucose is performed, and the result is 140 mg/dL.

- **What is your diagnosis?**

- **What is your next step?**

ANSWERS TO CASE 42: Type 2 Diabetes Diagnosis and Management

Summary: A 46-year-old woman presents for her yearly physical exam. Her past medical history is notable only for borderline hypertension and moderate obesity. She has a family history of diabetes and hypertension. The patient has not followed the recommended lifestyle changes. Today, her blood pressure is 140/92 mmHg and her BMI is 27 kg/m^2. Her exam is notable for acanthosis nigricans at the neck, suggesting insulin resistance. A fasting plasma glucose is 140 mg/dL, which is consistent with diabetes mellitus.

- **Most likely diagnosis:** Given her hypertension, obesity, family history, and the finding of acanthosis nigricans, this patient most likely has type 2 diabetes. Diabetes is defined by the American Diabetes Association as a fasting plasma glucose greater than or equal to 126 mg/dL.

- **Next step:** The fasting glucose level should be repeated to confirm the diagnosis. If the next result is less than 126 mg/dL, then an oral glucose tolerance test should be performed.

Analysis

Objectives

1. Know the diagnostic criteria for type 2 diabetes.
2. Understand the initial medical management of diabetes.
3. Understand cardiovascular risk modification in diabetic patients.
4. Understand the prevention of microvascular complications of diabetes.

Considerations

If this patient's diagnosis of diabetes is confirmed, she will require patient education, lifestyle modification, and medical therapy to prevent acute and chronic complications of diabetes. Strict glycemic control can reduce the incidence of microvascular complications such as retinopathy and nephropathy. In addition, patients with diabetes are among the highest at risk for cardiovascular disease, so risk factor modifications, such as smoking cessation and lowering of cholesterol, are essential. **Diabetes confers the same level of risk for coronary events, such as heart attack, as in patients with established coronary artery disease**. Thus, in this patient, the target blood pressure is <130/80 mmHg and the target low-density lipoprotein (LDL) cholesterol is <100 mg/dL.

APPROACH TO SUSPECTED DIABETES MELLITUS

Definitions

Type 1 diabetes: Caused by what is believed to be an autoimmune destruction of the pancreatic beta cells and complete loss of endogenous insulin production. The presentation of this type of diabetes is usually acute, with hyperglycemia and metabolic acidosis. These patients are dependent upon exogenous insulin delivery.

Type 2 diabetes: A heterogenous syndrome of insulin resistance caused by genetic factors and/or obesity, and relative insulin deficiency. Oral medications to enhance endogenous insulin production, or improve insulin sensitivity are useful. Exogenous insulin may be used when oral medications are no longer sufficient for adequate glycemic control.

Clinical Approach

As the prevalence of obesity increases in the American population, so does the prevalence of type 2 diabetes, especially in children and teenagers. Ninety percent of all new cases of diabetes diagnosed in the United States are type 2, and it is estimated that this disease affects approximately 7% of the population older than 45 years of age. **Diabetes is the leading cause of blindness, renal failure, and nontraumatic amputations of the lower extremities.** It is a major risk factor in coronary artery disease, peripheral vascular disease, and stroke.

Type 2 diabetes is believed to have a prolonged asymptomatic phase. During these years of asymptomatic hyperglycemia, however, organ damage begins to occur. Therefore, several organizations recommend screening of certain high-risk populations. The risk factors for diabetes include obesity or overweight, defined as a BMI >25 kg/m^2, other signs of an insulin-resistance syndrome or "metabolic" syndrome such as hypertension, or low high-density lipoproteins (HDLs) and triglycerides >250 mg/dL, a first-degree relative with diabetes, a history of gestational diabetes, or being a member of a high-risk ethnic group including African-Americans, Hispanics, American Indians, Asian Americans, or Pacific Islanders. Screening should begin at age 45 years, and be repeated every 3 years. Children with risk factors can be considered for screening at age 10 years and every 2 years after that.

Most patients with type 2 diabetes mellitus (DM) are insulin resistant and hyperinsulinemic for years before developing overt diabetes, are able to maintain normoglycemia for a long time, first develop postprandial hyperglycemia, and later develop both postprandial and fasting hyperglycemia (i.e., hyperglycemia all the time). Thus a **glucose tolerance test** to detect postprandial hyperglycemia would be most sensitive test for DM, but is time-consuming and difficult to perform in a clinical practice. The **fasting plasma glucose** is the most specific test. The **Hgb A_{Ic}** is not a recommended screening/diagnostic test because of a lack of standardization between laboratories, but is useful for monitoring glycemic control once diagnosis established (see Tables 42–1 and 42–2). Tests should be confirmed by a separate measurement on another day.

By using these tests, patients can be classified into three categories: normal, impaired glucose tolerance/impaired fasting glucose (i.e., "prediabetic"),

Table 42-1
TESTS TO DIAGNOSE DIABETES

TEST	NORMAL	IMPAIRED GLUCOSE TOLERANCE	DIABETES
Fasting plasma glucose	<110 mg/dL	110–126 mg/dL	>126 mg/dL
Random glucose			>200 mg/dL
Oral glucose tolerance test (75-g load)	Fasting <110 mg/dL 2-hour <140 mg/dL	110–126 mg/dL 140–200 mg/dL	>126 mg/dL >200 mg/dL

Source: Powers AC. Diabetes Mellitus. In: Braunwald E, Fauci AS, Kasper KL, et al, eds. Harrison's principles of internal medicine, 15th ed. New York: McGraw-Hill. 2001:1513-17

Table 42-2
CRITERIA FOR DIAGNOSIS OF DIABETES MELLITUS

1. Symptoms of diabetes plus casual glucose concentration ≥200 mg/dL (11.1 mmol/L). Casual is defined as any time of day without regard to time since last meal. The classic symptoms of diabetes include polyuria, polydispsia, and unexplained weight loss.

or

2. FPG ≥126 mg/dL (7.0 mmol/L). Fasting is defined as no caloric intake for at least 8 hours.

or

3. 2hPG ≥200 mg/dL during an OGTT. The test should be performed as described by WHO, using a glucose load containing the equivalent of 75-g anhydrous glucose dissolved in water.

Abbreviations: FPG = fasting plasma glucose; OGTT = oral glucose tolerance test; 2hPG = 2-hour plasma glucose.
Source: Powers AC. Diabetes Mellitus. In: Braunwald E, Fauci AS, Kasper KL, et al, eds. Harrison's principles of internal medicine, 15th ed. New York: McGraw-Hill. 2001:1513-17

or diabetic. Increased risk for microvascular complications of hyperglycemia are seen at a fasting glucose >126 mg/dL. Increased risk for macrovascular complications are seen at a fasting glucose >110 mg/dL. Once diabetes is diagnosed, therapy is instituted with three major goals.

1. Prevention of acute complications of hyperglycemia (e.g., diabetic ketoacidosis or nonketotic hyperosmolar hyperglycemia) or hypoglycemia.
2. Prevention of long-term complications of hyperglycemia, for example, microvascular disease such as retinopathy or nephropathy.

3. Prevention of long-term complications of macrovascular disease, for example, cardiovascular or cerebrovascular disease.

The foundation of diabetes therapy is dietary and lifestyle modifications. Randomized trials show that even small amounts of weight loss can lower blood pressure and improve glucose control. Patients should be given instruction in nutrition and encouraged to change sedentary lifestyles. Exercise that the patient finds enjoyable and possible should be encouraged. However, most people with diabetes will eventually require medications, and most patients will eventually require a combination of at least two medications. The United Kingdom Prospective Diabetes Study (UKPDS) followed almost 5000 patients over 20 years and compared intensive blood glucose control to conventional therapy in the prevention of **macrovascular** (coronary artery disease) and **microvascular** (retinopathy, nephropathy, and neuropathy) complications. Intensive therapy, with a Hgb A_{1c} of ≤7% resulted in fewer microvascular complications, but there was no significant differences in macrovascular complications between the two groups. Patients in the intensive therapy group had more episodes of hypoglycemia, so intensive therapy may not be appropriate for elderly patients or those patients with other comorbid conditions.

The UKPDS randomized patients to begin treatment either with sulfonylureas or insulin therapy. A subgroup of overweight patients was started on metformin. In the end, those on insulin tended to gain more weight each year, otherwise there were no differences between the groups. This has been interpreted to mean that any of these medications are appropriate first choices in a newly diagnosed diabetic patient. However, obese persons may benefit from metformin, as it has some effects on appetite, and is associated with modest weight loss. Sulfonylureas are very inexpensive and effective. Other medications developed since the UKPDS trial may be added if needed (see Table 42–3). If possible, introduction of insulin may be delayed as it leads to weight gain, which may worsen insulin resistance.

When diabetes is diagnosed, other cardiovascular risk factors should be assessed. Blood pressure and lipid levels should be measured. With regards to lipid therapy, the cardiovascular risk in diabetes is equivalent to those with known coronary artery disease, so that the desired LDL threshold is less than 100 mg/dL. Those with higher LDL should undergo dietary modification or be started on a statin.

The desired blood pressure threshold is also lower, with a goal of <130/80 mmHg. Several randomized trials have demonstrated a **benefit for angiotensin-converting enzyme (ACE) inhibitors** and **angiotensin receptor blockers (ARBs)** in preventing the progression of proteinuria and kidney disease. Because proteinuria and kidney disease are common in diabetes, an ACE inhibitor or ARB is a good first choice for treating hypertension in diabetics.

Other routine care in diabetic patients includes frequent physician visits, at least every 3–6 months depending on their glucose control, at least yearly ophthalmologic exams to screen for retinopathy, semiannual dental visits to

Table 42-3
MEDICATIONS AVAILABLE IN THE UNITED STATES FOR THE TREATMENT OF TYPE 2 DIABETES

MEDICATION	MECHANISM OF ACTION/INDICATIONS	SPECIAL CONSIDERATIONS	COST
Insulin	Supplement patient's own insulin production	Must check blood glucose frequently to monitor therapy and prevent complications	$
Sulfonylurea	Augments patient's own insulin production, works at the pancreatic β cells	Can cause hypoglycemia; can accumulate in renal insufficiency and cause prolonged hypoglycemia. Best for young patients with fasting plasma glucose <300 mg/dL	$
Metformin	Decreases gluconeogenesis in the liver; decreases insulin resistance	In patients with renal insufficiency or liver dysfunction may cause lactic acidosis	$$–$$$
Alpha-glucosidase	Inhibits breakdown of complex carbohydrates in the GI tract	Can cause GI distress, and must be taken TID with meals; dose-dependent hepatotoxicity	$$
Pioglitazone; rosiglitazone	Promote skeletal muscle glucose uptake and decrease insulin resistance	Hepatotoxicity; edema	$$$–$$$$
Repaglinide	Nonsulfonylurea, but works in a similar manner; rapid onset of action; monotherapy or in combination with metformin	Caution in elderly and in patients with renal or hepatic insufficiency; must dose TID with meals	$$

prevent periodontal disease, and yearly urine screens to detect microalbuminuria. Hemoglobin A_{Ic} should be checked at least every 3–6 months, depending on the patient's glucose control. This test allows the physician to know the general glucose control over the preceding 2–3 months. Patients without neuropathy should have a foot exam yearly to detect early neuropathic changes; however, those with neuropathy should be examined every 3 months and be instructed on daily self-examination and prevention of injury.

Comprehension Questions

[42.1] A patient comes in for a fasting plasma glucose test. On two separate occasions, the result has been 115 mg/dL and 120 mg/dL. Which of the following is the most appropriate next step?

A. Reassurance that these are normal blood sugars
B. Recommend weight loss, an American Diabetes Association diet, and exercise
C. Diagnose diabetes mellitus and start a sulfonylurea agent
D. Recommend cardiac stress testing
E. Obtain stat arterial blood gas and serum ketone levels

[42.2] A 45-year-old obese Hispanic woman presents for followup of her diabetes. She currently takes glipizide (sulfonylurea) 10 mg twice a day, and her fasting morning glucose runs about 170–200 mg/dL. Her last Hgb A_{Ic} was 7.9. She states that she conscientiously follows her diet and that she walks 30 minutes to 1 hour daily. What is the best next step in her care?

A. Add an insulin pump
B. Add metformin
C. Add NPH (neutral protamine Hagedorn) insulin
D. Hospitalize her urgently

[42.3] A 75-year-old woman with diabetes for about 20 years, diabetic retinopathy, and diabetic nephropathy is brought into the office by her daughter for followup. The patient currently takes a sulfonylurea for her diabetes, and an ACE inhibitor for her proteinuria. Her daughter reports that on three occasions in the past 2 weeks, her mother became sweaty, shaky, and confused, which resolved when she was given some orange juice. Which of the following conditions is most likely to be contributing to these episodes?

A. Excess caloric oral intake
B. Interaction between the ACE inhibitor and the sulfonylurea agents
C. Worsening renal function
D. Hyperglycemic amnesia

Answers

[42.1] **B.** By diagnostic criteria, this patient falls into the definition of impaired glucose tolerance. This means that her fasting glucose levels are not normal, but neither do they meet the criteria for diabetes. This places the patient at greater risk for developing diabetes in the future. Interventions such as weight loss will decrease her insulin resistance, and following a diet lower in simple sugars and fats may place less stress on her pancreas and increase the time to development of outright diabetes.

[42.2] **B.** Because this patient is obese and young, after reviewing her meal plan and exercise schedule, adding metformin is the next best step. Although insulin is just as beneficial in controlling blood sugar levels and vascular complications, it may be associated with weight gain, and most patients prefer to be maintained on oral agents rather than injections, if possible.

[42.3] **C.** Sulfonylureas have long half-lives and can cause prolonged hypoglycemia in elderly patients, as well in those with **renal insufficiency.** Another method, such as insulin, may be more appropriate in this patient, as well as less-intensive control, aiming for a Hgb A_{Ic} of 8 instead of 7.

CLINICAL PEARLS

❖ Type 2 diabetes has a prolonged asymptomatic stage during which microvascular disease, for example, retinopathy or nephropathy, can occur. Physicians should have a high index of suspicion and screen those patients with risk factors.

❖ Tight glycemic control (Hgb A_{Ic} <7.0) reduces the incidence and progression of microvascular complications of diabetes.

❖ The major cause of morbidity and mortality in patients with type 2 DM is macrovascular disease: coronary artery disease, stroke, and peripheral vascular disease.

❖ Aggressive treatment of other risk factors (hypertension, hyperlipidemia, smoking cessation) is necessary to reduce the incidence of macrovascular complications.

REFERENCES

American Diabetes Association. Standards of medical care for patients with diabetes mellitus. Diabetes Care 2003;26(Suppl 1):S33–50.

Baldeweg S, Yudkin J. Implications of the UKPDS. Prim Care 1999;26(4):809–27.

Florence J, Yeager B. Treatment of type II diabetes. Am Fam Physician 1999;59(10):2835-2849.

CASE 43

An 18-year-old woman is brought to the emergency room by her mother because she seems confused and is behaving strangely. Her mother reports the patient has always been healthy, and has no significant medical history, but has lost 20 pounds recently without trying, and has been complaining of fatigue for 2 or 3 weeks. The patient had attributed the fatigue to sleep disturbance, as she has been getting up several times at night to urinate recently. This morning, the mother found the patient in her room, complaining of abdominal pain, and she had vomited. She appeared confused, and did not know that today was a school day.

On examination, the patient is slender, lying on a stretcher with eyes closed, but is responsive to questions. She is afebrile, her heart rate is 118 bpm, with a blood pressure of 125/84 mmHg, and is breathing deeply 24 times per minute. Upon standing, her heart rate rises to 145 bpm, and her blood pressure falls to 110/80 mmHg. Her funduscopic exam is normal, her oral mucosa is dry, and her neck veins are flat. Her chest is clear to auscultation and her heart is tachycardic with a regular rhythm and no murmur. Her abdomen is soft with active bowel sounds and mild diffuse tenderness, but no guarding or rebound. Her neurologic exam reveals no focal deficits.

Laboratory studies include serum Na (131) mEq/L, K (5.3) mEq/L, Cl (95) mEq/L, CO_2 (9) mEq/L, blood urea nitrogen (BUN) (35) mg/dL, creatinine (1.3) mg/dL, and glucose (475) mg/dL. Arterial blood gas shows pH 7.12 with PCO_2 24 mmHg and PO_2 95 mmHg. A urine drug screen and urine pregnancy test are negative, and urinalysis shows no hematuria or pyuria, but 3+ glucose, and 3+ ketones. Chest radiograph is read as normal, and plain film of the abdomen has nonspecific gas pattern but no signs of obstruction.

- **What is the most likely diagnosis?**

- **What is your next step?**

ANSWERS TO CASE 43: Diabetic Ketoacidosis

Summary: A young woman presents with unintentional weight loss, nocturia, and polyuria, with hyperglycemia, which likely represents new-onset diabetes mellitus. She is hypovolemic as a result of osmotic diuresis, and has an anion gap metabolic acidosis, which is primarily caused by ketoacids. Her mental status and abdominal pain are probably manifestations of the metabolic acidosis and of hyperosmolarity.

◆ **Most likely diagnosis:** Diabetic ketoacidosis (DKA).

◆ **Next step:** Aggressive hydration to improve her volume status and insulin therapy to resolve the ketoacidosis.

Analysis

Objectives

1. Know how to diagnose patients with anion gap metabolic acidosis.
2. Be able to differentiate diabetic ketoacidosis, nonketotic hyperosmolar hyperglycemia, and alcoholic ketoacidosis.
3. Understand principles of DKA management: restoration of volume, electrolyte replacement, resolution of ketosis, and control of hyperglycemia.
4. Learn the complications of diabetic ketoacidosis and of improper management.

Considerations

Diabetic ketoacidosis (DKA) occurs as a result of severe insulin deficiency, and may be the initial presentation of diabetes mellitus, as in this patient. In all patients with DKA, one must be alert for precipitating factors such as infection, pregnancy, or severe physiologic stressors, such as myocardial infarction. Careful management and close monitoring will be required to correct fluid and electrolyte deficits, and to prevent complications such as hypokalemia and cerebral edema.

APPROACH TO SUSPECTED DKA

Diabetic ketoacidosis (DKA) is a clinical syndrome that results when the **triad of anion gap metabolic acidosis, hyperglycemia, and ketosis** is present, and is caused by a significant insulin deficiency. It is a medical emergency, with an overall mortality rate that is <5% so long as standard written therapeutic guidelines are followed. The majority of the episodes are preventable and many of the deaths are also avoidable with proper attention to detail during management.

Pathophysiology

In normal physiologic state, there is a fine balance between anabolic and catabolic hormones. In the fed state, anabolic actions of insulin predominate.

Glycogenesis, lipogenesis, and protein synthesis are all increased. This results in storage of energy reserves in the form of triglycerides and glycogen.

In the fasting state, insulin serves to inhibit lipolysis, ketogenesis, gluconeogenesis, glycogenolysis, and proteolysis. These effects are critical in controlling the rate of breakdown of energy stores under the influence of catabolic hormones. **Glucagon is the most important catabolic hormone.** In the fasting state, it maintains normal glucose levels by stimulating hepatic gluconeogenesis and glycogenolysis.

Diabetes is the condition of relative or absolute insulin deficiency. When there is a severe insulin deficiency and a relative excess of glucagon, lipolysis is enhanced, causing release of free fatty acids. Oxidation of the fatty acids produces ketones, such as acetoacetate and beta-hydroxybutyrate, which are organic acids, and are often referred to as **ketoacids**. The excess of these ketoacids can produce a life-threatening metabolic acidosis. In addition, the hyperglycemia produces an osmotic diuresis, which causes severe volume depletion, and electrolyte deficiencies by washing extracellular sodium, potassium, magnesium, phosphate and water out of the body. The combination of acidosis, hypovolemia, and electrolyte deficiencies can lead to **cardiovascular collapse, the most common cause of death in DKA**.

Clinical Presentation

Patients with diabetes have an underlying impairment in glucose metabolism and, when challenged by a stress, have an increase in insulin requirements. If they are unable to meet these insulin requirements, DKA may result. **The most common precipitating events are infections** such as pneumonia or urinary tract infection, vascular disorders such as myocardial infarction, or other stressors such as trauma. It may also be the presentation of new-onset diabetes, and commonly occurs in patients with established diabetes because of the failure to use insulin for whatever reason, or because of use of other medications (e.g., phenytoin, thiazides, glucocorticoids) that interfere with insulin action.

An episode of DKA evolves over a short period of time, typically <24 hours. The patient with DKA has the signs and symptoms of hyperglycemia, acidosis, and dehydration. Polyuria, polydipsia, weight loss, visual blurring, and decreased mental status are related to hyperglycemia and osmotic diuresis. Nausea, vomiting, abdominal pain, fatigue, malaise, and shortness of breath may be related to the acidosis.

Typical signs include reduced skin elasticity, dry mucous membranes, hypotension, and tachycardia related to volume depletion. **Kussmaul respirations**, deep and rapid breathing, represent hyperventilation in an attempt to generate a respiratory alkalosis to compensate for the metabolic acidosis. One may also note the fruity breath odor typical of ketosis.

Laboratory Diagnosis

The laboratory values show hyperglycemia (usually >250 mg/dL), acidosis (pH <7.3), anion gap (usually >15 mmol/L), and ketonemia. The most important laboratory parameters are the degree of acidosis, the anion gap, and the serum potassium level.

Patients with a very low pH <7.0 are severely acidotic and have a worse prognosis. The lower pH is a result of the higher concentration of ketoacids, which are estimated using the anion gap. The first step in evaluating any patient with metabolic acidosis should be the calculation of the **anion gap.** This concept is based on the principle of electrical neutrality, that is, all the cations must equal all the anions. The anion gap estimates those negatively charged particles that are not routinely measured, and can be calculated using the following calculation:

$$\text{Anion Gap} = [\text{Na}] - [\text{Cl} + \text{HCO}_3]$$

The normal anion gap is 10–12 mmol/L. When it is elevated, there is an excess of unmeasured anions, which typically occurs because of one of four causes, which are listed in Table 43–1.

Lactic acidosis can be a result of severe tissue hypoxia, as in septic shock or carbon monoxide poisoning, or a result of hepatic failure and subsequent inability to metabolize lactate. Ketoacidosis most commonly occurs as an acute complication of uncontrolled diabetes, but can also be seen in starvation and in alcoholism, which are discussed later in this chapter. The ingested toxins may be organic acids themselves, such as salicylic acid, or have acidic metabolites, such as formic acid from methanol. Renal failure leads to an inability to excrete organic acids as well as inorganic acids such as phosphates (often without an anion gap).

In patients with DKA, the total body potassium stores are depleted due to urinary losses and potassium replacement will always be necessary. Initially,

Table 43-1
HIGH ANION GAP METABOLIC ACIDOSIS

1. Lactic acidosis
2. Ketoacidosis
   a. Diabetic
   b. Alcoholic
   c. Starvation
3. Toxins
   a. Ethylene glycol
   b. Methanol
   c. Salicylates
4. Renal failure (acute or chronic)

Reproduced with permission from DuBose TD. Acidosis and alkalosis. Braunwald E, Fauci AS, Kasper KL, et al., eds. Harrison's principles of internal medicine 15th ed. New York: McGraw-Hill, 2001:289.

the measured potassium levels in serum may be high despite the total body deficit because of acidosis resulting in movement of potassium from the intracellular compartment to the extracellular compartment. As the acidosis is corrected, and with the administration of insulin, which drives potassium intracellularly, the serum levels will fall rapidly.

The serum sodium level can be variable. Hyperglycemia causes water to move extracellularly, which can lead to hyponatremia. Similarly, phosphate levels can be variable in the presence of body store deficits with the extracellular movement of phosphate caused by catabolic state. Blood urea nitrogen (BUN) and creatinine are elevated, reflecting dehydration. Serum acetoacetate may cause a false elevation in serum creatinine because of interference with the assay.

Management

The goal of treatment is to restore metabolic homeostasis with correction of precipitating events and biochemical deficits, which consists of

1. Replacement of fluid losses with improvement of circulatory volume.
2. Correction of hyperglycemia, and, in turn, plasma osmolality.
3. Replacement of electrolyte losses.
4. Clearance of serum ketones.
5. Identification and treatment of precipitating cause and complications.

Close monitoring of the patient is important. A flow sheet recording vital signs, input and output, insulin dosage, and metabolic progress is important. Serum glucose should be measured every 1 hour and serum electrolytes, and phosphate must be assessed every 3–5 hours. Urinalysis, urine and blood cultures, EKG and chest x-ray should be obtained to identify precipitating factors and complications. Other investigations should be pursued as symptoms and signs warrant.

Fluids **All patients with DKA are volume-depleted** as a consequence of osmotic diuresis, as well as from other ongoing losses such as vomiting. Hydration improves renal perfusion and cardiac output, facilitating excretion of glucose. Rehydration may also diminish insulin resistance by decreasing levels of counterregulatory hormones and hyperglycemia. Sudden reduction in hyperglycemia can lead to vascular collapse with shift of water intracellularly. To avoid this, initial replacement fluid should be isotonic normal saline (NS) to correct circulatory volume deficit. **Over the first hour, 1–2 L of NS should be infused**. Following this, total body water deficit is corrected at the rate of 250–500 mL/h, depending on state of hydration. The composition of fluid should be tailored according to serum sodium and chloride measurements.

Hydration should be gentler in patients with congestive heart failure or end-stage renal disease because such patients can easily get fluid overload.

Insulin The goal of therapy is a glucose reduction of 80–100 mg/dL/h. The use of continuous low-dose intravenous infusion of insulin is recommended because it reduces episodes of hypoglycemia and hypokalemia, and allows a more controlled reduction of serum glucose and osmolality. Intramuscular and subcutaneous routes can be used if tissue perfusion is adequate.

Insulin treatment may be initiated as an **intravenous bolus** of 0.1–0.15 U/kg. This should be followed by a **continuous infusion of 0.1 U/kg/h with hourly serum glucose determinations**. If blood glucose fails to decline at the desired rate, volume status should be reassessed and insulin infusion should be titrated. The rate of infusion should be decreased to 0.05 U/Kg/h when blood glucose decreases to 250–300 mg/dL. Glucose levels fall more quickly than ketones resolve. Insulin is necessary for resolution of the ketoacidosis and can be coadministered with a glucose infusion until the anion gap is resolved. A 5–10% dextrose solution should be added to the hydrating solution when plasma glucose is <300 mg/dL. One can judge the resolution of ketoacidosis when the bicarbonate is >18 mEq/L, the anion gap is <12, patient feels better, and the vital signs are stabilized. Serial measurement of serum ketones is not clinically useful in measuring response to therapy. Lab tests measure acetoacetate and acetone, but not beta-hydroxybutyrate. With the administration of insulin, beta-hydroxybutyrate is first oxidized to acetoacetate, so measured ketone levels may actually increase with effective therapy. Instead, one should be guided by normalizing the anion gap when making decisions about the rate of insulin infusion. Subcutaneous insulin should be given approximately 30 minutes before stopping insulin infusion to avoid rebound acidosis.

Bicarbonate Bicarbonate therapy is controversial, and should not be given to ketoacidotic patients unless their arterial pH is below 7.0 or other indications, such as cardiac instability or severe hyperkalemia, are present. Bicarbonate therapy can cause worsening hypokalemia, paradoxical central nervous system acidosis, and delay in ketone clearance.

Electrolytes In DKA, there is total-body deficit of potassium, phosphate, and magnesium. Patients frequently have hyperkalemia as a result of acidosis, insulin deficiency, and hypertonicity that cause a shift of potassium extracellularly. During treatment, plasma potassium concentration will fall as the metabolic abnormalities are corrected. Potassium should be added to initial intravenous fluids once the concentration is <5 mEq/L. Once adequate urine output is established, 20–40 mEq of potassium should be added to each liter of fluid. The goal is to maintain potassium in the range of 4–5 mEq/L. Cardiac monitoring is recommended in presence of hypokalemia or hyperkalemia.

Phosphate replacement should be given to patients if serum phosphate concentrations <1 mg/dL and to patients with moderate hypophosphatemia with concomitant hypoxia, anemia, or cardiorespiratory compromise. Careful monitoring of serum calcium is necessary with phosphate administration.

Magnesium and calcium may be supplemented as needed.

Precipitating Causes It is important to correct precipitating factors to restore metabolic balance. Identifiable sources of infection should be treated aggressively. Possible presence of ischemia and infarction should be evaluated and treated appropriately with help from specialists as needed.

Complications Cerebral edema, acute respiratory distress syndrome, thromboembolism, fluid overload, and acute gastric dilatation are rare, but serious, complications of DKA.

Prevention The major precipitating factors in development of DKA are inadequate insulin treatment and infection. These events can be prevented by patient education and effective communication with a health care team. Sick-day management regarding dosing of insulin, blood glucose monitoring, avoiding prolonged fasting, and preventing dehydration should be addressed. There are socioeconomic barriers that contribute to the high rates of admission for DKA. Appropriate allocation of health care resources toward preventive strategies is needed.

Other metabolic complications of deranged carbohydrate metabolism deserve mention at this point. The first is **hyperosmolar nonketotic diabetic coma**. This condition occurs mainly in patients with type 2 diabetes, who become profoundly dehydrated because of osmotic diuresis. However, these patients have sufficient insulin action to prevent the development of ketoacidosis. They may present with glucose levels >1000 mg/dL, serum osmolarity >320–370 osm, and neurologic symptoms ranging from confusion to seizures to coma. Compared to patients with DKA, they have a much larger fluid deficit, and therapy is primarily volume resuscitation with normal saline. Insulin is also used to reverse hyperglycemia, but usually in lesser doses than is required for clearance of ketosis in DKA.

Alcoholic ketoacidosis develops in chronic alcoholics who are malnourished, with depleted glycogen stores, and is often seen in the setting of binge drinking, which may shift the ratio of nicotinamide adenine dinucleotide (reduced form) (NADH) to nicotinamide adenine dinucleotide (NAD), inhibiting gluconeogenesis. They develop an anion gap metabolic acidosis as a result of ketoacidosis and lactic acidosis. They present with the same symptoms of acidosis as DKA patients, for example, abdominal pain, nausea, and vomiting, but with low, normal, or slightly elevated glucose levels (in contrast to DKA, where glucose is usually markedly elevated). Treatment is administration of volume in the form of normal saline and glucose solution. Insulin administration is typically unnecessary.

Comprehension Questions

[43.1] Which of the following most likely will lead to a non-anion-gap acidosis?

A. Diarrhea
B. Lactic acidosis
C. Diabetic ketoacidosis
D. Ethylene glycol ingestions

[43.2] An 18-year-old male is noted to be in diabetic ketoacidosis with a pH of 7.20 and serum glucose level of 400 mg/dL. Which of the following is the most accurate statement regarding this patient's potassium status?

A. Likely to have a potassium level of <3.0 mEq/L
B. Likely to have a potassium level of >5 mEq/L
C. Likely to have a total-body potassium deficit regardless of the serum level
D. The serum level is likely to increase with correction of the acidosis

[43.3] Which of the following is the most important first step in the treatment of diabetic ketoacidosis?

A. Replacement of potassium
B. Intravenous fluid replacement
C. Replacement of phosphorus
D. Antibiotic therapy

Answers

[43.1] **A.** Diarrhea leads to bicarbonate loss, and usually does not affect the anion gap.

[43.2] **C.** The total-body potassium is usually depleted regardless of the serum level.

[43.3] **B.** The basic tenets of treating DKA include intravenous fluid, insulin to control the glucose, correction of metabolic disturbances, and identification of the underlying etiology.

CLINICAL PEARLS

❖ All patients with DKA are volume-depleted and require significant replacement of salt solution, and later, free water in the form of glucose solutions.

❖ Despite sometimes elevated potassium concentrations, all patients with DKA have a total body potassium deficit, and will require substantial potassium replacement.

❖ Glucose levels fall more quickly than ketones resolve. Continuous insulin therapy is necessary for resolution of the ketoacidosis and can be coadministered with a glucose infusion until the anion gap is resolved.

❖ Cerebral edema can result from overly rapid correction of hyperglycemia, or possibly from rapid administration of hypotonic fluids.

❖ Occurrence of DKA requires a precipitating cause: either insulin deficiency or a physiologic stressor such as infection.

REFERENCES

Butkiewicz EK, Leibson CL, et al. Insulin therapy for diabetic ketoacidosis: bolus vs. continuous insulin infusion. Diabetes Care 1995;18:1187.

Delaney MF. Diabetic ketoacidosis and hyperglycemic hyperosmolar nonketotic syndrome. Endocrinol Metab Clin North Am 2000;129(4):683–705.

Fass B. Diabetic ketoacidosis and hyperosmolar coma. In: Manual of endocrinology and metabolism, 2nd ed. Norman Lavin, (ed.). Little, Brown: Boston 1994:543–562.

Fishbein HA, Palumbo PJ. Acute metabolic complications in diabetes. In: Diabetes in America. Bethesda, MD: National Diabetes Data Group, NIH 1995:283–91.

Kitabchi AE. Management of hyperglycemic crises in patients with diabetes. Diabetes Care 2001;24(1):131–53.

Lebovitz HE. Diabetic ketoacidosis. Lancet 1995;345:767–772.

Magee MF. Management of decompensated diabetes. Crit Care Clin 2001;117(1):75–107.

Okuda Y, Adrogue HJ, Field JB, et al. Counterproductive effects of sodium bicarbonate in diabetic ketoacidosis. J Clin Endocrinol Metab 1996;81:314–20.

Quinn L. Diabetes emergencies in the patient with type 2 diabetes. Nurs Clin North Am 2001;136(2):341–59.

CASE 44

A 37-year-old previously healthy woman presents to your clinic for unintentional weight loss. Over the past 3 months, she has lost approximately 15 lb without changing her diet or activity level. Otherwise, she feels great. She has an excellent appetite, no gastrointestinal complaints except for occasional loose stools, a good level of energy, and no complaints of fatigue. She denies heat or cold intolerance. On examination, her heart rate is 108 beats per minute, her blood pressure is 142/82 mmHg, and she is afebrile. When she looks at you, she seems to stare, and her eyes are somewhat protuberant. You note a large, smooth, nontender thyroid gland, a 2/6 systolic ejection murmur on cardiac exam, and that her skin is warm and dry. There is no tremor.

- **What is the most likely diagnosis?**

- **How could you confirm this?**

- **What are the options for treatment?**

ANSWERS TO CASE 44: Thyrotoxicosis/Graves Disease

Summary: A 37-year-old woman presents with weight loss without anorexia, tachycardia, borderline hypertension, exophthalmos, and a smooth, nontender goiter.

- **Most likely diagnosis:** Thyrotoxicosis/Graves disease.
- **Confirm diagnosis**: A low serum thyroid-stimulating hormone (TSH) and an increased free thyroxine (T4) with this clinical presentation would be confirmatory. However, other tests that might help would be thyroid stimulating immunoglobulins, or diffusely elevated uptake of radioactive iodine on thyroid scan.
- **Treatment options:** Antithyroid drugs, radioactive iodine ablation, or surgical ablation of the thyroid.

Analysis

Objectives

1. Understand the clinical presentation of thyrotoxicosis.
2. Be able to discuss the causes of hyperthyroidism, including Graves disease and toxic nodule.
3. Learn the complications of thyrotoxicosis, including thyroid storm.
4. Understand the evaluation of a patient with a thyroid nodule.
5. Know the available treatment options for Graves disease, and outcomes of treatment.

Considerations

This 37-year-old woman has unintentional weight loss, loose stools, and warm skin. These are all symptoms of hyperthyroidism. Her thyroid gland is diffusely enlarged and nontender, and she has exophthalmus (protuberant eyes), which is consistent with Graves disease. This is a systemic disease with many complications that affect the entire body, including osteoporosis and heart failure. Treatment can include elimination of the excess thyroid hormone, but definitive therapy may include radioactive (or, less commonly, surgical) ablative therapy.

APPROACH TO HYPERTHYROIDISM

Definitions

Hyperthyroidism is the hypermetabolic condition that results from the effect of excessive amounts of thyroid hormones produced by the thyroid gland itself. Because almost all cases of thyrotoxicosis are caused by thyroid overproduction, these terms are often used synonymously.

Thyrotoxicosis is usually used as a general term for biochemical and physiologic manifestations of excessive levels of thyroid hormones from any source, for example, exogenous ingestion.

Clinical Approach

Hyperthyroidism affects numerous body systems.

Neuromuscular system: Nervousness, tremors and brisk reflexes are common. Inability to concentrate, proximal muscle weakness emotional lability and insomnia might also be present.

Cardiac system: Wide pulse pressure, flow heart murmurs, and tachycardia are usually present. Atrial fibrillation is present in 10–20% of patients. Long-standing thyrotoxicosis can cause cardiomegaly and result in high output heart failure.

Gastrointestinal system: Despite increased food intake weight loss is common. Hyperdefecation is usually present as a result of increased gastrointestinal motility, but diarrhea is rare.

Eyes: Retraction of the upper eyelid as a consequence of increased sympathetic tone gives some patients a wide-eyed stare. Lid-lag might be found on physical examination (sclera can be seen above the iris as the patient looks downward).Exophthalmos is distinctive of Grave's disease.

Skin: The skin is warm, moist, and velvety. Sweating is usually present as a consequence of vasodilatation and heat dissipation.

Reproductive system: Hyperthyroidism impairs fertility in women and may cause oligomenorrhea. In men, the sperm count is reduced. Impotence and gynecomastia might also be present.

Metabolism: Weight loss is a common finding, especially in older patients who develop anorexia, but sometimes, especially in young adults, weight gain can occur as a consequence of markedly increased caloric intake. Many patients develop an aversion to heat and a preference for cold temperatures.

Apathetic hyperthyroidism: Older patients with hyperthyroidism may lack typical adrenergic features and present instead with depression or apathy weight loss atrial fibrillation worsening angina pectoris or congestive heart failure.

Thyroid Storm It is a dangerous condition of decompensated thyrotoxicosis. The patient has **tachycardia** (exceeding 140 beats per minute), **fever** (104–106°F), **agitation, delirium, restlessness or psychosis, vomiting, and/or diarrhea**. It usually results from long-neglected severe hyperthyroidism to which a complicating event (intercurrent illness—infection, surgery, trauma or iodine load) is added. Treatment includes supportive care with fluids, antibiotics if needed, and specific treatment directed at the hyperthyroidism: large doses of antithyroid medications to block new hormone synthesis, iodine solution to block the release of thyroid hormone, propranolol to control the symptoms induced by the increased adrenergic tone, and glucocorticoids to decrease T4 to T3 conversion.

Etiology of Thyrotoxicosis **Graves disease** is the most common cause of hyperthyroidism (80%) and is usually seen in women, especially between ages of 30 and 50 years. It is an autoimmune disease caused by autoantibodies that activate the TSH receptor of the thyroid follicular cell, stimulating thyroid hormone synthesis and secretion, as well as thyroid gland growth. These antibodies cross the placenta and can cause neonatal thyrotoxicosis. The disease might follow a relapsing and remitting course.

Graves disease is marked by **goiter** (enlarged thyroid gland), thyroid bruit, **hyperthyroidism, ophthalmopathy, and dermopathy**. These features are variably present. Ophthalmopathy is characterized by inflammation of extraocular muscles, orbital fat, and connective tissue, resulting in proptosis (exophthalmos), impairment of eye muscle function, and periorbital edema. Ophthalmopathy can progress even after the treatment of thyrotoxicosis. Graves dermopathy is characterized by raised hyperpigmented orange peel texture papules. The most common site is the skin overlying the shins (pretibial myxedema). A low serum thyroid-stimulating hormone (TSH) will confirm the diagnosis. The degree of elevation of serum free thyroxine (T4) and free triiodothyronine (T3) levels can give an estimate of the severity of the disease. Tests that might be of help for the etiology of thyrotoxicosis are the levels of thyroid-stimulating immunoglobulin (TSI), which is elevated in Graves, and a thyroid uptake and scan, which will reveal a diffusely elevated iodine uptake in our patient.

Treatment options for Graves disease are medications, radioactive iodine, or surgery. Medications include beta-blockers (which are used for symptom relief) and antithyroid drugs (methimazole, propylthiouracil). The antithyroid drugs work mainly by decreasing the production of thyroid hormone. They can be used for short-term (prior to treatment with radioactive iodine or surgery) or long-term (1–2 years) treatment, after which, chance for remission is 20–30%. Side effects can be rash, allergic reactions, arthritis, hepatitis and agranulocytosis. Radioactive iodine is the treatment of choice in the United States. It is administered as an oral solution of sodium ^{131}I which is rapidly concentrated in thyroid tissue, inducing damage that results in ablation of the thyroid, depending on the dose, within 6–18 weeks. At least thirty percent of patients will become hypothyroid in the first year after treatment and 3% each year after that, requiring thyroid hormone supplementation. Radioactive iodine is contraindicated in pregnancy, and women of reproductive age are advised to postpone pregnancy for 6–12 months after treatment. Graves ophthalmopathy might be exacerbated by radioactive iodine treatment, so in selected patients glucocorticoids can be used to prevent this.

Surgery is usually reserved for large goiters with obstructive symptoms (dyspnea, dysphagia). Complications might include laryngeal nerve injury and hypoparathyroidism (due to removal of parathyroids or compromise of the vascular supply to them).

For our patient, treatment with radioactive iodine or antithyroid medications seems the most reasonable way to proceed and a discussion regarding her options and our recommendations should take place after confirming the diagnosis.

Other causes of thyrotoxicosis include the following:

Toxic multinodular goiter: It is found mainly in elderly and middle-age patients. Treatment consists of radioactive iodine or surgery. Radioactive iodine uptake is normal to increased and the scan reveals irregular thyroid lobes and a heterogenous pattern.

Autonomous hyperfunctioning adenoma ("hot nodule" or Plummer disease): Hyperthyroidism is not usually present unless the nodule exceeds 3 cm in size. The iodine scan looks like the flag of Japan: it demonstrates the hot nodule as having increased uptake (dark) and the rest of the gland with suppressed uptake (white). Hot nodules are almost never malignant. Cold nodules (no increased thyroid hormone production and no demonstration of local uptake if thyroid scan is performed) have a 5–10% risk of malignancy, so fine-needle aspiration, surgical removal, or ultrasonographic followup is needed for these nodules.

Thyroiditis: It is caused by destruction of thyroid tissue and release of preformed hormone from the colloid space. Subacute (de Quervain's) thyroiditis is an inflammatory viral illness with thyroid pain and tenderness. The hyperthyroid phase lasts for several weeks to months and then recovery follows. Treatment with nonsteroidal antiinflammatory medications and beta-blockers is usually sufficient, but in severe cases, glucocorticoids might be used. Other forms include postradiation, postpartum, subacute (painless thyroiditis), and amiodarone-induced thyroiditis. In thyroiditis, the radioactive iodine uptake is invariably decreased.

Medications: Excessive ingestion of thyroid hormone (factitious or iatrogenic), amiodarone, and iodine load.

Other causes, such as TSH-secreting pituitary adenoma hydatidiform moles choriocarcinomas secondary to secretion of human chorionic gonadotropin (hCG), ovarian teratomas, and metastatic follicular thyroid carcinomas, are rare causes of thyrotoxicosis.

Comprehension Questions

[44.1] A 44-year-old woman is noted to be nervous and has heat intolerance. Her thyroid gland is diffusely enlarged, nontender, with an audible bruit. Her TSH is very low. Which of the following is the most likely etiology?

A. Lymphocytic thyroiditis
B. Hashimoto thyroiditis
C. Graves disease
D. Multinodular toxic goiter

[44.2] Which of the following distinguishes hyperthyroidism from thyroid storm?

A. Tachycardia
B. Weight loss
C. Autonomic instability
D. Large goiter

[44.3] A 33-year-old woman is noted to have Graves disease. Which of the following is the best therapy?

A. Long-term propranolol
B. Lifelong oral propylthiouracil (PTU)
C. Radioactive iodine ablation
D. Surgical thyroidectomy

Answers

[44.1] **C.** Graves disease is the most common cause of hyperthyroidism in the United States, and often includes the thyroid gland features described, as well as the distinctive eye findings

[44.2] **C.** Autonomic instability (hyperthermia) and CNS dysfunction, such as confusion or coma, are the hallmarks of thyroid storm. It is a medical emergency with a high motality.

[44.3] **C.** Radioactive iodine is the definitive treatment for Graves disease. Surgery is indicated for obstructive symptoms, or during pregnancy.

CLINICAL PEARLS

❖ The most common cause of thyrotoxicosis is Graves disease. No other diagnosis is likely if the patient has bilateral proptosis and a goiter.

❖ In patients with Graves disease, thyrotoxic symptoms may be treated with antithyroid medication, or by thyroid gland ablation by radioactive iodine or surgery, but the ophthalmopathy may not improve.

❖ Graves disease may remit and relapse; in patients treated medically, one-third to one-half will become asymptomatic within 1–2 years.

❖ After radioablation, most patients with Graves disease become hypothyroid and will require thyroid hormone supplementation.

❖ Hyperfunctioning thyroid nodules (excessive thyroid hormone production, suppressed TSH, "hot" on radionuclide scan) are almost never malignant.

❖ Most "cold" thyroid nodules are not malignant, but fine-needle aspiration should be used to evaluate the need for surgical excision.

REFERENCES

Davies DF, Larsen TF. Thyrotoxicosis. In: Wilson JD, Foster DW, Kronenberg HM, et al., (eds). Williams textbook of endocrinology, 9th ed. Philadelphia: WB Saunders. 2003:372–421.

Hershman JM. Hypothyroidism and hyperthyroidism. In: Norman Lavin, ed. Manual of endocrinology and metabolism. Boston. Little, Brown: 2002:396–409.

McDermott MT. Thyroid emergencies. In: Endocrine secrets. Hanley and Belfus: Philadelphia. 2002:302–05.

Ross DS. Diagnosis of hyperthyroidism. Disorders that cause hyperthyroidism. Overview of the clinical manifestations of hyperthyroidism in adults. Treatment of Graves' hyperthyroidism. UpToDate 2003 (last referenced Dec. 2003).

Singer PA. Thyroiditis. In: Norman Lavin, (ed). Manual of endocrinology and metabolism. Little, Brown: Boston. 2002:386–95.

Wingo ST, Burch HB. Hyperthyroidism. In: McDermott MT, (ed). Endocrine secrets. Hanley and Belfus: Philadelphia. 2002:273–78.

CASE 45

A 32-year-old woman presents to the hospital emergency room complaining of productive cough, fever, and chest pain for 4 days. She was seen 2 days ago in her primary care physician's office with the same complaints, was diagnosed clinically with pneumonia, and sent home with oral azithromycin. Since then, her cough is still productive of greenish sputum, although it has diminished in quantity. But the fever has not abated, and she still experiences right-sided chest pain, which is worse when she coughs or takes a deep breath. In addition, she has begun to feel short of breath when she walks around the house. She has no other medical history. She works as a parking lot attendant and does not smoke. She has not traveled outside of the United States and has no sick contacts.

On physical examination, her temperature is 103.4°F, her pulse is 116 bpm, her blood pressure is 128/69 mmHg, her respiratory rate is 24 breaths per minute and shallow, and her pulse oximetry is 92% saturation on room air. Her physical examination is significant for decreased breath sounds in the lower half of the right lung fields posteriorly, with dullness to percussion about halfway up. There are a few inspiratory crackles in the mid-lung fields, and her left side is clear to auscultation. Her heart is tachycardic but regular with no murmurs. She has no cyanosis. Figure 45–1 shows her chest x-ray.

- **What is your most likely diagnosis?**

- **What is your next step?**

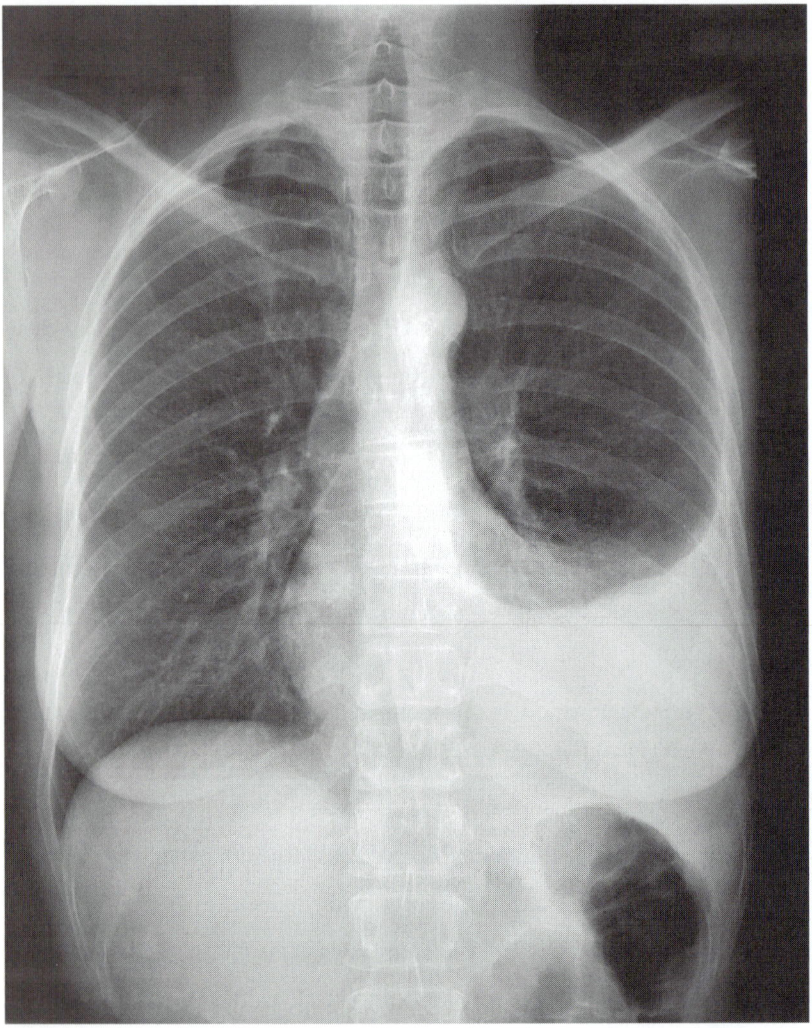

Figure 45–1. The PA film on the left reveals a left-side pleural effusion. The right image is a decubitus chest film of the same patient. **(Courtesy of Dr Jorge Albin)**.

ANSWERS TO CASE 45: Pleural Effusion, Parapneumonic

Summary: A previously healthy young woman comes in with a clinical diagnosis of community-acquired pneumonia that has not improved with outpatient treatment. She has diminished breath sounds and dullness to percussion on the left side of her chest, suggesting a large left-sided pleural effusion, which is confirmed by chest radiography. The effusion is likely caused by infection in the adjacent lung parenchyma, and may be the cause of her failure to improve on antibiotics.

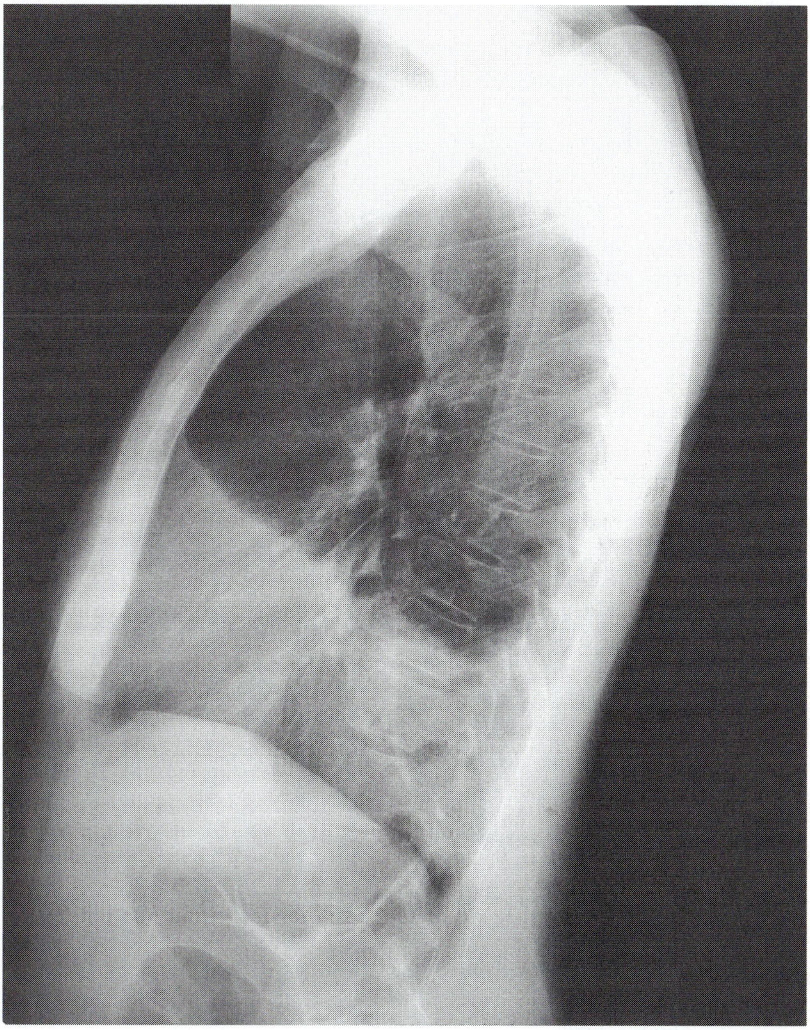

- **Most likely diagnosis:** Bacterial pneumonia with parapneumonic effusion.
- **Next step:** Diagnostic thoracentesis to help diagnose the cause of the pleural effusion and to determine the necessity for drainage of the fluid.

Analysis

Objectives

1. Understand the use of Lights criteria to distinguish transudative effusions from exudative effusions, as a guide to the etiology of the effusion.

2. Learn what pleural fluid characteristics suggest a complicated parapneumonic effusion or empyema, and the need for drainage.
3. Know the treatment of a complicated parapneumonic effusion that does not improve after thoracentesis.

Considerations

In this patient, the effusion is large and if free-flowing such as on a lateral decubitus film, then diagnostic thoracentesis can easily be accomplished. It is important to determine if the effusion is, in fact, caused by the pneumonia, and if so, whether it is likely to resolve with antibiotics alone, or will it need drainage with tube thoracostomy.

APPROACH TO PLEURAL EFFUSION

Definitions

Exudate: Effusion caused by inflammatory or malignant causes, usually with high protein or high lactate dehydrogenase (LDH) levels.
Pleural effusion: Accumulation of fluid in the pleural space.
Transudate: Effusion caused by alteration of oncotic forces, usually with low protein and low LDH levels.

Clinical Approach

Diagnostic thoracentesis should be considered on every patient that presents with a chest radiograph with evidence of pleural effusion. Possibly the only exception to this rule is if the patient is known to have congestive heart failure with equal bilateral effusions or if the effusion is too small, that is, less that 10 mm on lateral decubitus film. If the pleural effusion of congestive heart failure does not significantly improve after a trial of diuresis, however, a diagnostic tap should be performed. See Table 45-1 for correlation of pleural fluid appearance. About 50 mL of fluid is needed to be visible on a lateral decubitus film (more reliable in detecting smaller effusions) and fluid greater than 500 cc in volume usually obscures the whole hemidiaphragm.

Indications for thoracentesis:

- Uneven pleural effusion or unilateral pleural effusion.
- Evidence of infection, for example, productive cough, fever, or pleurisy.
- Normal cardiac silhouette (no heart failure).
- Alarming signs, for example, significant weight loss, hemoptysis, or hypoxia.
- Need to evaluate underlying lung parenchyma.

A simple "diagnostic" thoracentesis can be performed, but if the effusion is significant in size and patient is dyspneic, especially at rest, a "therapeutic" thoracentesis may also be done with a safe removal of up to 1500 mL. With removal of more fluid, the patient is at risk of developing reexpansion pulmonary edema.

Table 45-1
PLEURAL FLUID APPEARANCE

Clear yellow	Transudative, e.g., secondary to CHF, cirrhosis, nephrotic syndrome
Frank pus	Infectious process, empyema
Bloody	If the hematocrit of the pleural fluid is: <1% : Blood caused by traumatic tap 1–20%: Cancer, pulmonary embolus, tuberculosis >50%: Hemothorax: most commonly secondary to trauma but also seen in malignancy and pulmonary embolism
Milky, turbid	Chylothorax triglyceridws >110 mg/dL resulting from disruption of thoracic duct, cholesterol effusion
Dark green	Biliothorax

Transudate versus Exudate To appreciate the pathophysiology of the formation of a transudate versus an exudate is to understand the differential under each category. About 10 mL of pleural fluid is formed every day by the visceral pleura and absorbed by the parietal pleura (capillaries and lymphatics). Processes that disturb this "equilibrium" lead to the accumulation of fluid. Clinical settings in which the hydrostatic pressure is increased, for example, congestive heart failure (CHF) and constrictive pericarditis, or in which the oncotic pressure is decreased, for example, nephrotic syndrome and cirrhosis, or the intrapleural pressure is reduced, for example, atelectasis, leads to the formation of a "transudate." In contrast, "exudates" are more a result of local inflammation, for example, infection, malignancy, and connective-tissue diseases, which cause a protein leak into the pleural space. Less commonly, impaired lymphatic drainage, such as in chylothorax, or lymphangitic spread of a malignancy may also cause an exudative fluid. Pulmonary emboli can cause both exudative and transudative effusions. See Tables 45–2 and 45–3 for etiologies.

Pleural Fluid: Lights Criteria The most widely used criteria to distinguish between a transudative and exudative fluid is the Lights criteria first described in 1997. For a fluid to be labeled an **exudate**, it must meet **at least one of the following criteria** (transudates meet none of these criteria):

1. Pleural fluid protein/serum protein ratio greater than 0.5
2. Pleural fluid LDH/serum LDH ratio greater than 0.6
3. Pleural fluid LDH greater than two-thirds the upper limits of normal of the serum LDH

Pleural LDH correlates with the degree of **pleural inflammation**, and along with **fluid protein**, should always be sent in the initial evaluation.

Parapneumonic Effusions and Empyemas Pleural effusions occur in 40% of patients with an underlying bacterial pneumonia. Most of these effusions

Table 45-2
CAUSES OF TRANSUDATIVE PLEURAL EFFUSIONS

TRANSUDATE	CLINICAL OR RADIOGRAPHIC FEATURES
Congestive heart failure	Most commonly bilateral and symmetric, at times isolated right-sided effusion
Nephrotic syndrome	Bilateral and subpulmonic
Cirrhosis with ascites	Fluid should have characteristics similar to ascitic fluid
Malignancy	Secondary to decreased drainage of daily fluid by obstructed lymphatics
Pulmonary embolism	May also be exudative or bloody; rarely large
Hypothyroidism	Secondary to the thyroid hormone deficiency

Table45-3
CAUSES OF EXUDATIVE PLEURAL EFFUSIONS

EXUDATE	COMMENT
Infection	Bacterial pneumonia, viral etiology, fungal infection, parasitic (eosinophilic) involvement; subdiaphragmatic abscesses
Tuberculosis	A third have parenchymal involvement; lymphocytes >80%; adenosine deaminase >43 U/L; total protien >4.0 g/dL; diagnostic yield of fluid for acid-fast bacilli <10%; pleural biopsy increases yield to between 80 and 90%
Malignancy	Lymphocytic predominant and occasionally bloody; cytologic examination positive in >50% of cases; usually indicative of dismal prognosis
Connective-tissue disease	Rheumatoid pleurisy: very low glucose, Rheumatoid factor >1:320 and >serum titer and LDH >1000 IU/L; More common in men Lupus pleuritis: positive lupus erythematosus cells; pleural fluid/serum antinuclear antibody >1.0; usually responsive to steriod treatment
Pancreatitis	Elevated pancreatic amylase isoenzyme; salivary isoenzyme seen in esophageal rupture with associated low pH
Chylothorax	Triglycerides >110 mg/dL
Asbestos exposure	Spectrum of disease ranges from the presence of pleural plaques to effusion and malignancy; also usually eosinophilic

should resolve with appropriate antibiotic treatment, but if the fluid characteristics predict a **"complicated" parapneumonic** effusion, urgent tube drainage is indicated to prevent formation of fibrous peels which may need surgical decortication.

The following fluid characteristics suggest chest tube drainage is necessary:

- Empyema (frank pus in the pleural space)
- Positive Gram stain of fluid
- Presence of loculations
- pH <7.10
- Glucose <40 mg/dL
- LDH >1000 U/L

If the patient does not meet the criteria for immediate drainage, a 1-week trial of antibiotics is indicated with close reevaluation of those patients who do not respond or who clinically deteriorate.

If tube thoracostomy drainage is required, a chest tube is placed until drainage rate has fallen below 50 mL/d. Postdrainage imaging must be obtained to confirm complete drainage of fluid and to assess the need to place a second tube if the fluid has not been adequately drained (as is often seen if the effusion is loculated. Complete sterilization of the cavity is desirable when treating an empyema with 4–6 weeks of antibiotics, as is complete obliteration of the space by lung expansion. Multiloculated empyemas are treated further by administering fibrinolytic agents such as streptokinase or urokinase through the chest tube. Video-assisted thorascopic surgery (VATS) is another option to try to break up fibrinous adhesions.

Comprehension Questions

[45.1] A 55-year-old man with congestive heart failure develops bilateral pleural effusions. What is the most likely pleural fluid characteristic if thoracentesis is performed?

A. Pleural fluid LDH 39, LDH ratio 0.2, protein ratio 0.7
B. Pleural fluid LDH 39, LDH ratio 0.2, protein ratio 0.1
C. Pleural fluid LDH 599, LDH ratio 0.9, protein ratio 0.1
D. Pleural fluid LDH 599, LDH ratio 0.9, protein ratio 0.7

[45.2] A 39-year-old man develops a moderate free-flowing pleural effusion following a left lower lobe pneumonia. Thoracentesis reveals straw-colored fluid with Gram-positive diplococci on Gram stain, pH 6.9, glucose 32 mg/dL, and LDH 1890. Which of the following is the best next step?

A. Send the fluid for culture.
B. Continue treatment with antibiotics for pneumococcal infection.
C. Tube thoracostomy to drain the effusion.
D. Schedule a follow-up chest x-ray in 2 weeks to document resolution of the effusion.

[45.3] A 69-year-old man complains of gradually worsening dyspnea and a nagging cough over the past 4 weeks, and is found to have a right-sided pleural effusion, which is tapped and is grossly bloody. Which of the following is the most likely diagnosis?

A. Parapneumonic effusion
B. Malignancy in the pleural space
C. Rupture of aortic dissection into the pleural space
D. Pulmonary embolism with pulmonary infarction

Answers

[45.1] **B.** Congestive heart failure is commonly associated with bilateral pleural effusions, which are transudative, as a consequence of alteration of Starling forces. The elevated LDH or protein ratio in each of the other answers would be found in an exudative effusion. The effusions of heart failure are best managed by treating the heart failure, for example, with diuretics.

[45.2] **C.** The positive Gram stain, low pH, low glucose, and markedly elevated LDH all suggest that this parapneumonic effusion is "complicated," that is, it is unlikely to resolve with antibiotic therapy and is likely to produce loculated pockets of pus, which will require surgical intervention. Drainage by serial thoracentesis or tube thoracostomy is essential.

[45.3] **B.** The most common causes of a hemorrhagic pleural effusion are malignancy, pulmonary embolism, and tuberculosis. Pulmonary embolism would be suggested by an acute onset of dyspnea and pleuritic chest pain rather than this subacute presentation. Similarly, aortic rupture can produce a hemothorax, but would have an acute presentation with pain and hemodynamic compromise.

CLINICAL PEARLS

❖ Transudative effusions meet *none* of the following criteria (exudative effusions meet at least one):
 Pleural fluid protein/serum protein ratio >0.5
 Pleural fluid LDH/serum LDH ratio >0.6
 Pleural fluid LDH greater than two-thirds of the upper limit of normal for serum

❖ Tube thoracostomy or more aggressive drainage of parapneumonic effusion predict is usually required with gross pus (empyema), positive Gram stain or culture, glucose <40 mg/dL, pH <7.10, and loculations.

- ❖ The most common cause of pleural effusion is congestive heart failure, which typically gives bilateral symmetric transudative effusions and is best treated with diuresis.
- ❖ The most common causes of a bloody pleural effusion (in the absence of trauma) are malignancy, pulmonary embolism with infarction, and tuberculosis.

REFERENCE

Light RS. Disorders of the Pleura, Mediastinum and Diaphragm. In: Braunwald E, Fauci AS, Kasper KL, et al., eds. Harrison's principles of internal medicine, 15th ed. New York: McGraw-Hill. 2001:1513-1517.

CASE 46

A 25-year-old man presents to your clinic for a general checkup and cholesterol screening. He denies having medical problems, and takes no medications on a regular basis. He works as a computer programmer, exercises regularly at a gym, and does not smoke or use illicit drugs. He drinks two to three beers on the weekend. His father suffered his first heart attack at age 36 years, and eventually died of complications of a heart attack at 49 years of age. The patient's older brother was recently diagnosed with "high cholesterol."

The patient's blood pressure is 125/74 mmHg, with a heart rate of 72 bpm. He is 69 inches tall and weighs 165 pounds. His physical examination is unremarkable.

Fasting lipid levels are drawn. The next day, you receive the results: Total cholesterol 362 mg/dL, triglycerides 300 mg/dL, high-density lipoprotein (HDL) 36 mg/dL, and low-density lipoprotein (LDL) 266 mg/dL.

- **What is the most likely diagnosis?**
- **What is your next step?**
- **What are the possible complications if left untreated?**

ANSWERS TO CASE 46: Hypercholesterolemia

Summary: A healthy 25-year-old man presents for a physical examination and is found to have markedly elevated total and LDL cholesterol and triglycerides, and low HDL cholesterol. He has an unremarkable physical examination. He is normotensive, a nonsmoker, but with a strong family history of hypercholesterolemia and premature atherosclerotic coronary artery disease.

- **Diagnosis:** Familial hypercholesterolemia.
- **Next step:** Counsel regarding lifestyle modification with low-fat diet and exercise, and offer treatment with an HMG-CoA (beta-hydroxy-beta-methylglutaryl-coenzyme A) reductase inhibitor.
- **Complications if untreated:** The development of atherosclerotic vascular disease, including coronary heart disease.

Analysis

Objectives

1. Know the risk factors for developing coronary artery disease, and know how to estimate the risk for coronary events using the Framingham risk-scoring system.
2. Be familiar with the recommendations for cholesterol screening and for the treatment of low-, intermediate-, and high-risk patients.
3. Understand how the different classes of lipid-lowering agents affect lipid levels and the potential side effects of those agents.
4. Know the secondary causes of hyperlipidemia.

Considerations

A young man presents to the clinic for a checkup and is found to have markedly elevated total cholesterol (normal <200 mg/dL) and LDL levels (normal <100 mg/dL), and low HDL levels (normal >45 mg/dL). He does not have any apparent secondary causes of dyslipidemia, and no signs or symptoms of vascular disease. He does have a strong family history of hypercholesterolemia and premature death caused by myocardial infarction. The decisions regarding the method and intensity of lipid-lowering therapy are based on one's estimation of the patient's 10-year risk of major coronary events. Because of his very high lipid levels and his family history, he is a high-risk patient and, thus, should be counseled about lipid-lowering medical therapy. The very high cholesterol levels at a young age in the absence of secondary causes, leads one to suspect familial hypercholesterolemia, a condition caused by defective or absent LDL surface receptors, and subsequent inability to metabolize LDL particles. Meanwhile, the importance of lifestyle modification cannot be overemphasized.

APPROACH TO HYPERLIPIDEMIA

Atherosclerotic coronary artery disease is the leading cause of death of both men and women in the United States. Because of the association of hypercholesterolemia and development of atherosclerotic heart disease, most authorities recommend routine screening of average risk individuals at least every 5 years. Clinical laboratories usually measure total cholesterol, HDL, and triglycerides. The LDL cholesterol may be calculated by using the formula:

LDL = Total cholesterol – HDL – (Triglycerides/5)

A fasting sample should be measured, if possible, but the total cholesterol and HDL are still reliable in a nonfasting sample. The triglycerides and the calculated LDL levels are affected by recent dietary intake, and should be drawn in the fasting state.

Approximately 25% of American adults have a total cholesterol level >240 mg/dL, which the guidelines from the National Cholesterol Education Program consider as elevated. Management of patients with hypercholesterolemia involves assessment of other atherosclerotic risks to estimate the 10-year risk of coronary events such as fatal or nonfatal myocardial infarction. The LDL goal is set based on the estimated cardiovascular risk.

The **highest risk patients** already have **established coronary heart disease (CHD)** or other **atherosclerotic vascular disease**: their 10-year risk for future coronary events is **>20%**. The presence of **diabetes is now considered a "CHD risk equivalent"** because of their higher risk of vascular disease, as well as a higher mortality rate from myocardial infarction than nondiabetics. High-risk individuals have an **LDL goal <100 mg/dL.**

The LDL goal for individuals who do not have established CHD or CHD equivalents (diabetes or other vascular disease such as stroke) is based on a risk-stratification process. First, the number of risk factors for CHD is counted (Table 46–1). The absolute 10-year risk for patients with two or more risk factors may be estimated using a scoring system based on data from the Framingham heart study (Figure 46–1). Patients with multiple risk factors are then assigned to high risk (>20%), intermediate risk (10–20%), or low risk (<10%). Those in the intermediate risk category should have an LDL goal of **<130 mg/dL, whereas the lowest risk patients have an LDL goal of <160mg/dL.**

One should exclude a secondary cause of lipid disorder, either by clinical or laboratory evaluation. These underlying disorders include diabetes, hypothyroidism, obstructive liver disease, chronic renal failure/nephrotic syndrome, and medication side effects (progestins, anabolic steroids, corticosteroids). High cholesterol levels in young patients in the absence of secondary causes suggests familial hypercholesterolemia, a condition caused by defective or absent LDL surface receptors, and subsequent inability to metabolize LDL particles. Homozygotes for this condition may develop

Table 46-1
CHD RISK FACTORS

Cigarette smoking
Hypertension (elevated blood pressure when seen, or patient on antihypertensives)
Low HDL cholesterol (<40 mg/dL)
Family history of premature coronary artery disease (in men <55 years old, or in women <65 years old)
Age of the patient (men >45 years old, women >55 years old)

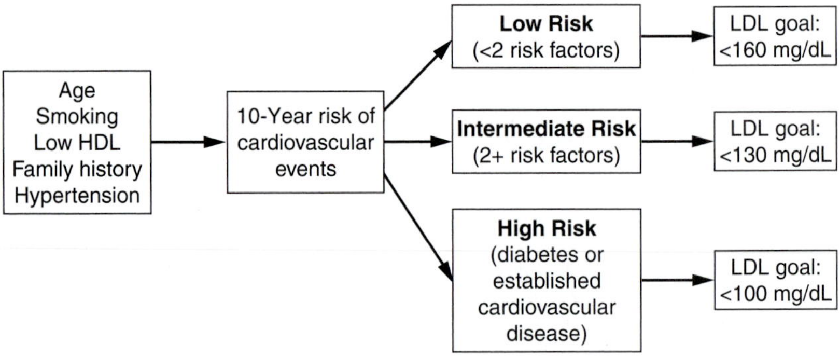

Figure 46–1. Risk of coronary heart disease based on risk factors.

atherosclerotic disease in childhood, and usually require intensive lipid-lowering drug therapy.

Lowering serum cholesterol levels decreases the risk of major coronary events and death in hypercholesterolemic patients without a prior history of coronary heart disease **(primary prevention),** as well as reducing the overall mortality and coronary disease mortality in patients who have established cardiovascular disease **(secondary prevention).** All patients should first be educated regarding therapeutic lifestyle changes. These changes include a diet low in saturated fat (<7% of total daily calories) and low in cholesterol (<200 mg/d), as well as exercise, which can help to lower cholesterol.

When lifestyle modifications are not enough to reach the LDL goal, multiple lipid-lowering medications are available. Table 46–2 lists their effects on lipids and their potential side effects. **Side effects of statins** are uncommon, but include **myopathy**, which may manifest as muscle tenderness with elevated creatine kinase levels, and may progress to rhabdomyolysis. Less commonly, **elevated liver enzymes**, or even severe hepatitis, has been reported. When these drugs are used, routine clinical or laboratory monitoring for these effects is advisable.

Table 46-2
DRUGS FOR HYPERLIPIDEMIA

DRUG CLASS	THERAPEUTIC EFFECTS	SIDE EFFECTS	MONITORING
HMG-CoA reductase-inhibitors ("statins")	Lower LDL 25–55% Lower TG 10–25% Raise HDL 5–10%	Hepatic injury, myositis	Monitor LFTs and creatine kinase
Nicotinic acid (e.g., niacin)	Lower TG 25–35% Lower LDL 15–25% Raise HDL 15–30%	Flushing, tachycardia	Flushing may be relieved by aspirin
Bile-acid resins (e.g., cholestyramine)	Lower LDL 20–30% Raise HDL 5%	Constipation, nausea, GI discomfort	Binds fat-soluble vitamins
Fibric-acid derivatives (e.g., gemfibrozil)	Lower TG 25–40% Raise HDL 5–15%	Gallstones, nausea, increased LFTs	Caution if used with statins

Abbreviations: LFT = liver function test; TG = triglycerides. Ginsberg HN, Goldberg IJ. Disorders of lipoprotein metabolism. In: Braunwald E, Fauci AS, Kasper KL, et al, eds. Harrison's principles of internal medicine, 15th ed. New York: McGraw-Hill; 2001:2254.

Comprehension Questions

[46.1] A 35-year-old man with no history of cardiac or other vascular disease asks how often he should have routine cholesterol screening. Which of the following is the best answer?

A. Every 3 months
B. Annually
C. Every 5 years
D. Every 7–10 years

[46.2] A 38-year-old man presents to your office following a health fair screening of his cholesterol because he was told that it is high. He watches his diet, plays tennis, exercises 3–5 times a week, and appears to be in good physical condition. He is a nonsmoker, and has no family history of cardiovascular disease. His profile is total cholesterol 202 mg/dL, HDL 45 mg/dL, LDL 128 mg/dL, and triglycerides 145mg/dL. Following a review of this patient's profile, which of the following would you recommend?

A. Administer gemfibrozil
B. Administer HMG-CoA reductase inhibitor

C. Administer low-dose niacin and slowly increase to achieve 3 g daily
D. Suggest he continue his current diet and exercise program

[46.3] Which of the following patients is the best candidate for lifestyle modification alone rather than lipid-lowering medications?

A. A 40-year-old man with a recent myocardial infarction: cholesterol 201, HDL 47, and LDL 138
B. A 62-year-old diabetic man: cholesterol 210, HDL 27, and LDL 146
C. A 57-year-old asymptomatic woman: cholesterol 235, HDL 92, and LDL 103
D. A 39-year-old man with nephrotic syndrome: cholesterol 285, HDL 48, LDL 195

Answers

[46.1] **C.** The recommended interval for cholesterol screening in this population of healthy adults is every 5 years. Cholesterol levels do not change rapidly over a person's lifetime. A rapid change should prompt investigation for an underlying secondary cause.

[46.2] **D.** In this scenario, this 38-year-old man's only risk factor for CHD is male sex, thus, his 10-year risk is <10%. His total cholesterol is barely in the borderline high category, fairly near the desirable level, his LDL is <130 mg/dL, and his HDL is acceptable.

[46.3] **C.** Patient A is the highest risk for future events because he has established CHD, so his 10-year risk for events is >20%. His goal LDL is <100 mg/dL. Patient B has diabetes, a CHD equivalent. Besides lifestyle modifications, he should start drug therapy to lower his LDL and raise his HDL. Patient C has very high HDL, which is protective, and probably contributes to her elevated total cholesterol. Patient D has nephrotic syndrome causing hyperlipidemia, which may be treated by reduction of proteinuria using angiotensin-converting enzyme (ACE) inhibitors, but often requires drug therapy such as statins.

CLINICAL PEARLS

❖ The intensity of lipid-lowering therapy is based on the patient's estimated 10-year risk for coronary events: high risk goal LDL is <100, intermediate risk goal LDL is <130, low-risk- goal LDL is <160 mg/dL.

❖ The highest risk patients are those with established coronary heart disease, other atherosclerotic vascular disease such as stroke or peripheral vascular disease, or diabetes, which is considered a "CHD equivalent."

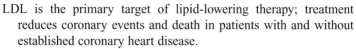

- ❖ LDL is the primary target of lipid-lowering therapy; treatment reduces coronary events and death in patients with and without established coronary heart disease.
- ❖ The major side effects of statins are myopathy and hepatocellular injury.

REFERENCE

Executive summary of the third report of the National Cholesterol Education Program Expert Panel on Detection, Evaluation, and Treatment of High Blood Cholesterol in Adults (ATP III). JAMA 2001;285(19):2486–97.

CASE 47

A 72-year-old man is admitted to the hospital because of an acute onset of a right facial droop, right arm weakness, and some difficulty speaking. These symptoms occurred this morning while he was sitting at the breakfast table. He had no headache, no diminishment of consciousness, and no abnormal involuntary movements. Two weeks ago, he had a transient painless loss of vision in his left eye, which resolved spontaneously within a few hours. His past medical history is significant for long-standing hypertension, and a myocardial infarction 4 years previously, which was treated with percutaneous angioplasty. His medications include a daily aspirin, metoprolol, and simvastatin. He does not smoke. When you see him 5 hours later, his symptoms have nearly resolved. He is afebrile, his heart rate is 62 bpm and his blood pressure is 135/87 mmHg. The corner of his mouth droops, with slight flattening of the right nasolabial fold, but he is able to fully elevate his eyebrows. His strength is 4/5 in his right arm and hand, and the rest of his neurologic exam is normal. He has no carotid bruits, his heart is regular with no murmur but with an S4 gallop. The remainder of his physical exam is normal. Laboratory studies including his renal function, liver function, lipid profile, and complete blood count are all normal. By the next morning, all of the patient's symptoms have resolved.

- **What is the most likely diagnosis?**

- **What is the next step?**

ANSWERS TO CASE 47: Transient Ischemic Attack

Summary: A 72-year-old man is admitted because of an acute right face and, right arm weakness, and some difficulty speaking, which resolves within 5 hours. He denies headache, diminishment of consciousness, or abnormal involuntary movements. Two weeks ago, he had a transient painless loss of vision in his left eye, which resolved spontaneously within a few hours. He has no carotid bruits, but he does have atherosclerotic coronary artery disease.

- **Most likely diagnosis:** Transient ischemic attack caused by atheroembolism from the left internal carotid artery.

- **Next step:** Perform a noninvasive study such as a high-resolution carotid ultrasonography or a magnetic resonance angiogram to evaluate for carotid artery stenosis.

Analysis

Objectives

1. Know the most common mechanisms for ischemic stroke: carotid stenosis, cardioembolism, lipohyalinosis, or other small vessel disease.
2. Understand the evaluation of a stroke patient with the goal of secondary prevention.
3. Learn which patients are best managed with medical therapy, and which patients benefit from carotid endarterectomy.

Considerations

This 72-year-old man has resolution of neurological deficits, the hallmark of transient ischemic attacks. He has established atherosclerotic coronary disease, but no known carotid artery disease. He denies headache, which is important because migraine headache may be associated with neurological deficits; it would be rare for an elderly man to have the first presentation of migraine headache. Various neurological diseases, such as multiple sclerosis, are characterized by complete resolution of neurological deficits, but the symptoms usually last longer than 24 hours. He does not have abnormal motor activity, which would suggest seizure disorder. Although this gentleman does not have carotid bruits, the distribution of the neurological deficits most likely corresponds to left carotid disease. Initially, noninvasive imaging of the carotid arteries should be performed to determine the extent of stenosis. With these symptoms, if there is >70% stenosis of the left internal carotid artery, the possibility of left carotid endarterectomy should be discussed.

APPROACH TO TRANSIENT ISCHEMIC ATTACK/STROKE

Definitions

Amaurosis fugax: Transient monocular blindness that is often described as a gray shade being pulled down over the eye caused by ischemia to the retinal artery.

Stroke: Acute onset of a focal neurologic deficit due to a cerebral infarction or hemorrhage.

Transient ischemic attack: Transient neurologic deficit secondary to ischemia in a defined vascular territory that lasts less than 24 hours (most commonly lasting < 1 hour).

Clinical Approach

Transient ischemic attacks (TIA), often referred to as "mini-strokes" refer to a sudden onset of a focal neurologic deficit, with spontaneous resolution within 24 hours (usually within the first hour). Not all transient focal neurologic events actually represent ischemia, however. The differential diagnosis includes classic migraine, postictal paralysis, seizures, cerebral hemorrhage, or even slow-evolving intracranial processes such as subdural hematoma, abscess, or tumors, which can suddenly produce symptoms because of edema, hemorrhage, or production of seizure activity. However, clinical evaluation and imaging studies of the brain should be sufficient to exclude most or all of these diagnoses.

The **focal neurologic symptoms** produced by ischemia depends on the **area of the cerebral circulation** involved, and may include (a) amaurosis fugax, (b) hemiparesis, (c) hemianesthesia, (d) aphasia, or (e) dizziness/vertigo as a result of vertebrobasilar insufficiency. The significance of a TIA is not the symptoms it produces, because by definition it is self-resolved, but of the risk for future events it portends. **The highest-risk patients for stroke are those with previous ischemic events such as TIA;** that is, it can be looked upon as a warning sign of impending potential disaster.

TIAs are produced by temporary ischemia to a vascular territory, usually caused by thrombosis or embolism, and less commonly caused by vasculitis, hematologic disorders such as sickle cell disease, or vasospasm. By far, the most common causes of stroke or TIA are **carotid atherosclerosis** (large vessel disease), **cardioembolism** usually to branches of the middle cerebral artery (medium-size vessel disease), or **lipohyalinosis** affecting small lenticulostriate arteries (small vessel disease). Table 47–1 lists the etiologies of TIA/stroke.

The workup for a transient ischemic attack begins with a history and physical examination. Pertinent historical factors include onset, course, and duration of symptoms, atherosclerotic risk factors, and relevant past medical history (i.e., atrial fibrillation). Physical examination should begin

Table 47-1
ETIOLOGY OF TRANSIENT ISCHEMIC ATTACKS

Emboli of cardiac origin
Intracardiac thrombus or mass
Myocardial infarction (anterior wall sputum, akinetic segment)
Cardiomyopathy (infectious, idiopathic)
Arrhythmia (atrial fibrillation)
Cardiac myxoma
Valvular heart disease
Rheumatic heart disease
Bacterial endocarditis
Nonbacterial endocarditis (carcinoma, Libman-Sacks disease)
Mitral valve prolapse
Prosthetic valve
Vasculitides
Primary central nervous system vasculitis
Systemic necrotizing vasculitis (polyarteritis nodosa, allergic angiitis)
Hypersensitivity vasculitis (serum sickness, drug-induced, cutaneous vasculitis)
Collagen vascular diseases (rheumatoid arthritis, scleroderma, Sjögren disease)
Giant cell (temporal arteritis, Takayasu arteritis)
Wegener granulomatosis
Lymphomatoid granulomatosis
Behçet disease
Infectious vasculitis (neurovascular syphilis, Lyme disease, bacterial and fungal meningitis, tuberculosis, acquired immunodeficiency syndrome, ophthalmic zoster, hepatitis B)
Hematologic disorders
Hemoglobinopathies (sickle cell, sickle-cell hemoglobin C [HbSC]
Hyperviscosity syndromes (polycythemia, thrombocytosis, leukocytosis, macroglobulinemia, multiple myeloma)
Hypercoagulable states (carcinoma, pregnancy, puerperium)
Protein C or S deficiency
Antiphospholipid antibodies (lupus anticoagulant, anticardiolipin antibody)
Drug related
Street drugs (cocaine, crack, amphetamines, lysergic acid, phencyclidine, methylphenidate, sympathomimetics, heroin, pentazocine)
Alcohol
Oral contraceptives
Other
Fibromuscular dysplasia
Arterial dissection (trauma, spontaneous, Marfan syndrome)
Homocystinuria
Migraine
Subarachnoid hemorrhage or vasospasm
Other emboli (fat, bone marrow, air)
Moyamoya

with blood pressures in four extremities, and should include a funduscopic exam. In this patient, the first symptom was amaurosis fugax due to cholesterol emboli, called Hollenhorst plaques, which can often be seen lodged in the retinal artery. Auscultation for carotid bruits, cardiac murmurs, assessment of cardiac rhythm, evidence of embolic events to other parts of the body, and a complete neurologic examination should also be assessed.

Laboratory data that should always be obtained include a complete blood count, fasting lipid profile, and serum glucose. Other laboratory data, such as an erythrocyte sedimentation rate in elderly populations to evaluate for temporal arteritis, should be tailored to the demographic of the patient. Generally, a 12-lead EKG must be obtained to evaluate for or atrial fibrillation. An echocardiogram can be useful to evaluate for valvular or mural thrombi. A noncontrast CT scan of the brain also must be done initially. Noncontrasted CT scans of the brain are very sensitive in detecting acute cerebral hemorrhage, but are relatively insensitive to acute ischemic strokes, particularly when the area of the stroke is less than 5 mm in diameter, in the region of the brainstem, or are <12 hours old. Further imaging with magnetic resonance may be considered.

Finally, imaging of the extracranial vasculature to detect severe **carotid artery stenosis is essential to guide further stroke prevention therapy.** The **gold standard** for imaging of extracranial and intracranial vasculature is **cerebral angiography**. However, carotid Doppler ultrasound and magnetic resonance angiography are effective noninvasive imaging studies, and are often used as a first-line diagnostic tools.

Stroke prevention begins with **antiplatelet therapy**, and **aspirin** should be used in all cases unless there is a contraindication to its use. Use of **clopidogrel** may be slightly superior to aspirin for stroke prevention, but at a substantially higher dollar cost. For patients with TIA/stroke as a consequence of carotid atherosclerosis, medical management includes antiplatelet agents, blood pressure control, treatment of hyperlipidemia, and smoking cessation. For patients with cardioembolic stroke, as a result of atrial fibrillation, long-term anticoagulation with Coumadin is recommended. For patients with small vessel disease producing lacunar infarctions, blood pressure control and antiplatelet agents are the mainstay of therapy.

Surgical endarterectomy for severe carotid artery stenosis has successfully reduced the long-term risk of stroke in both symptomatic and asymptomatic patients. The North American Symptomatic Carotid Endarterectomy Trial (NASCET) showed that in patients who have had a TIA or stroke and have ipsilateral **carotid artery stenosis >70%,** endarterectomy reduced the rate of stroke was reduced from 26% to 9% over 2 years, as compared with standard medical management. The Asymptomatic Carotid Artery Stenosis (ACAS) trial also showed benefit from carotid endarterectomy in asymptomatic carotid artery stenoses greater than 60%. However, the risk reduction was smaller than in symptomatic patients, from 11% to 5% over 5 years as compared to medical management. It should also be noted that the surgery is not without risk, and can actually cause strokes. In both trials, the stipulation was made that in order to achieve the risk reduction benefit, surgery should be performed in a center with a very low surgical morbidity and mortality.

Comprehension Questions

[47.1] A healthy 55-year-old man without prior history of stroke or TIA is seen for his annual physical examination. He is found to have a right carotid bruit. On Duplex ultrasound, he is found to have a 75% stenosis of the right carotid artery. Which of the following is the best therapy?

A. Aspirin
B. Coumadin
C. Carotid endarterectomy
D. Observation and reassurance

[47.2] One year ago, a 24-year-old woman had an episode of diplopia for 2 weeks duration. The symptoms resolved completely. Currently, she complains of left arm weakness but no headache. Which of the following is the most likely diagnosis?

A. Recurrent transient ischemic attacks
B. Subarachnoid hemorrhage
C. Complicated migraine
D. Multiple sclerosis

[47.3] A 67-year-old woman with extensive atherosclerotic cerebrovascular disease complains of dizziness and vertigo. Which of the following arteries is most likely to be affected?

A. Vertebrobasilar
B. Carotid
C. Aorta
D. Middle cerebral

Answers

[47.1] **C.** In this asymptomatic patient, carotid endarterectomy may be considered for severe stenosis (>70%), provided that it can be done in a center with very low surgical morbidity and mortality.

[47.2] **D.** Multiple neurologic deficits separated in space and time in a young patient are suggestive of multiple sclerosis.

[47.3] **A.** Vertigo and dizziness can be seen vertebrobasilar insufficiency.

CLINICAL PEARLS

- The most common causes of cerebral infarction are carotid atherosclerotic stenosis, cardioembolism, or small vessel disease such as lipohyalinosis.
- Cerebral infarction, TIA, and amaurosis fugax may all be symptoms of carotid stenosis.
- In symptomatic patients with severe stenosis >70%, carotid endarterectomy is superior to medical therapy in stroke prevention provided the surgical risk is low (<3%).
- For other patients, stroke prevention consists mainly of antiplatelet agents (aspirin, clopidogrel) and risk factor modification, for example, blood pressure, hypercholesterolemia, smoking cessation.

REFERENCES

Sacco RL. Extracranial Carotid Stenosis. N Engl J Med 2001;345(15): 1113–18.

Pulsinelli WA. Ischemic Cerebrovascular Disease. In: Goldman L, Bennett JC (eds). Cecil's textbook of medicine, 21st ed. Philadelphia: WB Saunders. 2000:2099-2109.

Chung CS, Caplan LR. Neurovascular Disorders. In: Goetz CG, Pappert EJ, (eds). Textbook of clinical neurology, 1st ed. Philadelphia: WB Saunders. 1999:907-932.

CASE 48

A 25-year-old man comes to an outpatient clinic complaining of low-grade fever and sore throat, and receives an injection of intramuscular penicillin for presumed streptococcal pharyngitis. He is otherwise healthy and takes no regular medications. Within 20 minutes, he begins to complain of swelling of his face and difficulty breathing. He looks dyspneic and frightened. His heart rate is 130 bpm, his blood pressure is 90/47 mmHg, and he has shallow respirations at 28 breaths per minute. His face and lips are edematous and he can barely open his eyes because of swelling. He is wheezing diffusely, and he has multiple raised urticarial lesions on his skin. An ambulance has been called.

- **What is the most likely diagnosis?**
- **What is your next step?**

ANSWERS TO CASE 48: Anaphylaxis/Drug Reactions

Summary: A 25-year-old man develops facial edema and difficulty breathing minutes after an injection of penicillin. He is tachypneic, tachycardic, with borderline hypotension. He is wheezing diffusely, his abdomen is nondistended with hyperactive bowel sounds, and his skin is warm with multiple raised urticarial lesions.

- **Most likely diagnosis:** Anaphylaxis as a result of penicillin hypersensitivity.

- **Next step:** Immediate administration of subcutaneous epinephrine, along with corticosteroids and H_1 and H_2 blockers. Close observation of the patient's airway and oxygenation, with possible endotracheal intubation if he becomes compromised.

Analysis

Objectives

1. Learn the clinical presentation and emergency management of anaphylaxis.
2. Understand the diagnosis and complications of serum sickness.
3. Be able to recognize and treat erythema multiforme minor and major.

Considerations

This young man developed manifestations of immediate hypersensitivity, that of "hives" of the skin, and swelling of the airway and bronchospasm. Penicillin is fairly allergenic, and leads to an immunoglobulin (Ig) E-mediated release of histamines and other vasoactive chemicals. Epinephrine is the agent of choice in acute anaphylaxis. Antihistamines may also help. Because the airway is vulnerable to compromise as a result of severe edema, intubation to protect the airway is sometimes indicated. The differential diagnosis should include these disease entities: anaphylactoid reactions, angioedema (hereditary and non-hereditary), urticaria–angioedema syndrome, serum sickness, systemic mastocytosis, erythema multiforme major and minor, and vasovagal reactions.

APPROACH TO SUSPECTED ANAPHYLAXIS

Definitions

Angioedema: Swelling of the lips, periorbital region, face, hands, or feet.

Anaphylactoid reactions: A similar clinical picture to anaphylaxis, but not caused by immunologic mechanisms.

Anaphylaxis: A syndrome with varied mechanisms, clinical presentations and severity that is an acute life-threatening reaction, mediated by an immunologic IgE-mediated mechanism.

Clinical Approach

Common causes of anaphylaxis include drugs, hymenoptera stings, radiographic contrast media (anaphylactoid), blood products, allergen immunotherapy injections, and foods. **The most common cause of drug-related anaphylaxis is beta-lactam antibiotics such as penicillins.** The **most common cause of food-related anaphylaxis is peanuts**, partly because of the frequency with which peanut products are included in other types of foods. However, it is important to note that almost any agent that can activate mast cells or basophils can cause an anaphylactic reaction. Approximately one-third of all cases of anaphylaxis are idiopathic.

The clinical presentation of anaphylactic reactions varies greatly, but the following guidelines are a good rule of thumb. Symptoms usually develop within 5–60 minutes following exposure, although a delayed reaction is possible. Symptoms and signs are variable and are listed in Table 48–1. The key fact to remember is that a **true anaphylactic reaction is life-threatening**. Angioedema may occur with or without urticaria, but is not anaphylaxis unless the reaction is associated with other life threatening processes, such as hypotension or laryngeal edema.

Treatment of anaphylaxis begins with first assessing the **ABCs** (airway, breathing, circulation). If intubation is required, this should not be delayed. Second, **epinephrine** should be administered to help control symptoms and blood pressure. Intramuscular epinephrine injected in the anterolateral thigh leads to more rapid and higher peak levels than either subcutaneous or deltoid intramuscular injection. Additional treatment measures include placing the patient in a recumbent position, elevating the legs, oxygen as needed, normal saline volume replacement and/or pressors as required, administration of diphenhydramine 50 mg oral or intravenously every 4 hours as needed. (see Table 48–2).

Other considerations in the differential diagnosis of anaphylaxis include erythema multiforme major and minor. **Erythema multiforme minor**, often occurs after herpes simplex virus (HSV) or other infections, and manifests itself as urticarial or bullous skin lesions. The pathognomonic finding is a target lesion, described as a lesion that is centrally inflamed, surrounded by an area of less inflamed skin. Treatment includes management of the underlying cause when known, withdrawal of suspected causative drugs, and acyclovir if HSV involvement is suspected. Erythema multiforme major (Stevens-Johnson Syndrome [SJS]) is similar to erythema multiforme minor, but is more severe and involves 2 or more mucosal surfaces. It is also more likely to be induced by drugs such as sulfonamides or NSAIDS than is erythema multiforme minor. The skin findings may include petechiae, vesicles, and bullae and can result in some desquamation of the skin. If the epidermal detachment involves less than 10% of the skin, it is considered SJS. If epidermal detachment involves more than 30% of the skin, it is considered **toxic epidermal necrolysis** (TEN). Other symptoms include fever, headache, malaise, arthralgias, corneal ulcerations, arrhythmia, pericarditis, electrolyte abnormalities,

Table 48-1
CLINICAL MANIFESTATIONS OF ANAPHYLAXIS

Pruritus
Flushing, urticaria, and angioedema
Diaphoresis
Sneezing, rhinorrhea, nasal congestion
Hoarseness, stridor, laryngeal edema
Dyspnea, tachypnea, wheezing, bronchorrhea, cyanosis
Tachycardia, bradycardia, hypotension, cardiac arrest, arrythmias
Nausea/vomiting, diarrhea, abdominal cramping
Dizziness, weakness, syncope
Sense of impending doom
Seizures

Table 48-2
SUGGESTED TREATMENT OF ANAPHYLAXIS

Address ABCs (airway, breathing, circulation); intubate if needed
Epinephrine either as intravenous solution (1:1000 0.1–0.3 mL in 10 mL of normal saline over several minutes) or intramuscularly (1:1000 0.3–0.5 every 5 minutes as needed).
Oxygen as needed
Placing the patient in a recumbent position, elevating the legs
Normal saline volume replacement and/or pressors as required
Diphenhydramine 50 mg orally or intravenously every 4 hours as needed
Other measures Ranitidine or other H_2 blockers Albuterol or levalbuterol for bronchospasm Glucagon if the patient is taking beta-blockers Systemic steroids to prevent delayed reactions

seizures, coma, and sepsis. The treatment involves withdrawal of the suspected offending agent, treatment of concurrent infections, aggressive fluid maintenance, and supportive treatment similar to burn care. The use of corticosteroids is controversial, but they are often prescribed.

Most drug rashes are maculopapular and occur several days after starting treatment with an offending drug. They are usually not associated with other signs and symptoms and resolves several days after removal of the offending agent. **Serum sickness** on the other hand, is an allergic reaction that occurs 7–10 days after primary administration or 2–4 days after secondary administration of a foreign serum or a drug (i.e., a heterologous protein or a nonprotein drug). It is characterized by fever, polyarthralgia, urticaria, lymphadenopathy and sometimes glomerulonephritis. It is caused by the formation of immune complexes of IgG and the offending antigen. Treatment is based on symptomatology and the disease is usually self-limiting. This may include antihistamines, aspirin/nonsteroidal antiinflammatory drugs (NSAIDs), and treatment of associated disease. Finally, there are several other types of drug reactions that do not fit into the above categories. Two of the most important ones are iodine allergy and phenytoin (Dilantin) hypersensitivity. "Iodine allergy" if often associated with radiologic contrast media. Reactions caused by contrast media are caused by the hyperosmolar dye causing degranulation of mast cells and basophils rather than a true allergic reaction. These reactions can be avoided by pretreatment with diphenhydramine, H_2 blockers, and corticosteroids beginning 12 hours prior to the procedure. Dilantin hypersensitivity can manifest itself in range from skin rash to TEN to hypotension and cardiovascular collapse. This is not IgE mediated and the exact mechanism remains unclear. Treatment is withdrawal of the offending agent.

Comprehension Questions

[48.1] A 55-year-old accountant complains of facial and tongue swelling. He notes that his firm recently changed its stationery and ink. His medical problems include osteoarthritis and mild hypertension, for which he takes acetaminophen and captopril, respectively. Which of the following is the most likely etiology?

A. Captopril
B. Paper and ink hypersensitivity
C. Hypothyroidism
D. Acetaminophen
E. Food-related allergy

[48.2] An 18-year-old male with epilepsy controlled with medication develops fever, lymphadenopathy, a generalized maculopapular rash, and arthralgias. He notes having been bitten by ticks while working on the yard outside. Which of the following is most likely etiology?

A. Severe poison ivy dermatitis
B. Reaction to epilepsy medication
C. Acute HIV infection
D. Lyme disease

[48.3] A 34-year-old man is brought into the emergency room for a severe allergic reaction caused by fire ant bites. He is treated with intramuscular epinephrine and intravenous corticosteroids. His oxygen saturation falls to 80% and he becomes apneic. Which of the following is the best next step?

A. Intravenous diphenhydramine
B. Intravenous epinephrine
C. Oxygen by nasal cannula
D. Endotracheal intubation
E. Electrical cardioversion

[48.4] A 57-year-old woman with congestive heart failure has a positive cardiac stress test. Cardiac catheterization is required to evaluate for coronary bypass grafting. She states that she has an allergy to iodine. Which of the following is the best next step?

A. Desensitization with increasing doses of oral iodine
B. Infusion of diphenhydramine during the procedure
C. Cancel the procedure, and proceed to surgery
D. Diphenhydramine and corticosteroids the night before the procedure

Answers

[48.1] **A.** Angiotensin-converting enzyme (ACE) inhibitors are often associated with angioedema.

[48.2] **B.** This is the typical presentation of phenytoin (Dilantin) hypersensitivity. Poison ivy is not associated with fever and lymphadenopathy.

[48.3] **D.** He has developed airway obstruction due to an anaphylactic reaction. He requires intubation and positive pressure ventilation to maintain oxygenation.

[48.4] **D.** Pretreatment with diphenhydramine, H_2 blockers, and corticosteroids beginning 12 hours prior to the procedure greatly decreases the reaction to contrast dye.

CLINICAL PEARLS

❖ Anaphylaxis is characterized by respiratory distress caused by bronchospasm, cutaneous manifestations such as urticaria or angioedema, and gastrointestinal hypermotility. Patients may die as a consequence of airway compromise or hypotension and vascular collapse caused by widespread vasodilatation.

❖ The treatment of anaphylaxis is immediate epinephrine, antihistamines and airway protection and blood pressure support as necessary. Corticosteroids may help prevent late recurrence of symptoms.

- ❖ Serum sickness is an immune-complex-mediated disease that may include fever, cutaneous eruptions, lymphadenopathy, arthritis, and glomerulonephritis. It is usually self-limited, but treatment may be necessary for the renal complications.
- ❖ Erythema multiforme minor is characterized by urticarial or bullous eruptions, often with target lesions, usually following HSV infections. Erythema multiforme major (Stevens-Johnson syndrome) is usually caused by drugs and includes cutaneous and mucosal involvement.

REFERENCES

Stern RS, Chosidow OM, Wintroub BU. Cutaneous Drug Reactions. In: Braunwald E, Fauci AS, Kasper KL, et al., eds. Harrison's principles of internal medicine, 15th ed. New York: McGraw-Hill, 2001:341; 1967.

Peters B. Anaphylaxis. In: Dambro et al. Griffith's 5-minute clinical consult 2001 (can access online at http://www.5mcc.com/content.html). Last accessed December 2003. New York: Lipincott Williams & Wilkins.

Kemp SF, Lockey RF. Anaphylaxis: a review of causes and mechanisms. J Allergy Clin Immunol 2002;110(3):342–48.

O'Dowd LC, Zweiman B. Up To Date. Anaphylaxis. http://www.utdol.com Updated December 8, 2003.

Simmons ER, Roberts JR, et al. Epinephrine absorption in children with a history of anaphylaxis. J Allergy Clin Immunol 1998;101:33–37.

Simmons ER, Xiaochen G, et al. Epinephrine absorption in adults: intramuscular versus subcutaneous injection. J Allergy Clin Immunol 2001;108:871–73.

CASE 49

A 68-year-old woman has been noted by her daughter to have memory loss and confusion. The daughter states that her mother has been going "downhill" for the past several months. The mother has lived on her own for many years, but recently she has begun to become unable to take care of herself. The daughter states that her mother has become withdrawn and has lost interest in her usual activities, such as gardening and reading. Her mother's memory is poor, and she is often fatigued. The patient states that she sleeps well at night and that her appetite is good, although she has lost 10 lb over the past 6 months. She denies bowel and urinary incontinence. The patient's past medical history is significant for hypertension for which she has been taking hydrochlorothiazide. The patient was last hospitalized 35 years ago when she underwent a total abdominal hysterectomy with bilateral salpingo-oophorectomy. The patient has enjoyed overall good health. She does not smoke or drink. On examination, her blood pressure is 116/56 mmHg, her heart rate is 78 bpm, her temperature is 98.7°F, and her respiratory rate is 18 breaths per minute. She weighs 160 lb and her height is 5 ft 3 in. The patient is a well-developed white women with a flat affect. She is oriented to person, but she is not oriented to time and place. Mini Mental Status Examinatin gives a score of 18 out of 30. The head and neck and cardiovascular examination are unremarkable. Abdomen is benign without hepatosplenomegaly. The extremities are without edema, cyanosis, or clubbing. The neurologic examination reveals that the cranial nerves are intact, and the motor and sensory exams are within normal limits. Cerebellum examination is unremarkable and the gait is normal.

- **What is the most likely diagnosis?**
- **What are the next diagnostic steps?**
- **What is the best treatment for this condition?**

ANSWERS TO CASE 49: Alzheimer Dementia

Summary: A 68-year-old woman has memory loss, confusion, and fatigue, and is withdrawn. She has a flat affect. She is oriented to person, but she is not oriented to time and place. The remainder of the examination, including neurological examination, is normal except for a low score on the MMSE.

- **Most likely diagnosis:** Alzheimer dementia.
- **Next diagnostic step:** Assess for depression and reversible causes of dementia.
- **Probable treatment:** Acetylcholinesterase inhibitor.

Analysis

Objectives

1. Know some of the common causes of dementia.
2. Understand the presentation and diagnosis of Alzheimer dementia.
3. Know the treatment for Alzheimer dementia is acetylcholinesterase inhibitor.

Considerations

This is an elderly woman without any significant past medical history except for hypertension who was brought to your office with a history of progressive functional decline and memory loss. The first step should be to rule out depression. Depression in the elderly may have a presentation very similar to that of dementia with withdrawal, apathy, irritability, memory impairment, and confusion. The next step should be to rule out all the possible causes of reversible or arrestable dementia, such as multi-infarct dementia, hypothyroidism, drugs, B_{12} deficiency, normal pressure hydrocephalus, alcoholism, HIV, and syphilis. Laboratory tests will help you to eliminate some of these common causes of reversible dementia: **complete blood count (CBC), comprehensive metabolic panel, thyroid-stimulating hormone (TSH), urinalysis, serologic test for syphilis, and a head CT (see table 49–1).** The possibility of HIV-induced dementia is not high on the differential in this case given the patient's age, but it would certainly be a consideration in younger people. Possible infectious causes of reversible dementia include not only HIV but also neurosyphilis. Therefore, a serologic test for syphilis is indicated. Because our patient does not have a history of chronic alcoholism, we can rule out this condition. The CBC and mean cell volume (MCV) are normal, as is the TSH, eliminating the possibilities of vitamin B_{12} deficiency and of hypothyroidism. The patient is only taking hydrochlorothiazide, which is not associated with the described mental status changes. A CT head scan can assess for brain lesions, multiple infarcts, and hydrocephalus. Therefore, in this case we are left with the possibility of multiinfarct dementia and

Table 49-1
ABBREVIATED WORKUP FOR DEMENTIA

Complete blood count and consider erythrocyte sedimentation rate (ESR)
Chemistry panel
Thyroid-stimulating hormone level
Venereal Disease Resaerch Laboratory (VDRL)
HIV assay
Urinalysis
Serum vitamin B_{12} and folate levels
Chest radiograph
Electrocardiogram
CT or MRI imaging of the head

Alzheimer disease. Multi-infarct dementia develops later in life and is caused by diffuse cerebrovascular disease. Most of the patients will have a history of transient ischemic attacks and strokes, and stepwise progression of dementia which our patient does not report. In this particular case, Alzheimer dementia becomes the most likely diagnosis.

APPROACH TO DEMENTIA

Definitions

Alzheimer disease: The leading cause of dementia, accounting for half of the cases involving elderly individuals, correlating to brain atrophy with ventricular enlargement.

Dementia: Progressive and generalized decline of intellectual ability from a previously attained level, usually without alteration of consciousness.

Multiinfarct dementia: Numerous small cerebral vascular accidents, most commonly caused by atherosclerotic disease, leading to dementia.

Normal pressure hydrocephalus: Reversible form of dementia where the cerebral ventricles slowly enlarge as a result of disturbances to cerebral spinal fluid resorption. The classic triad is dementia, gait disturbance, and urinary or bowel incontinence.

Clinical Approach

A patient who presents with memory and functional impairment should be approached from the perspective that many etiologies can be causative. A thorough description of the patient's cognitive, adaptive, memory, and behavioral ability over time is critical. Multiple family members are often needed to construct a complete and accurate picture. The time frame (months to years versus days to weeks) is important. A history of head trauma, neurological symptoms, a stepwise decline (multi-infarct dementia) versus a insidious gradual decline may be helpful. A record of all medications, habits, alcohol use (even remote), can potentially cause mental status changes in the elderly. A resting tremor of Parkinson disease, cold intolerance suggestive of hypothyroidism, or vitamin deficiencies may be helpful.

The other intracranial diseases that could cause a dementia-like picture include subdural hematoma and normal pressure hydrocephalus. Usually, a CAT (computed axial tomography) scan will allow you to rule out these disease processes. Also, remember, that normal pressure hydrocephalus is usually accompanied by gait disturbances and urinary incontinence which our patient does not have. Parkinson disease is also associated with the development of dementia but patients with Parkinson disease have symptoms and physical findings that will alert you to the diagnosis. Table 49–2 lists the neurological diseases that impair cognitive ability.

The etiology of Alzheimer dementia is an unknown but Alzheimer disease has a genetic component. The risk of developing the disease for an individual in a family with Alzheimer disease increases by a factor of 3 or 4. The gene that codes for apoprotein E seems to be associated with some prediction. The pathologic changes in the brains of Alzheimer disease patients include neurofibrillary tangles with a deposition of abnormal amyloid in the brain. The disease onset can be very insidious and the average life expectancy after diagnosis is 7–10 years. The clinical course is characterized by the progressive decline of cognitive functions (memory, orientation, attention and concentration) and the development of psychological and behavioral symptoms (wandering, aggression, anxiety, depression and psychosis) (see Table 49–3).

Treatment

The goals of treatment in Alzheimer disease are to (a) improve cognitive function, (b) reduce behavioral and psychological symptoms, and (c) improve the quality of life. Donepezil (Aricept) and rivastigmine (Exelon) are cholinesterase inhibitors that are effective in improving cognitive function and global clinical state. Risperidone reduces psychotic symptoms and aggression in patients with dementia. Other issues include wakefulness, nightwalking and wandering, aggression, incontinence, and depression. A structured environment, with predictability, and judicious use of pharmacotherapy, such as selective serotonin reuptake inhibitor (SSRI) for depression or a short-acting benzodiazepine for insomnia, are helpful. The primary caregiver is often overwhelmed and needs support. The Alzheimer Association is a national organization developed to give support to family members, and can be contacted through www.alz.org.

Table 49-2
NEUROLOGICAL DISEASES IMPAIRING COGNITIVE ABILITY

DISEASE	CLINICAL FEATURES	TREATMENT
Alzheimer disease	Slow decline in cognitive and behavioral ability; pathology: neurofibrillary tangles, enlarged cerebral ventricles, and atrophy	Cholinesterase inhibitors such as donepezil or rivastigmine
Normal-pressure hydrocephalus	Gait disturbance, dementia, incontinence; enlarged ventricles without atrophy	Ventricular shunting process
Multi-infarct dementia	Focal deficits, stepwise loss of function; multiple areas of infarct usually subcortical	Address atherosclerotic risk factors, identify and treat thrombus
Parkinson disease	Extrapyramidal signs (tremor, rigidity), slow onset	Dopaminergic agents
HIV infection	Systemic involvement; risk factors for acquisition; positive HIV serology	Treat specific infection
Neurosyphilis	Optic atrophy, Argyll-Robertson pupils, gait disturbance; positive cerebro-spinal fluid serology	High dose intravenous penicillin
Multiple sclerosus	Brainstem signs, optic atrophy, long-standing disease with exacerbations and remissions; MRI showing white matter abnormalities	Recombinant interferon, corticosteroids
Intracranial tumor	Focal signs, papilledema, seizures	Corticosteroids to reduce intracranial pressure, treat the lesion

Table 49-3
ALZHEIMER DISEASE CLINICAL COURSE

CLINICAL STAGE	MANIFESTATIONS
Early	Mild forgetfulness, poor concentration, fairly good function, denial, occasional disorientation
Intermediate	Drastic deficits for recent memory, can travel to familiar locations, suspicious, anxious, aware of confusion
Late	Cannot remember names of family members or close friends; may have delusions or hallucinations, agitation, aggression, wandering, disoriented to time and place, need for substantial care
Advanced	Totally incapacitated and disoriented, incontinent, personality and emotional changes; eventually all verbal and motor skills deteriorate, leading to need for total care

Comprehension Questions

[49.1] A 78-year-old female is diagnosed with Alzheimer disease. Which of the following agents is most likely to help with the cognitive function?

A. Haloperidol
B. Estrogen replacement therapy
C. Donepezil
D. High dose Vitamin B_{12} injections

[49.2] A 74-year-old male was noted to have excellent cognitive and motor skill 12 months ago. His wife noted that 6 months ago, his function deteriorated in a noticeable way, and, again, 2 months ago, another level of deterioration was noted. Which of the following is most likely to reveal the etiology of his functional decline?

A. HIV Antibody test
B. Magnetic resonance imaging of the brain
C. Cerebrospinal fluid VDRL test
D. Serum thyroid-stimulating hormone (TSH)

[49.3] A 55-year-old man is noted by his family members to be forgetful and become disoriented. He also has difficulty making it to the bathroom in time, and complains of feeling as though "he is walking like he was drunk." Which therapy is most likely to improve his condition?

A. Intravenous penicillin for 21 days
B. Rivastigmine
C. Treatment with fluoxetine for 9 to 12 months

D. Ventriculoperitoneal shunt
E. Enrollment into Alcoholic Anonymous

[49.4] Which of the following commonly seen in brain imaging of patients with Alzheimer disease?

A. Normal cerebral ventricles and atrophic brain tissue
B. Enlarged cerebral ventricles and atrophic brain tissue
C. Enlarged cerebral ventricles and no atrophy of brain tissue
D. Normal cerebral ventricles and normal brain tissue, acetylcholine deficiency

Answers

[49.1] **C.** Cholinesterase inhibitors help with the cognitive function in Alzheimer disease and may slow the progression somewhat.

[49.2] **B.** The stepwise decline in function is typical for multi-infarct dementia, diagnosed by viewing multiple areas of the brain infarct.

[49.3] **D.** The classic triad for normal pressure hydrocephalus is dementia, incontinence, and gait disturbance; one treatment is shunting the cerebrospinal fluid.

[49.4] **B.** Alzheimer disease typically has enlarged cerebral ventricles and brain atrophy, whereas normal pressure hydrocephalus has enlarged brain ventricles without brain atrophy.

CLINICAL PEARLS

❖ Alzheimer disease is the most common type of dementia, followed by multi-infarct (arteriosclerotic) dementia.

❖ Approximately 5% of people older than age 65 years and 20% older than age 80 years have some form of dementia.

❖ Depression and reversible causes of dementia should be considered in the evaluation of a patient with memory loss and functional decline.

❖ A cholinesterase inhibitor such as donepezil is effective in improving cognitive function and global clinical state in patient's with Alzheimer disease.

REFERENCES

Bird TD. Alzheimer's Disease and other Primary Dementias. In: Braunwald E, Fauci AS, Kasper KL, et al., eds. Harrison's principles of internal medicine, 15th ed. New York: McGraw-Hill, 2001:2391-2398.

❖ CASE 50

A 59-year-old woman comes into your office because she is concerned that she might have a brain tumor. She has had a fairly severe headache for the last 3 weeks (she rates it as an 8 on a scale of 1–10). She describes the pain as constant, occasionally throbbing but mostly a dull ache, and localized to the right side of her head. She thinks the pain is worse at night, especially when she lies with that side of her head on the pillow. She has had no nausea, vomiting, photophobia, or other visual disturbances. She has had headaches before, but they were mostly occipital and frontal, which she attributed to "stress," and they were relieved with acetaminophen. Her past medical history is significant for hypertension, which is controlled with hydrochlorothiazide, and "arthritis" of her neck, shoulders, and hips for which she takes ibuprofen when she feels stiff and achy. On physical examination, her temperature is 100.4°F, her heart rate is 88 bpm, her blood pressure is 126/75 mmHg, and her respiratory rate is 12 breaths per minute. Her visual acuity is normal, visual fields are intact, and her funduscopic exam is significant for arteriolar narrowing, but no papilledema or hemorrhage. She has moderate tenderness over the right side of her head but no obvious scalp lesions. Her chest is clear, her heart is regular with a normal S1 and S2, and with an S4 gallop, and her abdominal exam is benign. She has no focal deficits on neurologic exam. She has no joint swelling or deformity, but is tender to palpation over her shoulders, hips, and thighs.

◆ **What is the most likely diagnosis?**

◆ **Which serum test will confirm the diagnosis?**

ANSWERS TO CASE 50: Headache/Temporal Arteritis

Summary: A 59-year-old woman complains of a 3-week history of severe right-side headaches, which are worse at night, when she lies with that side of her head on the pillow. Her past medical history is significant for hypertension and "arthritis" of her neck, shoulders, and hips, for which she takes ibuprofen. She has a temperature is 100.4°F and normal neurological and eye examinations. She has moderate tenderness over the right side of her head but no obvious scalp lesions.

- **Most likely diagnosis:** Temporal arteritis.
- **Test to confirm diagnosis:** Erythrocyte sedimentation rate (ESR).

Analysis

Objectives

1. Be familiar with the clinical features that help to distinguish a benign headache from one representing a serious underlying illness.
2. Know the clinical features and diagnostic tests for temporal arteritis.
3. Know the clinical features of migraine and cluster headaches and of subarachnoid hemorrhage.

Considerations

Although headaches are a very common complaint, this patient has features that are of greater concern: older age of onset, abrupt onset and severe in intensity, and unlike previous milder headaches. These are three of the nine factors of concern for significant underlying pathology outlined in Table 50–1. She is very concerned about the headaches and is worried that it is a brain tumor. She has no meningeal signs and her neurologic exam is nonfocal. She also has stiffness and achiness of the shoulder and hip girdles. Together these factors make the diagnosis of temporal arteritis a strong possibility. Temporal arteritis usually has its onset in a woman age 50 years or older, and involves inflammation of the medium- or large-sized vessels. Her low-grade fever and generalized body aches may represent polymyalgia rheumatica, which is closely associated with temporal arteritis. The diagnosis would be confirmed by an elevated erythrocyte sedimentation rate or temporal artery biopsy. Although temporal arteritis is not a common cause of headache, untreated patients often progress to permanent visual loss as a consequence of involvement of the ophthalmic artery, so a high index of suspicion is necessary to begin investigation. An elevated ESR necessitates further diagnostic testing, such as a temporal artery biopsy. In the meantime, empiric corticosteroids may help prevent complications.

APPROACH TO HEADACHES

Headache is one of the most common complaints of patients in the Western world, periodically afflicting 90% of adults and almost 25% have recurrent

Table 50-1
RED FLAGS FOR SECONDARY HEADACHE DISORDERS

Fundamental change or progression in headache pattern
First severe and/or worst headache
Abrupt-onset attacks, including those awakening one from sleep
Abnormal physical examination findings (general or neurological)
Neurological symptoms lasting >1 hour
New headache in individuals aged <5 years or >50 years
New headache in patients with cancer, immunosuppression, pregnancy
Headache associated with alteration in or loss of consciousness
Headache triggered by exertion, sexual activity, or Valsalva maneuver

severe headaches. As with many common symptoms, there is a broad range of conditions, from trivial to life-threatening, that might be responsible. The **majority of patients** presenting with **headache** will have **tension-type, migraine, or cluster**, and fewer than 1 in 20 will have significant underlying pathology. Because headache symptoms are usually accompanied by a paucity of associated findings, including on laboratory examination, the clinician must depend largely upon a thorough history with a general and focused neurological examination as the initial workup. Careful inquiry and meticulous physical examination keeping in mind the "red flags" of headaches (see Table 50–1) will serve the clinician well. Differentiating serious underlying causes of headache from more benign causes may be difficult. Table 50–2 lists some typical features of serious causes of headache.

One of the most catastrophic secondary cause of headache is **subarachnoid hemorrhage,** usually secondary to a ruptured intracerebral (berry) aneurysm. Up to 4% of patients presenting to an emergency center with severe headache, or the classic "worst ever headache," will have a subarachnoid bleed. The initial hemorrhage may be fatal, may result in severe neurologic impairment, or may only produce minor symptoms such as headache. A high index of suspicion is needed because no neurologic findings may be present initially, and the patient who will benefit the most from intervention will often have the mildest symptoms. The first diagnostic study should be a noncontrast CT scan with thin imaging cuts at the region of the brain base. This study will be positive in more than 90% of cases on the first day, with decreasing sensitivity over the next several days. If hemorrhage is suspected, but the CT is negative, lumbar puncture should be performed as soon as possible to assess for the presence of red cells or xanthochromia (yellowish discoloration of cerebrospinal fluid [CSF]); this finding indicates presence of bilirubin, and differentiates subarachnoid hemorrhage from a traumatic lumbar puncture.

Table 50-2
CAUSES OF PATHOLOGIC HEADACHES

DISEASE	CLINICAL FEATURES	DIAGNOSTIC FINDINGS
Meningitis	Nuchal rigidity, headache, photophobia, and prostration; may not be febrile	Lumbar puncture is diagnostic
Intracranial hemorrhage	Nuchal rigidity and headache; may not have clouded consciousness or seizures	Hemorrhage may not be seen on CT scan; lumbar puncture shows "bloody tap" that does not clear by the last tube; a fresh hemorrhage may not be xanthochromic
Brain tumor	May present with prostrating pounding headaches that are associated with nausea and vomiting; should be suspected in progressively severe new "migraine" that is invariably unilateral	CT or MR imaging
Temporal arteritis	May present with a unilateral pounding headache; onset generally in older patients (>50 years) and frequently associated with visual changes	The erythrocyte sedimentation rate is the best screening test and is usually markedly elevated (i.e., >50); definitive diagnosis can be made by arterial biopsy
Glaucoma	Usually consists of severe eye pain; may have nausea and vomiting; the eye is usually painful and red; the pupil may be partially dilated	Elevated intraocular pressure
Migraine headache	Unilateral throbbing headache with preceding aura, photophobia, and nausea, that is relieved with sleep	
Cluster headache	Male predominance; precipitated by alcohol; occurs with rhinorrhea and lacrimation	
Tension headache	Occipital-frontal headache; constant; "band-like"; relieved with relaxation	

Reproduced with permission from Raskin NH, Peroutka SJ. Headache, including migraine and cluster headache. Braunwald E, Fauci AS, Kasper KL, et al., eds. Harrison's principles of internal medicine 15th ed. New York: McGraw-Hill, 2001:72.

Giant cell arteritis, or **temporal arteritis** (TA), is a chronic vasculitis of large- and medium-size vessels, usually involving the cranial branches of the arteries arising from the aortic arch. The clinical criteria for diagnosis includes an age of onset greater than 50 years, a new onset or type of headache pattern, tenderness or decreased pulsation of the temporal artery, an elevated erythrocyte sedimentation rate (ESR), and abnormal findings on biopsy of the temporal artery. The presence of three or more criteria yields a greater than 90% sensitivity and specificity for the diagnosis. TA is closely related to **polymyalgia rheumatica** (PR), a condition with bilateral aching and stiffness of neck, torso, shoulders or proximal parts of the arms and thighs, as well as with an elevated ESR. Both conditions are probably polygenic diseases in which varying environmental and genetic factors influence susceptibility and severity. Clinical symptoms may also include jaw claudication and the most worrisome complication is permanent or partial loss of vision in one or both eyes, which can occur as an early manifestation in up to 20% of patients. Temporal artery biopsy is recommended in all patients suspected of having TA and long segments of the artery may have to be excised to find the typical areas of segmental inflammation. Corticosteroids are the drugs of choice to treat both PR and TA, with daily doses of 10–20 mg of prednisone for the former and 40–60 mg for the latter. Steroids may prevent, but usually do not reverse, visual loss. Steroid dosage is gradually tapered, but relapse is common, as are complications of corticosteroid therapy.

Migraine headache is much more common than TA, but is more variable in its presentation. It is the most common cause of initial office visits for headache because of its frequency, disabling qualities, and associated multiorgan symptoms. More common in women, migraine attacks may or may not have a preceding aura, may be unilateral or bilateral, and may have either throbbing or nonpulsatile pain, including the neck. They may have cranial autonomic features such as tearing or nasal congestion, leading to the misdiagnosis of sinus disease. A number of evidence-based guidelines are available for managing migraine headaches. In general, preventive therapies include tricyclic antidepressants and beta-blockers, while treatment of acute episodes involves the initial use of nonsteroidal antiinflammatory drugs (NSAIDs), followed by dihydroergotamine or sumatriptan if symptoms persist.

Episodic **cluster headache** is much less common, but more easily diagnosed by its distinctive pattern of grouped attacks of intense, unilateral, periorbital pain with nasal or ocular watering lasting only minutes to hours but recurring over several weeks or months. Acute attacks may be treated with oxygen or subcutaneous sumatriptan.

Comprehension Questions

Match the headache type (A to E) to the clinical presentation [50.1 to 50.3].

A. Common migraine headache
B. Classic migraine headache
C. Cluster headache
D. Subarachnoid hemorrhage
E. Meningitis

[50.1] A 42-year-old man with polycystic kidney disease who complained of a sudden onset of severe headache and then lost consciousness.

[50.2] A 22-year-old college student with fever, headache, photophobia, and 25 white blood cells per high-power field but no red blood cells or xanthochromia in CSF.

[50.3] A 31-year-old woman with a long history of intermittent severe unilateral headache lasting hours to days associated with nausea and photophobia, but no preceding symptoms, and no visual disturbance.

Answers

[50.1] **D.** The sudden onset of severe headache with diminution in level of consciousness is classic for subarachnoid hemorrhage. This patient likely had rupture of a cerebral artery aneurysm, which is associated with polycystic kidney disease.

[50.2] **E.** The presence of white blood cells but no red blood cells in the CSF is indicative of meningeal inflammation, the most common cause of which is viral infection.

[50.3] **A.** The patient's history is strongly suggestive of migraine (common type), which is not associated with a preceding aura or visual symptoms as seen in classic-type migraine.

CLINICAL PEARLS

❖ Temporal arteritis usually involves one or more branches of the carotid artery, and almost always occurs in patients older than age 50 years. Diagnosis is suggested by an elevated ESR and confirmed by temporal artery biopsy.

❖ Visual loss is a common complication of temporal arteritis and can be prevented by initiation of high-dose corticosteroids when the diagnosis is suspected.

- ❖ Subarachnoid hemorrhage typically presents as a sudden onset of severe headache and is diagnosed by visualization of blood on a CT scan, or by finding red blood cells or xanthochromic fluid on a lumbar puncture.
- ❖ Migraine is the most common type of headache for which patients seek medical attention in an office setting. The classic variety has a preceding aura, whereas the common type does not.

REFERENCES

Edlow J, Caplan L. Avoiding pitfalls in the diagnosis of subarachnoid hemorrhage. N Engl J Med 2000;342:29–36.

Kaniecki R. Headache assessment and management. JAMA 2003;289:1430–33.

Raskin N, Peroutka S. Headache, including migraine and cluster headache. In: Braunwald E, Fauci AS, Kasper KL, et al., eds. Harrison's principles of internal medicine, 15th ed. New York: McGraw-Hill, 2001:70-79.

Salvarani C, Cantini F, Boiardi L, Hunder G. Polymyalgia rheumatica and giant cell arteritis. N Engl J Med 2002;347:261–78.

Snow V, Weiss K, Wall E, Mottur-Pilson C. Pharmacologic management of acute attacks of migraine and prevention of migraine headache. Ann Intern Med 2002;137:840–52.

CASE 51

A 75-year-old white woman presents to the emergency room with right wrist pain after a fall at home. She tripped and fell while preparing dinner, and says that she tried to stop her fall with her outstretched right hand. She heard a "snap" and immediate pain. Her past medical history is remarkable only for three normal pregnancies, menopause at age 50 years, and hypertension that is well controlled with diuretics. She does have a 50 pack-year history of smoking. Her weight is 100 lb, and her height is 5 ft 6 in. Her exam is remarkable for normal vital signs, and a swollen, deformed right distal forearm and wrist, with limited mobility because of pain, and good radial pulses and capillary refill in the right fingernail beds. An x-ray confirms a fracture of the right radial head and the radiologist notes osteopenia.

- **What risk factor for fracture is this woman likely to have?**
- **What are the causes of this condition?**
- **What can her physician offer her to prevent future fractures?**

ANSWERS TO CASE 51: Osteoporosis

Summary: A 75-year-old white woman tried to stop her fall with her outstretched right hand, heard a "snap," and had immediate pain. Her past medical history is remarkable only for menopause at age 50 years and hypertension that is well controlled with diuretics. She does have a 50 pack-year history of smoking. She has a swollen, deformed, right distal forearm and wrist, with limited mobility because of pain, and good radial pulses and capillary refill in the right fingernail beds. An x-ray confirms a fracture of the right radial head and the radiologist notes osteopenia.

- **Risk factor for fracture:** Osteoporosis.
- **Causes of this condition:** Decreased bone strength as a consequence of demineralization and increased bone turnover as a result of decreased levels of sex steroids (estrogen and testosterone), medications, other hormonal conditions, or diseases of decreased calcium absorption.
- **Preventive measures:** Several medications are available to increase bone density, which may decrease the risk of future fractures. Also, her physician would want to work with her to prevent future falls, by limiting unnecessary medications that may cause instability, making changes in the home environment, evaluating her gait, visual acuity, and peripheral sensory system. The patient should also be advised to quit smoking.

Analysis

Objectives

1. Understand the pathophysiology of osteoporosis.
2. Learn the risk factors that predispose both men and women to osteoporosis.
3. Be familiar with the tests used to evaluate bone density.
4. Know the treatment options for osteoporosis.

Considerations

This 75-year-old woman with a fracture after a fall, likely had the fracture because of osteoporosis. Her risk factors for the osteoporosis are her race, smoking history, postmenopausal state without hormone replacement therapy, and thin physique. Osteoporosis puts her at risk for future fractures with substantial morbidity, such as painful vertebral compression fractures or incapacitating hip fractures. She needs intervention to reduce her risk of fractures as well as her risk of falls.

APPROACH TO OSTEOPOROSIS

Definitions

Bisphosphonates: Synthetic carbon phosphate compounds (alendronate, risedronate) act to build bone mass by binding to pyrophosphatase in bone and by inhibiting osteoclast bone resorption.

Osteopenia: T score between –1.0 and –2.5 standard deviations below the mean.

Osteoporosis: Decrease in bone mass leading to increased bone fragility and predisposing to fracture of the hip, vertebrae, and long bones, with a defined bone mineral density of less than 2.5 standard deviations below the mean of young healthy adults.

T score: Bone mineral density comparison against young healthy adults in standard deviations from the mean.

Clinical Approach

Osteoporosis is an important health issue because the resultant bone fractures cause a great deal of morbidity in chronic pain, loss of independence, and loss of function, as well as mortality. Risk factors for the development of osteoporosis include a low peak skeletal density reached in young adulthood, increasing age, loss of steroid hormone production (menopause or hypogonadism), smoking, nutritional deficiencies, and genetically low bone density. Approximately 14% of white women and 3–5% of white men will develop osteoporosis in their lifetime. The prevalence is lower in other ethnic groups.

Osteoporosis can either be idiopathic or a manifestation of another underlying disease process. Probably the most common form of secondary osteoporosis is that caused by glucocorticoid excess, usually iatrogenic steroid use for an inflammatory disease such as rheumatoid arthritis. Patients, both men and women, with rheumatoid arthritis, are susceptible to accelerated bone loss with even low doses of glucocorticoids. Gonadal deficiency is another common cause, which is seen physiologically in menopausal women, but pathologically in women who are amenorrheic, for example, in women athletes such as gymnasts or marathon runners, or as a result of hyperprolactinemia. Men with gonadal failure for whatever reason are also prone to develop osteoporosis.

Osteoporosis is a common feature of several endocrinopathies. Patients with hyperparathyroidism will develop osteoporosis because of increased calcium mobilization from bone. Long-standing hyperthyroidism, either naturally occurring, as in Graves disease, or as a result of excessive replacement of levothyroxine in patients with hypothyroidism, will also lead to accelerated bone loss. Malnutrition and nutritional deficiencies are also causative and are often seen in patients with malabsorption; for example, most patients, both men and women, with celiac sprue have osteoporosis. Certain medications, such as cyclosporine, antiepileptics, heparin, and gonadotropin-releasing hormone (GnRH) inhibitors, among others, may accelerate bone loss.

The peak bone density occurs in young adulthood under the influence of sex steroid hormone production. Other influential factors include genetics, which may account for 80% of total bone density, adequate calcium intake, and level of physical activity, especially weight-bearing activity. The type of bone growth at this stage is called modeling. After skeletal maturation is reached, the bone growth enters a new phase, termed remodeling, in which repairs are made to damaged bone, existing bone is strengthened, and calcium is released to maintain serum levels under the influence of estrogens, androgens, parathyroid hormone, vitamin D, and various cytokines and other hormones. The activity of the osteoclasts approximates the activity of the osteoblasts, in that overall bone density remains stable. However, after age 35 years, bone breakdown begins to exceed bone replacement, and this increases **markedly after menopause**, as a consequence of **increased osteoclast activity**.

Diagnostic Approach The benefits and costs of universal screening for osteoporosis are unclear. Rather, a targeted approach is advocated. Those with a family history or other risk factors should be offered screening, as well as those patients on a chronic drug (steroid) therapy that may lead to osteoporosis. **Currently, all women older than age 65 years, or those who have had a fracture before age 65 years, are recommended to have bone mineral density (BMD) testing.** Dual-energy x-ray photometry (DEXA scan) is the technique used to define diagnostic thresholds; however, whether the hip, spine, or forearm is the best site for screening is not clearly established. DEXA scan results can be expressed as a Z score, which compares bone mineral density to persons of the same age, and a T score, compares to the young adult normal range. **T scores are more useful for predicting fracture risk**. Every 1 standard deviation (SD) decrease in bone mineral density below the mean doubles the fracture risk. As mentioned, osteoporosis is defined as a T score of –2.5 SD.

Other laboratory evaluation should also routinely be considered in patients with osteoporosis. The serum levels of calcium, phosphorus, and alkaline phosphatase should be normal in patients with osteoporosis, although alkaline phosphatase is sometimes mildly elevated in the presence of a healing fracture. Laboratory abnormalities should prompt one to consider alternative diagnoses for the bone disease: hypercalcemia in hyperparathyroidism, or hypocalcemia in osteomalacia.

If a patient suffers a pathologic fracture, that is, one with minimal trauma, one needs to exclude other diagnoses. **Osteomalacia** is defective mineralization of bone matrix with accumulation of unmineralized osteoid, and is most often caused by vitamin D deficiency or phosphate deficiency. Patients with osteomalacia frequently have diffuse bone pain and tenderness, proximal muscle weakness, and laboratory abnormalities such as elevated alkaline phosphatase, and low or low-normal calcium. In the absence of fractures, patients with osteoporosis should have no bone pain or lab abnormalities. Both of these disease processes can coexist. A less-common bone disease is **Paget disease**, which is characterized by disorganized bone remodeling with a high alkaline phosphatase, causing weakened and enlarged bones with skeletal deformities. Other important causes of pathologic fracture which must be considered include **malignancy** such as multiple myeloma or metastatic disease, or vertebral osteomyelitis.

Treatment

Treatment takes a multifaceted approach. Adequate calcium intake, 1000–1200 mg/d for premenopausal women and adult men to prevent bone loss, and 1500 mg with 400–800 IU of vitamin D per day for postmenopausal women leads to decreased fractures. Estrogen replacement can also increase bone density and reduce fracture, as can the use of bisphosphonates, both in combination with calcium and vitamin D. **Bisphosphonates** can lead to **severe esophagitis** and must be used with caution in individuals with gastric reflux disease; they should be taken on an empty stomach, with a large quantity of water, and the patient should remain in the upright position for at least 30 minutes. Selective estrogen receptor modifiers are used in the treatment of osteoporosis as well.

Weight-bearing physical activity decreases bone loss and improves coordination and muscle strength, which may prevent falls. Making sure that patients can see adequately, that they use a cane or walker if needed, take up throw rugs, have railings to hold on to in the shower or bath, or wear hip protectors can further decrease the risk of life-altering bone fractures.

Comprehension Questions

[51.1] Which of the following patients is most likely to be a candidate for bone mineral density screening?

A. A 65-year-old, thin, white woman who smokes and is 15 years postmenopausal
B. A 40-year-old white woman who exercises daily and still menstruates
C. A healthy 75-year-old white man who is sedentary
D. A 60-year-old overweight African American woman
E. A 35-year-old asthmatic woman who has taken prednisone 40 mg dialy for a two-week course a week ago.

[51.2] Which of the following times in a woman's life is the most bone mass being accumulated?

A. Ages 15–25
B. Ages 25–35
C. Ages 35–45
D. Ages 45–55

[51.3] A 60-year-old woman presents with the results of her DEXA scan. She has a T score of –1.5 standard deviations at the hip and –2.5 at the spine. How do you interpret these results?

A. She has osteoporosis at the spine and osteopenia at the hip.
B. She has osteoporosis in both areas.
C. This is a normal examination.
D. She has osteoporosis of the hip and osteopenia at the spine.
E. You need to know the Z score.

[51.4] You see a 70-year-old woman in your office for a routine checkup, and you order a DEXA scan for bone mineral density screening. The T score returns as –2.5 in the spine and –2.6 for the hip. Which of the following statements is most accurate?

A. This patient has osteopenia.
B. Estrogen replacement therapy should be started with an anticipated rebuilding of bone mass to near normal within 1 year.

C. Swimming will help build bone mass.
D. Bisphosphonates would reduce the risk of hip fracture by 50%.

Answers

[51.1] **A.** Of the choices, this woman is the only one with risk factors. Risk factors include white race, age, postmenopausal status, smoking, positive family history, poor nutritional status, and chronic treatment with a drug known to predispose to bone loss.

[51.2] **A.** During adolescence is the time of greatest accumulation of bone mass in women.

[51.3] **A.** The T score is the number of standard deviations of a patient's bone mineral density from the mean of young, adult, white women. It is the standard measurement of bone mineral density used by the World Health Organization. A score of –2.5 standard deviations is the definition of osteoporosis. A Z score is the number of standard deviations from the mean bone mineral density of women in the same age group as the patient.

[51.4] **D.** Estrogen primarily inhibits loss of bone mass, although it can help to build a modest amount of bone mass. Weight-bearing exercise, and not swimming, is important in preventing osteoporosis. Bisphosphonates decrease the incidence of hip fractures by 30–50%.

CLINICAL PEARLS

❖ Bone mineral density screening should be offered to patients with risk factors for osteoporosis, and to all women older than age 65 years.

❖ Every 1 standard deviation (SD) decrease in bone mineral density below the mean of young adults doubles the fracture risk. Osteoporosis is defined as a T score of –2.5 SD.

❖ Patients with osteoporosis should have a normal serum calcium, phosphorus, and alkaline phosphatase. Lab abnormalities should prompt a search for an alternative diagnosis.

❖ Fractures can have a devastating effect upon a patients quality of life, and a multifaceted approach through nutritional counseling, home improvements, gait stabilization through exercise and with canes or walkers, and medical interventions to improve eyesight or with medications to improve bone density should be offered to patients at risk.

❖ In patients with a pathologic fracture, osteoporosis is a diagnosis of exclusion: one must also consider osteomalacia, Paget disease, and metastatic malignancies.

REFERENCES

Lindsay R, Cosman F. In: Braunwald E, Fauci AS, Kasper KL, et al., eds. Harrison's principles of internal medicine, 15th ed. New York: McGraw-Hill, 200:2226-2237.

NIH Consensus Development Panel on Osteoporosis Prevention, Diagnosis, and Therapy. JAMA 2001;285(6):785–95.

CASE 52

A 57-year-old man was admitted to the hospital 2 days previously following a motor vehicle accident. He suffered multiple contusions and a femur fracture that was surgically repaired 24 hours ago. He also had a laceration on his forehead, but had a CT scan of his head on admission that showed no intracranial bleeding. His hospital course has been uncomplicated, and his only medications currently are morphine as needed for pain and subcutaneous enoxaparin for prophylaxis of deep venous thrombosis. This evening he has been agitated and combative, having pulled out his IV line. He is cursing at the nurses, and trying to get out of bed to leave the hospital. When you see him, he is febrile with a temperature of 100.8° F; his heart rate is 122 bpm, his blood pressure is 168/110 mmHg, and his respiratory rate is 28 breaths per minute with oxygen saturations of 98% on room air. He is awake, fidgety, staring around the room nervously. He is disoriented to place and time, and seems to be having auditory hallucinations and is brushing off unseen objects from his arms. On examination, his forehead wound is bandaged, his pupils are dilated but reactive, and he is mildly diaphoretic. Auscultation of the chest reveals few inspiratory crackles in the left base, his heart is tachycardic but regular, his abdomen is benign, and he is tremulous. You are able to contact family members by phone. They confirm that prior to his car accident, the patient had no medical problems, no dementia or psychiatric illness, and was employed as an attorney. They report that he took no medications at home, did not smoke or use illicit drugs, and drank three to four mixed drinks every day after work.

- **What is your most likely diagnosis?**
- **What should be your next step?**

ANSWERS TO CASE 52: Delirium/Alcohol Withdrawal

Summary: A 57-year-old man has been hospitalized for 2 days for multiple contusions, and surgery for a femur fracture 24 hours ago from a motor vehicle accident. He had a normal CT scan of his head. His only medications are morphine and subcutaneous enoxaparin. This evening he is agitated, combative, and trying to leave the hospital. His temperature is 100.8° F; heart rate is 122 bpm, his blood pressure is 168/110 mmHg, and his respiratory rate is 28 breaths per minute with oxygen saturations of 98% on room air. He is awake, fidgety, disoriented, and seems to be having auditory and tactile hallucinations. His pupils are dilated, and he is mildly diaphoretic and tremulous. Family members confirm that the patient had no medical problems and no dementia or psychiatric illness. He took no medications, did not smoke or use illicit drugs, and drank three to four mixed drinks every day after work.

- **Most likely diagnosis:** Delirium as a result of an acute medical illness, or possibly alcohol withdrawal.

- **Next step:** Look for serious or reversible underlying medical causes for the delirium. If no other medical problems are identified, based on the patient's daily alcohol use, a possible diagnosis is alcohol withdrawal syndrome.

Analysis

Objectives

1. Be able to recognize delirium in a hospitalized patient.
2. Know the most common causes of delirium.
3. Understand the management of an agitated, delirious patient.
4. Know the special considerations applicable to an elderly demented patient with delirium.
5. Learn the stages, treatment, and complications of the alcohol withdrawal syndrome.

Considerations

This 57-year-old man had been in a normal physical and mental state prior to hospitalization. He then developed an acute change in mental status, with fluctuating consciousness and orientation, the hallmark of delirium. There are many possible causes for his delirium: pulmonary embolism, acute electrolyte disturbances, occult infection, CNS hemorrhage or infection, or drug intoxication or withdrawal. These require investigation before ascribing the symptoms to alcohol withdrawal, because they are potentially very serious or even fatal. In addition, further investigation to quantify his alcohol intake is necessary. Although the patient in the clinical scenario has all the features of alcohol withdrawal—agitation, hyperalert, confusion, possible hallucinations, and the gamut of signs of adrenergic stimulation, dilated pupils, fever, tachycardia, tachypnea, hypertension, tremor, peripheral vasodilatation—there are so many possibilities that it is mandatory to approach his care aware of the many etiologies of delirium.

APPROACH TO DELIRIUM

Delirium is an acute confusional state that is one of the most common mental disorders encountered in hospitalized or otherwise medically ill patients. The *Diagnostic and Statistical Manual of Mental Disorders, 4th Edition* (DSM-IV) defines delirium as having the following features:

- Disturbance of consciousness with impairment of attention.
- Change in cognition or the development of perceptual disturbances, for example, hallucinations.
- Symptoms developing over a short period of time.
- Evidence that the above are caused by a medical condition, medications, or intoxicants.

One of earliest signs of a disturbance of consciousness is an inability to focus or sustain attention, which may be evident as distractibility in conversation. There is also usually disturbance of the sleep–wake cycle. As symptoms progress, patients may become lethargic or even stuporous (arousable only to painful stimuli). In alcohol withdrawal, signs of autonomic hyperactivity predominate, and patients may go to the opposite extreme, becoming hypervigilant and agitated.

Regarding changes in cognition or perception, patients may have difficulty with memory, orientation, or speech. It is important to ascertain from family members whether these impairments were chronic, as in dementia, or developed acutely. Delirious patients may also have hallucinations or vague delusions of harm, but hallucinations are not a mandatory feature of the condition. Delirium is an acute process, with **symptoms developing over a period of hours to days**. Additionally, the patient's mental status fluctuates, with symptoms often becoming most severe in the evening and at night. It is not uncommon for hospitalized patients to appear relatively lucid on morning rounds, especially if mental status is only superficially assessed, only to have night staff report severe confusion and agitation.

Finally, delirium is a manifestation of an underlying medical disorder. Sometimes, the underlying condition is apparent. At other times, especially with elderly demented patients, delirium may be the first or only sign of an acute illness, or a serious decompensation or complication of a stable medical condition. Table 52–1 lists conditions that should be considered as causes of delirium. Of these conditions, the most common are drug toxicity (especially anticholinergics, sedatives, or narcotics in elderly patients), infection, electrolyte disturbances (most commonly hyponatremia or hypoglycemia), and withdrawal from alcohol or other sedatives.

Table 52-1
MEDICAL CAUSES OF DELIRIUM

Discrete CNS lesion present
- Head injury; stroke or intracranial bleed
- Infection: meningitis, meningoencephalitis, brain abscess
- Mass lesion: hematoma, tumor
- Seizure, postictal

No discrete CNS lesion
- Metabolic encephalopathy
  - Anoxia: any cause, heart or respiratory failure, pulmonary embolus, sleep apnea, etc.
  - Hepatic encephalopathy
  - Uremic encephalopathy
  - Hypo-hyperglycemia
  - Hyponatremia/hypercalcemia
  - Hypo-hyperthermia
- Toxic encephalopathy
  - Drug withdrawal, especially alcohol and benzodiazepines, but also demerol and many others
  - Drug toxicity, dilantin, for example
  - Substance abuse
  - Infections, especially pneumonia, urinary tract infections, intraabdominal infection, bacteremia, all more frequent in the elderly

Regardless of etiology, delirium produces a profound disturbance of brain function, and all etiologies are serious and potentially fatal illnesses. **Delirium has to be approached as an acute medical emergency.** A detailed history, aggressively pursued, is mandatory, and because these patients' responses cannot be relied upon, information from family, friends, or other caregivers is essential. A thorough physical examination with emphasis on neurological status, clarity of speech, level of awareness, attention span, facial droop, and weakness of an extremity must be established because changes in these must be carefully and frequently assessed. Basic laboratory studies should focus on chemical abnormalities (glucose, creatinine, bilirubin, serum sodium) and evidence of hypoxia. The two threatening and potentially easily reversible conditions—hypoxia and hypoglycemia—should be immediately investigated and treated.

Delirium develops more commonly in those with an underdeveloped brain (e.g., the febrile delirium of young children) and in those with involuting or diseased brains (many of the elderly). Delirium in the geriatric population can be the presenting manifestation of any acute illness with an incidence of up to 10% on admission and up to 30% during an acute hospitalization. Causes of delirium in the elderly include pneumonia, urinary tract infection, myocardial infarction, gastrointestinal hemorrhage, traumatic injury, or virtually anything else that precipitates an acute hospitalization. This is even more of a problem after major surgery; nearly half of individuals (usually elderly) who suffer hip fractures develop delirium postoperatively.

Persons at any stage of dementia may develop delirium with any superimposed acute illness or injury, or additional pharmaceutical agent or agents. Dementia is a chronic illness and in its earlier stages with no impairment of awareness, whereas delirium is an acute event with alteration of consciousness. Additionally an acute delirium may "unmask" an early underlying, undetected dementia. The confused and disoriented geriatric patient cannot be dismissed as one or the other, and the history on which this differential diagnosis is dependent, should concentrate on any changes from the behavioral status of the patient before the acute event.

The management of delirium is first and foremost the identification and treatment of the acute underlying illness. Adequate hydration, oxygenation, good nursing care, and round the clock careful supervision are always the initial measures. Management of agitation and disruptive behavior is the most challenging aspect of care of the delirious patient. If no specific treatable problem is identified, physical restraint should be used as a last resort. Frequent reassurance and orientation from familiar persons, or constant supervision from a nurse or hospital aide are preferable. **Agitation with psychotic symptoms (hallucinations and delusions) can be treated with a neuroleptic such as low-dose haloperidol.** Older patients are more likely to experience extrapyramidal side effects, however, so newer atypical antipsychotics such as **risperidone** may be used. Benzodiazepines have a rapid onset of action, but may worsen confusion and sedation.

Alcohol Withdrawal There are no absolute numbers, but ethanol intakes of less than 60 g/d (6 or 7 oz of distilled spirits or almost a bottle of wine) usually are not medically significant in adult men (less in women). If other causes of delirium cannot be found, and a history of heavy alcohol intake has been obtained, one still cannot assume our patient's delirium is caused by only alcohol withdrawal. Risk factors for the development of delirium tremens (DTs) include a history of sustained drinking, prior withdrawal symptoms, age >30 years, and a concurrent illness. Withdrawal can coexist with or mimic other conditions such as infection, intracranial bleeding, hepatic failure, gastrointestinal bleeding, or other drug overdose. DTs is a diagnosis of exclusion; one must look for and exclude other serious diagnoses before attributing the patient's mental status and autonomic signs to withdrawal. There should be a search for infection (blood cultures), pneumonia (chest radiograph), and hypoxia (blood gases or oximetry), and although it is early in his course, the possibility of pulmonary embolus kept in mind. It is important to understand the temporal course of the spectrum of alcohol withdrawal syndromes (Table 52–2).

In contrast to other causes of delirium, **benzodiazepines are the drugs of choice in alcohol withdrawal**. They can be given on a fixed schedule in high-risk patients (previous history of DTs or withdrawal seizures) to prevent withdrawal symptoms. If symptoms have already developed, they can be given according to one of two strategies. Long-acting benzodiazepines such as

Table 52-2
ALCOHOL WITHDRAWAL

STAGE	SYMPTOMS
Tremulousness	Earliest symptom occurring within 6 hours of abstinence, caused by CNS and sympathetic hyperactivity, often referred to as the "shakes" or "jitters," and can occur even when patients still have a significant blood alcohol level. In addition to the typical 6–8 Hz tremor, which can be violent or subtle, insomnia, anxiety, gastrointestinal upset, diaphoresis, and palpitations can occur. Tremor typically diminishes over 48–72 hours, but anxiety, easy startling, and other symptoms can persist for 2 weeks.
Withdrawal seizures	Also called "rum fits" and typically generalized tonic–clonic seizures, often occurring in clusters of two to six episodes, and almost always within 6–48 hours of abstinence. These are typically seen in patients with a long history of chronic alcoholism.
Alcoholic hallucinosis	Typically develops within 12 hours of abstinence, and resolves within 48 hours. The hallucinations are most often visual (e.g., bugs, pink elephants), but can be auditory or tactile. When auditory, they are often maligning or reproachful human voices. Despite the hallucinations, patients maintain a relatively intact sensorium.
Delirium tremens (DTs)	The most dramatic and serious form of alcohol withdrawal, but only occurs in 5% of patients with withdrawal symptoms. DTs typically begin within 48–72 hours after the last drink, and can last several days, often with a resolution as abrupt as its onset. It is characterized by hallucinations, agitation, tremor, and sleeplessness, as well as signs of sympathetic hyperactivity: dilated pupils, low-grade fever, tachycardia, hypertension, diaphoresis, and hyperventilation. Delirium tremens is a serious condition with an in-hospital mortality of 5–10%, usually from arrhythmias or infection, which is often unsuspected.

diazepam can be given in high doses until withdrawal symptoms cease, and then allow the slow clearance of the drug to prevent further withdrawal symptoms. Alternatively, shorter-acting agents such as lorazepam can be given as needed only when the patient has symptoms. Both strategies are effective. In either case, the key to successful management is aggressive upward titration of dosage initially until the patient is heavily sedated but responsive, followed by rapid downward titration as agitation decreases, usually over 48–72 hours.

Supportive measures are also important, such as adequate hydration, replacement of electrolytes, and supplementation with thiamine and other B vitamins in malnourished, chronic alcoholics to prevent the development of Wernicke encephalopathy.

Comprehension Questions

[52.1] Which of the following agents most closely resembles the action of alcohol in the brain?

A. Amphetamines
B. Marijuana
C. Cocaine
D. Benzodiazepine
E. Acetaminophen

[52.2] As compared with dementia, which of the following is a characteristic of delirium?

A. Fluctuating level of consciousness
B. Slow onset
C. Can be due to deficiencies of thiamine or cyanocobalamin
D. Decreased memory ability

[52.3] A 34-year-old man is brought to the emergency room for extreme tremors and auditory hallucinations. Which of the following statements is most likely to be correct?

A. The auditory hallucinations are unique to alcohol withdrawal and cannot be caused by a brain tumor.
B. If the serum blood alcohol level is higher than legal limits of intoxication, these symptoms cannot be alcohol withdrawal.
C. This patient should receive glucose intravenously for possible hypoglycemia.
D. If the patient also has hypertension, fever, and tachycardia, he has a 5-15% chance of mortality.

Answers

[52.1] **D.** Alcohol and benzodiazepines both interact with the gamma-aminobutyric acid (GABA) system, and thus benzodiazepines are the drugs of choice to treat acute alcohol withdrawal.

[52.2] **A.** A fluctuating level alertness and consciousness is typical of delirium.

[52.3] **D.** DTs with autonomic instability and sympathetic overactivity is associated with a 5–15% mortality. Auditory hallucinations can occur from a number of illicit agents or even brain tumors, the fall in serum blood alcohol level and not the absolute level may induce symptoms of withdrawal. An individual who abuses alcohol should first be given thiamine, before glucose is administered, to avoid an acute Wernicke encephalopathy.

CLINICAL PEARLS

- Delirium is characterized by an acute onset of impaired attention and cognition, fluctuating levels of consciousness, often with psychomotor and autonomic hyperactivity.
- Delirium requires urgent investigation to look for serious underlying systemic or metabolic causes.
- Frequent reassurance and orientation, and constant observation are useful in managing the agitated delirious patient. Low-dose haloperidol may be used to control agitation or psychotic symptoms. Physical restraint is used as a last resort.
- Delirium tremens is the most severe and dramatic form of alcohol withdrawal, with an abrupt onset 2–4 days after cessation of drinking, and with a sudden resolution several days later, and a mortality of 5%.
- Therapy for alcohol withdrawal syndromes includes benzodiazepines, hydration, electrolyte replacement, and B vitamins to prevent Wernicke encephalopathy.

REFERENCES

Shuckit MA. Alcohol and Alcoholism. In: Braunwald E, Fauci AS, Kasper KL, et al., eds. Harrison's principles of internal medicine, 15th ed. New York: McGraw-Hill. 2001:2561-2566.

CASE 53

A 66-year-old woman comes in for a routine physical examination. She volunteers that her menopause occurred at age 51 years, and that she is currently taking an estrogen pill along with a progestin pill each day. The past medical history is unremarkable. Her family history includes one maternal cousin with ovarian cancer. On examination, she is found to have a blood pressure of 120/70 mmHg, a heart rate of 70 beats per minute, and temperature of 98°F. She weighs 140 lb and is 5 ft 4 in tall. The thyroid is normal to palpation. Examination of her breasts reveals no masses or discharge. The abdominal, cardiac, and lung evaluations are within normal limits. The pelvic examination shows a normal multiparous cervix, a normal-size uterus, and no adnexal masses. She had undergone a mammogram 3 months previously.

- **What is your next step?**

- **What would be the most common cause of mortality for this patient?**

ANSWERS TO CASE 53

Summary: A 66-year-old woman presents for health maintenance. A mammogram had been performed 3 months previously.

- **Next step**: Each of the following should be performed: Papanicolaou (Pap) smear, stool for occult blood, colonoscopy or barium enema, pneumococcal vaccine, influenza vaccine, tetanus vaccine (if not within 10 years), cholesterol screening, fasting blood sugar, and urinalysis.
- **Most common cause of mortality:** Cardiovascular disease.

Analysis

Objectives

1. Understand which health maintenance studies should be performed for a 66-year-old patient.
2. Know the most common cause of mortality in a woman in this age group.
3. Understand that preventive maintenance consists of immunizations, cancer screening, and screening for common diseases.

Considerations

The approach to health maintenance includes three parts: (a) cancer screening, (b) immunizations, and (c) addressing common diseases for the particular patient group. For a 66-year-old woman, this includes Pap smear screening for cervical cancer, annual mammography for breast cancer screening, colon cancer (annual stool for occult blood and either periodic colonoscopy or barium enema), tetanus booster every 10 years, the pneumococcal vaccine, and yearly influenza immunization. Screening for hypercholesterolemia every 5 years up to age 75 years and fasting blood sugar levels every 3 years are also recommended. Finally, the most common cause of mortality is cardiovascular disease.

APPROACH TO HEALTH MAINTENANCE

Definitions

Cost-effectiveness: A comparison of resources expended (dollars) in an intervention versus the benefit, which may be measured in life years, or quality-adjusted life years.

Primary prevention: Identifying and modifying risk factors in subjects who have never had the disease of concern.

Screening test: A device used to identify asymptomatic disease in the hope that early detection will lead to an improved outcome. An optimal screening test has high sensitivity and specificity, is inexpensive, and is easy to perform.

Secondary prevention: Actions taken to reduce the morbidity or mortality once a disease has been diagnosed.

Clinical Approach

When the patient does not have an apparent disease or complaint, the goal of medical intervention is prevention of disease. One method of targeting diseases is by patient's age. For example, the most common cause of death in a 16-year-old is by motor vehicle accident; hence the teenage patient is well-served by the physician encouraging her to wear seat belts and to avoid alcohol intoxication when driving. In contrast, a 56-year-old woman is most likely to die of cardiovascular disease so that the physician might focus on exercise and weight loss, and screen for hyperlipidemia.

In each age group, particular screening tests are recommended (Table 53–1).

Comprehension Questions

For each of the patient scenarios listed below (53.1 to 53.4), assign one or more answers (A to I) pertaining to health maintenance.

A. Influenza vaccine
B. Pneumococcal vaccine
C. Barium enema or colonoscopy
D. Mammography every year
E. Cholesterol screening
F. Chest radiograph
G. Urinalysis
H. Papanicolaou smear
I. None of above

[53.1] A 16-year-old girl engaged in one episode of sexual intercourse 2 year ago, but is currently not sexually active.

[53.2] A 44-year-old woman denies any health problems.

[53.3] A 59-year-old woman has mild osteoarthritis.

[53.4] A man, aged 69 years, has mild hypertension that is controlled with an antihypertensive agent.

Answers

[53.1] **H.** Cervical cancer screening via Pap smear is indicated when a woman is sexually active or at age 18-21.

[53.2] **H, E.** Again, a Pap smear is indicated as well as cholesterol screening.

[53.3] **A, C, D, E, H.** At age 59 years, breast, cervical, and colon cancer screening is indicated.

[53.4] **A, B, C, D, E, H.** At age 69, cancer screening, vaccination including pneumococcal and influenza immunization, and urinalysis are recommended.

Table 53-1
SCREENING BASED ON AGE

	13–18 YEARS	19–39 YEARS	40–64 YEARS	65+ YEARS
Cancer screening	Pap smear if sexually active	Annual Pap smear	Annual Pap smear Age 50: stool for occult blood, barium enema every 5 years, or colonoscopy every 10 years, annual mammography	Annual Pap smear, Annual stool for occult blood; colonoscopy or barium enema every 5 years; annual mammography
Immunizations	Tetanus booster once between ages 11 and 16 years	Tetanus every 10 years	Tetanus every 10 years Age 50: annual influenza vaccine	Tetanus every 10 years; pneumococcal vaccine; annual influenza vaccine
Other diseases	Depression; firearms	Cardiovascular diseases	Cholesterol screening every 5 years beginning at age 45 years	Cholesterol screening every 5 years beginning at age 45 years
Most common causes of mortality	1. Motor vehicle accidents 2. Homicide 3. Suicide	1. Motor vehicle accidents 2. Cardiovascular disease 3. AIDS	1. Cardiovascular disease 2. Cancer	1. Heart disease 2. Cancer 3. Cerebrovascular disease

Adapted from American College of Obstetricians and Gynocologists. Primary and Preventive Care: periodic assessments. ACOG Committee Opinion 246 Washington DC: Author, 2000

CLINICAL PEARLS

- ❖ The basic approach to health maintenance is age-appropriate immunizations, cancer screening, and screening for common diseases.
- ❖ The most common cause of mortality in a woman younger than 20 years of age is motor vehicle accidents.
- ❖ The most common cause of mortality for a woman greater older 39 years of age is cardiovascular disease.
- ❖ Major conditions in women aged 65 years and older include osteoporosis, heart disease, breast cancer, and depression.

REFERENCES

American College of Obstetricians and Gynecologists. Primary and preventive care: periodic assessments. ACOG Committee Opinion 246. Washington, DC: 1999.

Peterson HB. Principles of screening. In: Holzman GB, Rinehart RD, Dunn LJ, eds. Precis: primary and preventive care. Washington, DC: American College of Obstetricians and Gynecologists, 1999:15–21.

CASE 54

You are the intern on call in the hospital, when the emergency room resident calls up a new admission. She describes an 84-year-old Alzheimer patient who was brought to the emergency department by ambulance from her long-term care facility for increased confusion, combativeness, and fever. Her past medical history is significant for Alzheimer disease and well-controlled hypertension; she otherwise has been very healthy. The resident states that the patient is "confused" and combative with staff, which, per her family, is not her baseline mental status. Her temperature is 100.5°F, her pulse is 130 bpm, her blood pressure is 76/32 mmHg, her respiratory rate is 24 breaths per minute with oxygen saturations of 95% on room air. On examination, she is lethargic but agitated when disturbed, her neck veins are flat, her lung fields are clear, and her heart is tachycardic but regular with no murmur or gallops. Her abdominal exam is unremarkable, and her extremities are warm and pink.

After administration of 2 L of normal saline over 30 minutes, her blood pressure is now 95/58 mmHg, and the initial lab work returns. Her white blood cell count is 14,000/mm^3, with 67% neutrophils, 3% bands, and 24% lymphocytes. No other abnormalities were noted. Chest x-rays obtained in the emergency room are normal. Her urinalysis shows 2+ leukocyte esterase, negative nitrite, and trace blood. Microscopy shows 20–50 white blood cells per high-power field, 0–3 red blood cells, and many bacteria.

What is your diagnosis?

What is your next step?

ANSWERS TO CASE 54: Urosepsis in the Elderly

Summary: An 84-year-old woman, a nursing home resident with Alzheimer disease, is brought to the emergency room for agitation and confusion, and is found to be febrile, tachycardic, and hypotensive. Examination shows flat neck veins, clear lung fields, no cardiac murmur or gallops, and her extremities are warm and well-perfused. Her hemodynamic status has improves with a fluid bolus. Laboratory examination shows evidence of a urinary tract infection.

- **Most likely diagnosis:** Shock, most likely as a consequence of urosepsis.
- **Next step:** Continued administration of blood pressure support with intravenous fluids, or vasopressors as necessary. Broad-spectrum antibiotics should be started as soon as possible.

Analysis

Objectives

1. Know how to diagnose a urinary tract infection (UTI).
2. Know effective treatments for UTI.
3. Recognize and know how to manage asymptomatic bacteruria.
4. Know how to recognize and treat septic shock.

Considerations

In this patient presenting with shock, that is, hypotension leading to inadequate tissue perfusion, it is essential to try to determine the underlying cause and, thus, appropriate treatment. She has no history of hemorrhage or extreme volume losses, so hypovolemic shock is unlikely. She has flat neck veins and clear lung fields, suggesting she does not have right- or left-heart failure, respectively, so cardiogenic shock (e.g., after a myocardial infarction) also seems unlikely. Additionally, both hypovolemic and cardiogenic shock typically cause profound peripheral vasoconstriction, resulting in cold clammy extremities. This patient's extremities are warm and well-perfused (inappropriately so) despite serious hypotension, suggesting a distributive form of shock. With the elevated white blood cell count with immature forms, as well as the urine findings, septic shock as a consequence of urinary tract infection seems most likely.

APPROACH TO SUSPECTED UROSEPSIS

Definitions

Asymptomatic bacteriuria: Condition in which urine Gram stain or culture is positive but no clinical signs or symptoms of infection are present.

Leukocyte esterase: Neutrophils within the urine release this enzyme, which can be detected in a urinalysis.

Nitrite: Nitrites are converted from nitrates by some bacteria, particularly Gram-negative organisms, and can be detected in a urinalysis.

Clinical Approach

Urinary tract infections (UTIs) are a common affliction of the elderly, affecting both debilitated and healthy adults. In fact, UTIs are second only to respiratory infections as the most common infections in patients older than age 65 years. Risk factors that contribute to the high incidence of UTIs in the elderly, as well as in institutionalized patients, include incontinence, a history of prior UTIs, neurological impairment, polypharmacy (namely anticholinergics), immunosuppression, poor nutrition, and comorbid disease states. These conditions may confer functional abnormalities within the urinary tract or altered defenses against infection. Furthermore, frequent hospitalizations expose these patients to nosocomial pathogens and invasive instrumentation such as indwelling catheters.

Urinary tract infections are typically diagnosed based on a combination of symptoms and urinary findings. In symptomatic patients, bacteria are typically found in high concentrations in the urine, and **>10^5 colony-forming units (CFU)/mL are typically recovered from a clean-catch** specimen. If the specimen is obtained by a **catheterization, finding >10^2 CFU/mL** is considered significant. In **women with symptoms of acute cystitis**, urine cultures are often not obtained, but empiric treatment can be initiated based on the **dipstick findings of leukocyte esterase** (used as a marker for pyuria) **or nitrites** (used as a marker for bacteriuria).

Most UTIs can be described as one of three clinical syndromes: **acute uncomplicated cystitis** (lower tract infection**), acute uncomplicated pyelonephritis** (upper tract infection), and **complicated UTI** (associated with urinary catheterization or instrumentation, or anatomic or functional abnormalities). Symptoms of cystitis reflect bladder irritation and generally include dysuria, frequency, urgency, or hematuria. **Pyelonephritis** typically presents with **systemic symptoms such as fever, chills, or nausea,** with or without symptoms of cystitis. Another clinical finding that deserves mention is **asymptomatic bacteriuria.** Asymptomatic bacteriuria is characterized by positive urine cultures without clinical symptoms. Outside of pregnancy or immunocompromised patients such as transplant recipients, no adverse outcomes have been reported as a result of asymptomatic bacteriuria, and no benefits of treatment have been demonstrated. Up to 50% of women and 30% of men older than age 65 years are reported to have asymptomatic bacteriuria. While in younger patients fever, dysuria, urgency, or flank pain may be presenting symptoms for a urinary tract infection, elderly and institutionalized patients often present with less-obvious symptoms. These patients may be febrile or hypothermic. Common manifestations include confusion or combativeness. **Mental status or behavioral changes in the elderly** should be considered **strong indicators for serious illness**, and a thorough workup should consider etiologies beyond infections. Even with localizing symptoms suggestive of a UTI, other sources of infection should still be investigated. Both urine and blood cultures should be sent in addition to a urinalysis and complete blood count. The results of the urine and blood cultures may take 2–3 days to yield an organism. If the clinical picture suggests a UTI, antibiotic treatment should not await these results and should be initiated immediately.

Antimicrobial therapy should not be directed solely at Gram-negative organisms as in younger patients. The elderly and institutionalized patients commonly acquire Gram-positive and mixed infections, so broad-spectrum antibiotics pending culture results are recommended. For uncomplicated UTIs, fluoroquinolones such as ciprofloxacin and gatifloxacin are considered first-line therapy. Treatment can range from 3 days in uncomplicated cystitis to 10 days in pyelonephritis. In patients presenting with a clinical picture of sepsis, broad-spectrum antibiotic coverage against enterococci and pseudomonas is recommended until cultures are available to guide therapy. Suggested regimens include ampicillin with gentamicin, imipenem, or piperacillin with tazobactam. The duration of therapy should be dictated by the patient's clinical status. In cases where UTIs have progressed to bacteremia, aggressive and prompt treatment is necessary to prevent the onset of septic shock. This life-threatening state may develop with little warning in elderly and institutionalized patients with multiple comorbidities, as it did in the patient in the scenario, who presents with hypotension and altered mental status because of infection, that is, in septic shock.

Septic Shock **Shock** is the clinical syndrome that results from inadequate tissue perfusion. It can be classified in a variety of ways, but one useful schema divides the causes into hypovolemic shock. cardiogenic shock, or distributive shock, usually caused by sepsis**. Hypovolemic shock** is the most common form, and results from either hemorrhage or by profound vomiting or diarrhea, resulting in loss of 20–40% of blood volume. **Cardiogenic shock** results from a primary cardiac insult, such as a myocardial infarction, arrhythmias, or end-stage heart failure such that the heart no longer pumps effectively. Hypovolemic and cardiogenic shock both cause a marked fall in cardiac output, and may appear clinically similar with tachycardia, hypotension, and cold clammy extremities. It is essential to differentiate between the two, however, because the treatment is markedly different. Patients with **hypovolemic shock** should have **flat neck veins** and **clear lung fields**; those with **cardiogenic shock** are more likely to have markedly **elevated jugular venous pressure and pulmonary edema**. The treatment of hypovolemic shock is aggressive volume resuscitation, either with crystalloid solution or with blood products as necessary. Treatment of cardiogenic shock focuses on maintaining blood pressure with dopamine or norepinephrine infusions, relief of pulmonary edema with diuretics, and reducing cardiac afterload, for example, with an intraaortic balloon pump.

Distributive shock, in contrast, is characterized by and an ***increase*** **in cardiac output**, but an inability to maintain systemic vascular resistance; that is, there is **inappropriate vasodilatation**. Clinically, it appears different than the other forms of shock in that despite the hypotension, the **extremities are warm and well-perfused**, at least initially. If septic shock continues, the cardiac output falls as a consequence of myocardial depression, multiorgan dysfunction ensues, and **intense vasoconstriction** occurs in an attempt to maintain blood pressure, the so called, **"cold phase."** These findings portend a poor prognosis; hence, prompt recognition of septic shock in the early (warm) phase is paramount.

While distributive shock may occur in neurogenic shock as a consequence of spinal cord injury or adrenal crisis, the most common cause is **septic shock**, most commonly from **Gram-negative sepsis**. Gram-negative organisms may release **endotoxins**, which cause a decrease in systemic vascular resistance and cardiac contractility. The primary treatment is isotonic fluid replacement to maintain blood pressure. Other cornerstones of therapy include broad-spectrum antibiotics to attack the underlying infection and removal of the infection source. Patients often require vasopressor support (dopamine being the most commonly used agent), and mechanical ventilation to optimize tissue oxygenation. All types of shock are associated with high mortality rates exceeding 50%. Early diagnosis and prompt treatment are imperative, in that untreated shock progresses to an irreversible point that is refractory to volume expansion or other medical therapies.

Comprehension Questions

[54.1] Which of the following asymptomatic patients would most benefit from treatment of the finding of $>10^5$ CFU/mL of *E. Coli* on a urine culture?

A. A 23-year-old asymptomatic sexually active woman
B. A 33-year-old asymptomatic pregnant woman
C. A 53-year-old asymptomatic diabetic woman
D. A 73-year-old asymptomatic woman in a nursing home

[54.2] Which of the following is the best treatment for a 39-year-old woman with fever to 103°F, nausea, flank pain, and $>10^5$ CFU/mL of *Escherichia coli* in a urine culture?

A. Oral trimethoprim-sulfamethoxazole for 3 days
B. Single-dose ciprofloxacin
C. Intravenous and then oral gatifloxacin for 14 days
D. Oral ampicillin for 21–28 days

[54.3] A 57-year-old man is noted to have a blood pressure 68/50 mmHg, a heart rate of 140 bpm, elevated jugular venous pressure, inspiratory crackles on exam, and cold clammy extremities. Which of the following is the most likely etiology?

A. Septic shock
B. Adrenal crisis
C. Cardiogenic shock
D. Hypovolemic shock

[54.4] A 45-year-old man is noted to have a blood pressure of 80/40 mmHg, a heart rate of 130 bpm, and a fever of 102°F. His abdomen is tender, particularly in the right lower quadrant, and acute appendicitis is diagnosed. Three liters of 0.9% normal saline are infused, and intravenous antibiotics are administered as he is prepared for surgery. His blood pressures persist in the 76/36 mmHg range. Which of the following is the most appropriate step?

A. Administer a beta-blocker
B. Administer corticosteroids
C. Infuse fresh-frozen plasma
D. Initiate dopamine intravenous infusion
E. Delay surgery for 24 hours until blood pressure can be stabilized

Answers

[54.1] **B.** All of these patients are asymptomatic and no benefit of treatment in terms of reduction in symptomatic UTIs or hospitalization has been shown for any of the other cases mentioned, except for pregnancy. Treatment is undertaken to prevent upper tract infection, preterm delivery, and possible fetal loss.

[54.2] **C.** The patient in the scenario has symptoms of upper tract infection, for example, pyelonephritis, and is moderately ill with nausea. She will need a 14-day course of treatment and may not be able to take oral antibiotics initially, so hospitalization and treatment with intravenous antibiotics is likely to be necessary. Single-dose and 3-day regimens are only useful for acute uncomplicated cystitis in women. Ampicillin is likely to have substantial resistance from *E. coli* at this point.

[54.3] **C.** The patient is hypotensive with signs of left- and right-heart failure; that is, this is probably cardiogenic shock. Septic shock and adrenal crisis are both forms of distributive shock, which would produce warm extremities. Hypovolemic shock should have flat neck veins and no pulmonary edema.

[54.4] **D.** When septic shock is refractory to intravenous fluids, then vasopressors such as dopamine are generally the next step. Delaying surgery for 24 hours would likely lead to death.

CLINICAL PEARLS

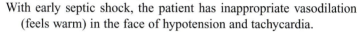

- Urosepsis is the most common cause of sepsis in the older patient.
- Urinary tract infections may be diagnosed by the presence of urinary symptoms and $>10^5$ CFU/mL in a clean-catch specimen, and $>10^2$ CFU/mL in a catheterized specimen.
- In healthy women with symptoms of acute uncomplicated cystitis, cultures are not routinely sent, and treatment can be initiated based on symptoms and on a urine dipstick finding of leukocyte esterase or nitrites.
- Asymptomatic bacteriuria is a common finding among elderly patients and requires no treatment; it is only routinely treated in pregnancy and in transplant recipients.
- With early septic shock, the patient has inappropriate vasodilation (feels warm) in the face of hypotension and tachycardia.

REFERENCES

Murphy PA. Genitourinary infections. In: Barker LR, Burton JR, Zieve PD, eds. Principles of ambulatory medicine, 5th ed. Lippincott, Williams & Wilkins. New York; 1999:331-41.

Shortliffe LMD, McCue JD. Urinary tract infection at the age extremes: pediatrics and geriatrics. Am J Med 2002;113:55S–66S.

Tierney LM, McPhee SJ, Papadakis MA. Current medical diagnosis & treatment 2001, 40th ed. New York: McGraw-Hill. 2001;501–02, 932–36, 1369–70.

❖ CASE 55

A 28-year-old man is brought to the emergency room by EMS after being found sitting at the side of the road, incoherent and disoriented. In the emergency room, he is uncooperative and combative. He is not oriented to self, place, or time. Security is called to help restrain him, and he is placed in five-point leather restraints for his own and the staff's protection. No specific complaints can be elicited from the patient, he continues to yell at the staff and seems to have auditory and visual hallucinations. His temperature is 100.5°F, his heart rate is 120 bpm, and his blood pressure is 150/100 mmHg. A Foley catheter is placed and the urine is noted to be tea-colored. A urine dipstick is reads 4+ for blood, but no red blood cells are seen on the microscopic examination. A urine drug screen is positive for cocaine and phencyclidine.

◆ **What is your most likely diagnosis?**

◆ **What is your next step?**

ANSWERS TO CASE 55: Rhabdomyolysis, Cocaine-Induced

Summary: An uncooperative, disoriented, and combative 28-year-old man is brought to the emergency room and placed in five-point leather restraints. He seems to have auditory and visual hallucinations. His temperature is 100.5°F, his heart rate is 120 bpm, and his blood pressure is 150/100 mmHg. A Foley catheter is placed and the urine is noted to be tea-colored, with 4+ for blood, but no red blood cells on microscopy. A urine drug screen is positive for cocaine and phencyclidine.

- **Most likely diagnosis:** Rhabdomyolysis secondary to cocaine and phencyclidine (PCP or angel dust) intoxication.

- **Next step:** Aggressive IV hydration with normal saline. To prevent further damage to muscle, chemical restraint of the patient may be advised, rather than physical restraint alone.

Analysis

Objectives

1. Know the clinically important toxic syndromes associated with cocaine and other drugs of abuse.
2. Learn the causes and natural history of untreated rhabdomyolysis.
3. Recognize the signs of myoglobinemia and myoglobinuria.
4. Learn the treatment of rhabdomyolysis.

APPROACH TO ILLICIT DRUG EFFECTS

Drug abuse is common and pervasive in our society. Contrary to popular belief, many highly educated and socioeconomically advantaged persons are involved in the illicit use of street drugs, legal drugs, or prescribed medications. The physician must have a high index of suspicion to be able to offer appropriate therapy and to prevent the disastrous consequences of such use. Alcohol and tobacco are the most commonly abused drugs; this discussion, however, focuses on common "street" drugs that are known to have serious medical consequences with both acute and chronic use.

Heroin, or opiate addiction, although less popular now than in the past, has seen something of a resurgence recently in some areas of the country. Acute intoxication causes hypotension, sedation or coma, nausea, and vomiting. The severity of the symptoms is dose dependent. Long-term secondary effects include infections such as HIV or hepatitis through sharing of contaminated needles and infectious endocarditis. Benzodiazepine or barbiturate intoxication can cause a similar presentation of respiratory, cardiovascular, and CNS depression. Phencyclidine (PCP), also called "angel dust," is a veterinary anesthetic that can be smoked or taken orally or intravenously. In a dose-dependent manner, people will develop agitation, excitability, acute psychosis, and convulsions when intoxicated with this drug.

Cocaine is a stimulant, vasoconstrictor, and local anesthetic derived from the leaves of the coca plant. The drug can be snorted, administered intravenously, or smoked. It blocks the reuptake of norepinephrine, serotonin, and dopamine at the receptor, which leads to elevated mood, heart rate, blood pressure, and temperature. Cocaine has a short half-life of about 1 hour, and its metabolites are detectable in the urine for about 3–5 days following use. Chronic use leads to tolerance of the effects, but high doses can be fatal. The resultant tachycardia, hypertension, and peripheral vasoconstriction may lead to ischemic stroke, subarachnoid hemorrhage, myocardial infarction, and hepatic or intestinal ischemia. Inhaling the cocaine or the chemicals used for purification can cause pneumonitis or the adult respiratory distress syndrome. Alteration of dopamine levels can lead to impotence and infertility.

Rhabdomyolysis, the breakdown of striated muscle, can also be caused by cocaine effect, through direct myotoxicity or vasoconstrictive ischemia. Other chemicals used to "cut" the cocaine may also be myotoxic. PCP can also cause myoglobinemia because of muscle breakdown from the overexertion the drug causes. Together, these effects may be additive and more toxic to the patient. Table 55–1 lists multiple other causes of rhabdomyolysis, ranging from injury to infection to genetic diseases.

Whatever the cause, the breakdown of muscle tissue leads to release of myoglobin into the blood, which is then bound up by the serum haptoglobin. This system, however, saturates at low levels of myoglobinemia. The **free**

Table 55-1
ETIOLOGIES OF RHABDOMYOLYSIS

Alcohol Abuse
Drug Abuse (Cocaine, amphetamines, LSD, heroin, phencyclidine)
Medications (Diuretics, narcotics, theophyllline, corticosteroids, benzodiazepines, phenothiazides, tricyclic antidepressants)
Trauma
High temperatures
Strenuous exercise
Seizures
Toxin ingestion
Infection

Seaman SR. Rhabdomyolysis. In: Cline DM, Ma OJ, Tintinalli JE, Kelen GD, Stapczynski JS eds. Just the Facts in Emergency Medicine. McGraw-Hill: New York; 2001: pp25-527.

myoglobin is then filtered by the kidneys, where it can **precipitate in the tubules and cause obstruction and acute renal failure**. The damaged muscle itself can also sequester liters of fluid, leading to intravascular depletion and hypovolemia, poor renal perfusion, and further renal damage. Finally, the free iron released from the myoglobin also has some renal tubule toxicity.

Often patients with rhabdomyolysis are asymptomatic early in the course of the illness. Patients may complain of muscle pain and discolored urine. Many patients with rhabdomyolysis are acutely ill and unable to communicate. Therefore, in relevant clinical situations, the clinician needs to maintain a high index of suspicion to make the diagnosis, because early intervention can avert renal failure and possible multiorgan failure. One key finding is urine dipstick showing blood but urine microscopy not identifying red blood cells. Then serum markers, such as creatinine kinase can be measured. The level of creatinine kinase elevation directly correlates with the risk of renal failure. If left untreated, early complications include hyperkalemia, hypocalcemia, possible cardiac arrest, and arrhythmia. Later on, approximately 15% of patients develop acute renal failure, which carries a high risk of future morbidity and mortality. **Early institution of aggressive IV hydration** with normal saline can reverse the hypovolemia and prevent precipitation of the myoglobin within the tubules. Some experts advocate the addition of **IV sodium bicarbonate to alkalinize the urine**, which may decrease the toxicity and precipitation of the myoglobin to the tubules even further. Others advocate the use of mannitol, an osmotic agent. Some patients may require hemodialysis. Diuretics, however, may worsen the situation, and are not indicated.

Comprehension Questions

[55.1] A 32-year-old man presents to the emergency room 30 minutes after smoking crack cocaine with the complaint of crushing substernal chest pain. His EKG shows >2 mm of ST elevation in the lateral leads, and his cardiac troponin levels are elevated. His urine drug screen is positive for cocaine. Which of the following is the best next step?

A. Give the patient acetaminophen for pain and discharge home
B. Admit to the hospital and observe until the cocaine wears off
C. Administer aspirin, sedation, and nitrates.
D. Give morphine and observe overnight in the emergency room
E. Give flumazenil to reverse the action of the cocaine

[55.2] A 35-year-old construction worker is pinned under a fallen beam that entraps his arm from the shoulder distally. He is conscious. Besides evaluating his airway, breathing, and circulatory status, which of the following is the best next action for the paramedics to take while awaiting removal of the beam?

A. Immediate aggressive IV hydration with normal saline
B. Immediate tourniquet placement on his upper arm

C. Immediately start IV antibiotics
D. Immediately take photos to document the accident
E. Immediately intubate the patient for airway protection

Answers

[55.1] **C.** This patient is having a myocardial infarction, most likely secondary to cocaine intoxication. Thrombolytics are relatively contraindicated. The patient should be given oxygen, aspirin, sedation and nitrates. If there are ST elevations greater than 1 mm in contiguous leads, intervention should be considered.

[55.2] **A.** Investigations performed in patients who sustained crush injuries following building collapses illustrated that the earlier the fluid resuscitation with IV saline was begun, the less risk there was of developing acute renal failure from rhabdomyolysis.

CLINICAL PEARLS

❖ Cocaine intoxication causes hypertension, tachycardia, agitation, excitation, and vasoconstriction. These effects can cause organ ischemia that manifests as myocardial infarction, stroke, hepatic or intestinal necrosis, or subarachnoid hemorrhage.

❖ Rhabdomyolysis is the breakdown and necrosis of striated (skeletal) muscle.

❖ The positive urine dipstick for blood in the absence of red blood cells by microscopy on a spun fresh urine sample should raise suspicion of rhabdomyolysis.

❖ Rhabdomyolysis can cause acute renal failure, possible permanent renal damage, and hypovolemia as a result of sequestration of fluid in the necrotic muscle tissue.

❖ The treatment of rhabdomyolysis is aggressive intravenous normal saline administration to prevent renal failure.

REFERENCES

Mendelson JH, Mello NK. Cocaine and Other Commonly Abused Drugs. In: Braunwald E, Fauci AS, Kasper KL, et al., eds. Harrison's principles of internal medicine, 15th ed. New York: McGraw-Hill, 2001:2570-2574.

Sauret JM, Marinides G, Wang G. Rhabdomyolysis. Am Fam Physician 2002;65(5):907–12.

❖ CASE 56

A 56-year-old woman presents to her doctor's office complaining of gradually progressive, nonpainful enlargement of the terminal joint on her left hand over a 9-month period. She has some stiffness with typing but not first thing in the morning. She also reports pain in her right knee, which also occasionally "locks up." The right knee also hurts after long walks. On examination, her blood pressure is 130/85 mmHg, her heart rate is 80 bpm, and her weight is 285 lb. Examination reveals only a nontender enlargement of her left distal interphalangeal (DIP) joint and the right knee is noted to have crepitus and slightly decreased range of motion. There is no redness or swelling.

◆ **What is your next step?**

◆ **What is the most likely diagnosis?**

◆ **What is the best initial treatment?**

ANSWERS TO CASE 56: Osteoarthritis/Degenerative Joint Disease

Summary: Patient is a 56-year-old obese woman with complaints of activity-related joint disease in the left DIP and right knee. There is no evidence of synovitis on exam.

- **Next step:** Obtain ESR, plain x-rays of the hand and knee.
- **Most likely diagnosis:** Osteoarthritis.
- **Best initial treatment:** Acetaminophen up to 4 g qd.

Analysis

Objectives

1. Know the major clinical characteristics of osteoarthritis.
2. Be familiar with management approaches to osteoarthritis.
3. Understand the major classes of medications used for osteoarthritis.
4. Know how to differentiate osteoarthritis from inflammatory arthritis.

Considerations

This patient's history and exam are characteristic for osteoarthritis. The lab work, typically negative for inflammatory arthritis, and x-rays will confirm the diagnosis. The most important features are the gradual onset, the lack of active synovitis, and the fact that her symptoms worsen with activity. If there were evidence of inflammation or joint effusion, then the best next step would be to aspirate the fluid from the joint and send it for various studies, including Gram stain and culture to assess for infection, crystal analysis to assess for gout or pseudogout, and cell count to assess for inflammation.

APPROACH TO OSTEOARTHRITIS

Definitions

Bouchard nodes: Bony enlargement of proximal interphalangeal (PIP) joints, often asymptomatic.

Crepitus: A creaking or Velcro-like sound made by a joint in motion. Typically not painful.

Heberden nodes: Bony enlargement of DIP joints, often asymptomatic.

Synovitis: Inflammation of the joint space characterized by redness, swelling, and tenderness to touch.

Clinical Approach

Osteoarthritis (OA) is the most common joint disease in adults. The disease affects women more often than men, and incidence increases sharply in the fifth and sixth decades of life. OA begins insidiously, progresses slowly, and may eventually lead to disability, recurrent falls, inability to live independently, and significant morbidity.

Patients with OA often experience joint stiffness that occurs with activity or after inactivity ("gel phenomena"), which lasts less than 15–30 minutes. This is in contrast to the morning stiffness of patients with an inflammatory arthritis such as rheumatoid arthritis, which often lasts for 1–2 hours, and often requires warming such as soaking in a hot tub, to improve. Early in the disease, there are no obvious findings. There may be some crepitus (creaking sound) in the joint and, unlike inflammatory arthritis, there is often no or minimal tissue swelling (except in the most advanced disease). Later, bony prominences, especially in the DIP/PIP joints, can occur. Figure 22–1 shows a typical joint involvement in OA versus rheumatoid arthritis. Pain seen in OA can typically be reproduced with passive motion of the joint. Table 56–1 lists the patterns of typical joint involvement.

Laboratory examination is typically unremarkable, as inflammatory markers such as erythrocyte sedimentation rate (ESR), creatinine phosphokinase (CPK), and white blood cell (WBC) are all normal. Likewise, autoimmune studies such as antinuclear antibody (ANA), rheumatoid factor, and complement levels are also normal. If the joint is aspirated then examination of the synovial fluid also reflects a lack of inflammation: WBC <2000 mm^3, protein <45/dL without crystals, and glucose equal to serum. X-ray evaluation in OA may show osteophytes which are the most specific finding in the disease, but might not be found early. Other characteristics seen on x-rays include joint space narrowing, subchondral sclerosis, and subchondral cysts.

It is critical to differentiate OA from other conditions that may present similarly. Periarticular pain that is not reproduced with passive motion suggests bursitis or tendonitis. Prolonged pain lasting more than 1 hour points

Table 56-1

JOINT INVOLVEMENT IN OSTEOARTHRITIS

JOINTS AFFECTED IN OA (IN ORDER OF INVOLVEMENT/FREQUENCY)	JOINTS SPARED
Hands (often asymmetric	
DIP (Heberden nodes)	Hands (all except DIP/PIP/CMP)
PIP (Bouchard nodes)	Wrist
Carpal metacarpophalangeal (CMP)	Elbow
of thumb	Shoulder
Knee	Spine
Hip	
Feet (usually first toe metatarsophalangeal joint)	

toward an inflammatory arthritis. Intense inflammation suggests one of the microcrystalline diseases (gout/pseudogout) or infectious arthritis. Systemic constitutional symptoms such as weight loss, fatigue, fever, anorexia, or malaise indicate an underlying inflammatory condition such as polymyalgia rheumatic, rheumatoid arthritis, systemic lupus erythematosus, or a malignancy, and generally demands aggressive evaluation. Table 56–2 lists the American College of Rheumatology's diagnostic criteria for OA.

Management Education is critical to patient staying active, because not using the joint can cause further immobility. Multiple short periods of rest throughout the day are better than one large period.

Equipment such as canes and/or walkers are helpful for patients with advanced disease because those patients are less stable and, as a result, have frequent falls. Physical therapy in the form of heat applied to the affected joints in early disease is often helpful. Perhaps the most important intervention is to have the patient maintain full/near-full range of motion with regular exercise.

Pharmacotherapy early in the course of the disease consists primarily of acetaminophen, the mainstay of therapy. It is well tolerated and as effective as nonsteroidal antiinflammatory medications (both nonprescription and prescription strength NSAIDs.) The nutraceutical agents, glucosamine and chondroitin, are as effective as NSAIDs, but the onset of action is a bit slower. NSAIDs inhibit the enzyme cyclooxygenase in the prostaglandin catabolism pathway, and either work as cyclooxygenase (COX)-1 or COX-2 inhibitors. For a long time COX-1-type NSAIDs were the most commonly prescribed

Table 56-2

AMERICAN COLLEGE OF RHEUMATOLOGY DIAGNOSTIC CRITERIA FOR OSTEOARTHRITIS

HAND OA	KNEE OA	HIP OA
Pain, aching +/–stiffness and 1. hard tissue enlargement of ≥2 bones and 2. x-ray of femoral or ≤3 swollen MCP and 3. ≥2 DIP hard tissue enlargements or 4. other joint deformity	Knee pain and Radiographic osteophytes and One or more of: age ≥50; morning stiffness ≤30 min; crepitus on motion	Hip pain and two or more of: • ESR<20^{mm}/hr • Acetabular osteophytes; • Joint space narrowing on x-rays

drug for OA. However, COX-1 NSAIDs have well-documented side effects of gastrointestinal irritation and bleeding and renal damage. The COX-2 inhibitor class has the same antiinflammatory potential but with significantly fewer side effects. Oral steroids are generally not used to treat osteoarthritis. Intraarticular steroids may be rarely useful for long-term treatment, and can be helpful for the rare inflammation of a loose cartilage fragment, which may cause the joint to "lock up."

Surgery is reserved for most severe cases only. These are seen in patients who have major instability, a loose body in the joint, intractable pain of advanced disease, or severe functional limitation. Joint replacement is the typical procedure.

Comprehension Questions

[56.1] Which of the following is most likely to be associated with advanced OA?

A. Disability with recurrent falls and inability to live alone
B. Joints with redness and effusion
C. Best treated with oral steroids
D. Improves throughout the day after about 1–2 hours of "unfreezing the joint"

Match the following disease processes (A to E) to the clinical setting [56.2 to 56.5].

A. Gonococcal arthritis
B. Gout
C. Pseudogout
D. Osteoarthritis
E. Rheumatoid arthritis
F. Systemic lupus erythematosus

[56.2] Symmetric bilateral ulnar deviation of both hands in a 42-year-old woman.

[56.3] Painful, swollen metatarsophalangeal great toe (unilateral) with redness and warmth, after eating steak and shrimp dinner in a 45-year-old man.

[56.4] Acute onset of unilateral elbow swelling, warmth, and tenderness and cervical discharge in a 25-year-old woman.

[56.5] Unilateral nontender bony enlargement of first DIP, along with activity-related right hip pain in a 68-year-old woman.

[56.6] A 72-year-old man complains of painful joints in his hips and knees, which you have diagnosed as osteoarthritis. Which of the following is the best agent to prescribe for this patient?

A. COX-1 NSAID
B. COX-2 NSAID

C. Oral prednisone
D. Intraarticular prednisone
E. Acetaminophen

Answers

[56.1] **A.** Degenerative joint disease is a major cause of decreased functional status in elderly patients and requires ongoing treatment and evaluation by the physician to try to improve symptoms and to promote mobility. Oral steroids are not helpful in this condition.

[56.2] **E.** Rheumatoid arthritis gives the ulnar deviation of the fingers.

[56.3] **B.** Gouty arthritis often affects the toes, and can be susceptible to diet (uric acid).

[56.4] **A.** The cervical discharge and inflammatory joint are consistent with gonococcal arthritis, which can also present as a migratory arthritis.

[56.5] **D.** The location and asymmetry of the joint involvement, lack of inflammatory signs, and worsening with exertion are all characteristic of OA.

[56.6] **E.** Acetaminophen is the first agent of choice in the treatment of early osteoarthritis.

CLINICAL PEARLS

- OA is the most common articular disease of adults and most often affects the DIP > PIP > knees > hip joints.
- Pain is worse with activity worsened in osteoarthritis, and is not associated with morning stiffness.
- There are no disease markers and no agents available that modify or stop the disease progression.
- Initial pharmacologic therapy should be **acetaminophen**. Joint replacement for severe OA is reserved for patients with intractable pain despite medical therapy and for those with severe functional limitation.

REFERENCES

Brandt KD. Osteoarthritis. In: Braunwald E, Fauci AS, Kasper KL, et al., eds. Harrison's principles of internal medicine, 15th ed. New York: McGraw-Hill, 2001:1987-1994.

CASE 57

A 62-year-old man presents to the emergency room with the sudden onset of abdominal discomfort, and passage of several large, black, tarry stools. He became diaphoretic and began to experience chest pain, similar to that of his recent myocardial infarction. Three weeks ago, he suffered an uncomplicated non-ST elevation myocardial infarction. He underwent a submaximal exercise treadmill test prior to discharge, which revealed no ischemia. He was discharged home with aspirin, clopidogrel, and metoprolol. On examination, his heart rate is 104 beats per minute and his blood pressure is 124/92 mmHg while lying down, but drops to 95/70 mmHg upon standing. He appears pale, uncomfortable, and is covered with a fine layer of sweat. His neck veins are flat, his chest is clear to auscultation, and his heart is tachycardic but regular, with a soft systolic murmur at the right sternal border, and an S4 gallop. His apical impulse is focal and nondisplaced. His abdomen is soft with active bowel sounds and mild epigastric tenderness, but no guarding or rebound tenderness, and no masses or organomegaly appreciated. Rectal exam shows black, sticky stool, which is strongly positive for occult blood. His hemoglobin level is 5.9 g/dL, his prothrombin time (PT) and partial thromboplastin time (PTT) are both normal, and he has normal renal function and liver function tests. EKG reveals sinus tachycardia with no ST segment changes, but T-wave inversion in the anterior precordial leads, and no ventricular ectopy. Creatine kinase is 127 with a normal CK-MB (myocardial) fraction, and troponin I and serum myoglobin levels are normal.

- **What is the most likely diagnosis?**

- **What is your next step?**

ANSWERS TO CASE 57: Transfusion Medicine

Summary: A man with a recent myocardial infarction but a negative postinfarction stress test, signifying no critical coronary artery stenosis, is now admitted with angina pectoris at rest and EKG changes consistent with recurrent cardiac ischemia. In addition, he has melena and epigastric tenderness, indicating an upper gastrointestinal hemorrhage, likely caused by his use of aspirin. He is tachycardic and has orthostatic hypotension, indicating significant hypovolemia as a result of blood loss.

- **Most likely diagnosis:** Unstable angina, which has been precipitated by anemia because of acute GI blood loss.
- **Next step:** Transfusion with packed red blood cells.

Analysis

Objectives

1. Understand the indications for transfusion of red blood cells.
2. Know the complications of transfusions.
3. Be aware of alternatives to transfusion.
4. Know the indications for transfusion of platelets and of fresh-frozen plasma.

Considerations

This patient has two urgent problems. He has suffered an upper gastrointestinal hemorrhage, with enough blood loss to cause hemodynamic compromise. In addition, he has unstable angina, because he has severe prolonged chest pain at rest but without definitive EKG or cardiac enzyme evidence of myocardial infarction. Rather than being a primary problem with his coronary arteries, such as thrombosis or vasospasm, the cardiac ischemia is secondary to his acute blood loss and consequent tachycardia and loss of hemoglobin and its oxygen-carrying capacity. He should be treated with urgent replacement of blood volume.

APPROACH TO SYMPTOMATIC ANEMIA

Symptoms attributable to anemia are manifold and depend primarily on the patient's underlying cardiopulmonary status and the chronicity with which the anemia developed. For a slowly developing, chronic anemia, in patients with good cardiopulmonary reserve symptoms may not be noted until the hemoglobin level falls to very low levels, e.g., 3–4 g/dL. For patients with serious underlying cardiopulmonary disease who depend upon adequate oxygen-carrying capacity, drops in hemoglobin can be devastating. Such is the case with the man in the scenario, who is suffering a cardiac complication as a consequence of his anemia, in this case, **unstable angina. Unstable angina is defined as** ischemic chest pain **at rest, of new onset or occurring at a lower**

level of activity. Unstable angina does not cause elevation of cardiac markers or a myocardial infarction tracing on EKG. The Braunwald classification defines patients into both class and clinical circumstance (Table 57–1).

In this case of secondary angina, the anemia must be corrected, which requires an understanding of transfusion medicine. Anemia is generally considered to be a hemoglobin of less than 12 g/dL in women or 13 g/dL in men. While lower values can often be tolerated or underlying etiologies treated, blood transfusions have been both necessary and lifesaving at times. In addition to packed red blood cells (PRBC), there are other components of whole blood, including platelets, fresh-frozen plasma (FFP), cryoprecipitate, and intravenous immunoglobulin (IVIg).

The indications for transfusion of PRBCs are for acute surgical or nonsurgical blood loss or anemia with end-organ effects (e.g., syncope, angina pectoris) or hemodynamic compromise, and in critical illness to improve oxygen-carrying capacity or delivery to tissues. There are no absolute guidelines or thresholds for transfusion, however. Many believe that a hemoglobin of 7 g/dL is adequate enough in the absence of a clearly defined increased need, such as cardiac ischemia, where we may wish to have a hematocrit of at least 30. In the absence of ongoing bleeding or destruction of red cells, we typically expect that each unit of PRBC will result an increase of 1 g/dL in the hemoglobin, or 3% in the hematocrit, level.

Transfusion also carries a small but definite risk, including transmission of infections, and reactions or consequences. Viruses, which we screen for, that can be passed, include hepatitis C virus (1 in 103,000 units), human T-cell lymphocyte virus types I and II, human immunodeficiency virus (1 in 700,000), hepatitis B Virus (1 in 66,000), parvovirus B19, and others. Rarely, bacterial contamination (e.g., *Yersinia enterocolitica*) can cause fevers, sepsis, and even death during or soon after transfusion. Parasites (e.g., malaria) are screened for by questioning a donors' medical and travel history.

Table 57-1
UNSTABLE ANGINA CLASSIFICATION

Class
- I. New or worsened angina not at rest
- II. Angina at rest, last occurred more than 48 hours ago
- III. Angina at rest within last 48 hours

and

Clinical circumstance
- A. Secondary angina—noncoronary precipitant (i.e., anemia, thyrotoxicosis, infection)
- B. Primary angina—in the absence of an extracardiac condition
- C. Postinfarction angina—within 2 weeks after a myocardial infarction, with those in III. C. having the worst prognosis.

Source: Braunwald E. Unstable angina: a classification. Circulation 1989; 80(2):410-4.

There are also noninfectious concerns, both immune and nonimmune mediated. With respect to immune mechanisms, it is possible that a recipient has preformed natural antibodies that lyse foreign donor erythrocytes, which can have to do with the major A and/or B or O blood types or others (e.g., D, Duffy, Kidd). Hemolysis can ensue, which is why a "type and cross" is first performed, where blood samples are tested for compatibility prior to transfusion. The most common cause of this reaction is actually clerical (i.e., mislabeling). **Acute hemolytic reactions** may present **with hypotension, fever, chills, hemoglobinuria, and flank pain**. The transfusion must be immediately halted and fluid and diuretics (or even dialysis) should be given to protect the kidney from failure via immune-complex deposits. Lab work for intravascular hemolysis should be checked (lactate dehydrogenase [LDH], indirect bilirubin, haptoglobin), as well as coagulation tests for disseminated intravascular coagulopathy (DIC). Less predictably, milder delayed hemolytic reactions involving amnestic responses from the recipient can occur. Febrile nonhemolytic transfusion reactions can also occur and may be helped by antipyretics. Reactions range from urticaria treated with diphenhydramine and transfusion interruption to even anaphylaxis where the transfusion must be stopped and epinephrine and steroids are needed. Sometimes seen is transfusion-related acute lung injury (TRALI), where bilateral interstitial infiltrates appear in the lung, representing noncardiogenic pulmonary edema.

Considering nonimmune consequences, the transfusion itself gives 300 cc per unit of PRBC intravascularly, so patients can easily become volume overloaded. Adjusting the volume and rate, and using diuretics will avoid this complication. With each unit of blood also comes 250 mg of iron. Multiple and frequent transfusions can cause iron overload and deposition, leading to cirrhosis, cardiac problems (i.e., arrhythmia, heart failure), or diabetes. Finally, a transfusion confers a mild immunosuppression to patients, which is potentially important in already compromised populations such as cancer or AIDS patients.

Alternatives to transfusion have shown us a role for **erythropoietin**, a hormone that promotes red cell production. It is often used in the treatment of patients with **renal failure** related anemia. It can also be used in patients who are banking a presurgical autologous transfusion to encourage quicker recovery of their hemoglobin levels prior to surgery. Cell savers salvage some intraoperative blood losses which are then transfused back into the patient. A Jehovah's Witness often does not wish to have foreign blood products transfused based upon religious convictions. We can, in some cases, increase baseline hemoglobin level by using, erythropoietin and iron before planned surgery, minimize lab testing, and use cell savers. Ultimately, however, a competent patient's wishes are to be respected.

Thrombocytopenia can frequently be treated with platelet transfusion. When a person has a platelet count less than 50,000/mm^3 and is bleeding, or when a patient is at risk for spontaneous bleeding at a level somewhere below

10,000/mm^3, platelets can be transfused. Each unit increases the platelet count from 5000 to 10,000/mm^3. In cases such as immune thrombocytopenic purpura (ITP) where the platelets are being destroyed, however, transfusion is generally not helpful unless there is active bleeding occurring.

FFP replaces clotting factors and is often given to reverse **Coumadin anticoagulation**. Cryoprecipitate from FFP replaces fibrinogen and some clotting factors, making it useful in hemophilia A and von Willebrand disease.

IVIg is administered in immune thrombocytopenia to temporarily block the reticuloendothelial system and thus elevate platelets counts quickly, albeit temporarily. One caution is that IgA deficiency in a recipient can cause anaphylaxis when IVIg or FFP is administered.

Comprehension Questions

[57.1] A 32-year-old man is brought into the emergency room after a motor vehicle accident. He is noted to be in hypovolemic shock with a blood pressure of 60/40mmHg and is active bleeding from a femur fracture. The patient's hemoglobin level is 7 g/dL. His wife is positive that the patient's blood type is A-positive. Which of the following is the most appropriate type of blood to be transfused?

A. Give AB-positive blood, uncross-matched
B. Await cross-matched A-positive blood
C. Give type specific A-positive blood, uncross-matched
D. Give O-negative blood, uncross-matched

[57-2] A 45-year-old woman is noted to have severe menorrhagia over 6 months and a hemoglobin level of 6 g/dL. She feels dizzy, weak, and fatigued. She receives 3 units of packed erythrocytes intravenously. Two hours into the transfusion, she develops fever to 103 F and shaking chills. Which of the following lab tests would most likely confirm an acute transfusion reaction?

A. Lactate dehydrogenase (LDH) level
B. Leukocyte count
C. Direct bilirubin level
D. Glucose level

[57-3] A 57-year-old man has a prosthetic aortic valve for which he takes coumadin 10 mg each day. He is noted to have an INR of 7.0 and is actively bleeding large clots from his gums, rectum, and when urinating. Which of the following is the best management for this patient?

A. Administer vitamin D
B. Transfuse with fresh frozen plasma
C. Administer intravenous immunoglobulin (IV IG)
D. Discontinue the coumadin and observe

Answers

[57-1] **D.** This patient needs a blood transfusion immediately as evidenced by his dangerously low blood pressure. He does not have the 45-minutes required for crossmatched blood. Even with the patient's wife being "absolutely sure" about the blood type, history is not completely reliable, and in an emergent situation such that uncrossmatched blood must be given, O-negative blood (universal donor) is usually administered.

[57-2] **A.** Elevated LDH and indirect bilirubin levels, or decreased haptoglobin levels would be consistent with hemolysis.

[57.3] **B.** When life-threatening acute bleeding occurs in the face of coagulopathy due to coumadin use, the treatment is fresh frozen plasma. The INR is extremely high, consistent with a severe coagulopathy. Sometimes vitamin K administration can be helpful if the bleeding is not severe.

CLINICAL PEARLS

❖ The symptoms of anemia are related to the rapidity or chronicity with which the anemia developed, as well as the patients' underlying cardiopulmonary status.

❖ Myocardial ischemia or infarction may be precipitated by factors not related to the coronary arteries, such as tachycardia or severe anemia with loss of oxygen-carrying capacity.

❖ Transfusion of blood carries certain risks such as hemolytic reaction, infection such as HIV or hepatitis C, and transfusion-related lung injury.

❖ Platelet transfusions are indicated for severe thrombocytopenia with bleeding symptoms, but are frequently not useful in immune-mediated ITP, and are definitely contraindicated in thrombotic thrombocytopenic purpura (TTP).

❖ Fresh-frozen plasma is used to correct coagulopathy by providing clotting factors.

REFERENCES

Dzieczkowski JS, Anderson KC. Transfusion Biology and Therapy. In: Braunwald E, Fauci AS, Kasper KL, et al., eds. Harrison's principles of internal medicine, 15th ed. New York: McGraw-Hill, 2001:733–739.

Goodnough LT, Brecher ME, Kanter MH, AuBuchon JP. Transfusion medicine (part 1). N Engl J Med 1999:340(6):438–47.

CASE 58

A 26-year-old woman presents herself to the emergency department on a Saturday afternoon with complaints of bleeding from her nose and mouth since the previous night. She has also noticed small, reddish spots on her lower extremities when she got out of the bed in the morning. She denies fever, chills, nausea, vomiting, abdominal pain, or joint pain. The patient reports developing an upper respiratory infection 2 weeks prior to the emergency room visit, which has now resolved. She denies significant medical problems. Her menses have been normal, and her last menstrual period was about 2 weeks ago. She denies excessive bleeding in the past, even after delivering her baby. She never had epistaxis prior to this episode, easy bruisability, or bleeding into her joints. There is no family history of abnormal bleeding. The patient does not take any medication.

On examination she is alert, oriented, somewhat anxious. Her blood pressure is 110/70 mmHg, her heart rate is 90 bpm, and she is afebrile. No pallor or jaundice is noted. There is bright red oozing from the nose and the gingiva. Skin exam reveals multiple 1-mm flat reddish spots on her lower extremities. The rest of the exam is normal. There is no lymphadenopathy or hepatosplenomegaly. Her CBC is normal except for a platelet count of $12{,}000/mm^3$. The PT and PTT are normal.

- **What is your most likely diagnosis?**

- **What is the best initial treatment?**

ANSWER TO CASE 58: Immune Thrombocytopenic Purpura.

Summary: A 26-year-old woman is seen in the emergency room because of persistent nasal bleeding since the previous night. She has also noticed small, reddish spots on her lower extremities this morning. She denies fever, chills, nausea, vomiting, abdominal pain, or joint pain, but did have an upper respiratory infection 2 weeks previously. She denies excessive bleeding with menses, childbirth, prior epistaxis, easy bruisability, or bleeding into her joints. There is no family history of abnormal bleeding. The patient does not take any medication. Her blood pressure is 110/70 mmHg, her heart rate is 90 bpm, and she is afebrile. There is bright red oozing from the nose and the gingiva. The skin reveals multiple 1-mm reddish spots on her lower extremities. There is no lymphadenopathy or hepatosplenomegaly.

- **Most likely diagnosis:** Immune thrombocytopenia purpura.
- **Best initial treatment:** Oral corticosteroids.

Analysis

Objectives

1. Learn the clinical approach to bleeding disorders, specifically platelets disorders versus coagulation disorders.
2. Learn about the differential diagnosis of thrombocytopenia, specifically thrombocytopenic purpura versus other platelet disorders, such as thrombotic thrombocytopenic purpura (TTP), hemolytic uremic syndrome (HUS), or disseminated intravascular coagulation (DIC).
3. Learn about the treatment of ITP.

Considerations

This is a young woman who has no prior bleeding episodes, no family history of bleeding diathesis, who presents with persistent mucosal bleeding, and who has suspicious lesions of petechiae, suggesting thrombocytopenia. She is hemodynamically stable. Because the patient in the clinical scenario has superficial petechiae and mucosal bleeding, we suspect she has disordered primary hemostasis, which is confirmed by laboratory testing showing thrombocytopenia, with normal measures of coagulation time. The most common causes of impaired primary hemostasis are thrombocytopenia, iatrogenic impairment of platelet function (e.g., use of aspirin, clopidogrel, or other antiplatelet agents), or von Willebrand disease. The initial step in establishing a diagnosis is to check the complete blood count, prothrombin time (PT), and partial thromboplastin time (PTT). Further laboratory exams may be needed, but this is a satisfactory initial screening. Bone marrow processes such as leukemia or HIV infection can cause thrombocytopenia, so assessment of the red blood cell and white blood cell lines are important.

APPROACH TO SUSPECTED THROMBOCYTOPENIA

A careful history is the most effective way to determine the presence and significance of a bleeding disorder. Abnormal hemostasis may result from liver disease, uremia, malignancy, systemic lupus erythematous. The history should include medications, including over-the-counter products (aspirin), family history of abnormal bleeding, history of epistaxis, menorrhagia, excessive prolonged bleeding from minor cuts, bruising, prolonged or profuse bleeding after dental extraction, excessive bleeding after major surgery or obstetric delivery, trauma followed by bleeding considered excessive relative to the injury. The timing and type of bleeding have diagnostic significance. For example, if bleeding following dental extraction is immediate and lasts for longer than 24 hours, a problem with primary hemostatic plug formation may be present. Therefore, this may suggest a platelet disorder. If initial hemostasis seemed normal but prolonged bleeding developed 2–3 days later, a problem in the coagulation phase is suspected. Spontaneous mucus membrane bleeding, such as gum bleeding, nose bleeding, and petechiae are suggestive of a vascular disorder, thrombocytopenia, or abnormal platelet function. On the other hand, hemarthrosis, deep hematomas, and retroperitoneal bleeding are more likely to reflect a severe coagulation abnormality, such as hemophilia, if problems have been lifelong, or spontaneous inhibitor of factor VIII, if problems appear later in life. Vascular disorders such as vascular purpura present with bleeding from mucus membranes and the appearance of petechiae, but usually the platelet count and the coagulation profile (PT and PTT) are normal. Another possible cause of bleeding is hereditary hemorrhagic telangiectasias, which is inherited as an autosomal trait of high penetrance. The disease is the most common hereditary vascular disorder and is associated with a hemorrhagic diathesis. The physical exam will show the presence of telangiectasias.

The causes of **thrombocytopenia can be divided** into **(a) decreased platelet production, (b) decreased platelet survival, (c) sequestration (hypersplenism), and (d) dilutional**. Automated cell counters report spurious thrombocytopenia in approximately 0.1% of patients. This is generally a result of platelet clumping after drawing blood into the anticoagulant ethylene diamine tetra acetate (EDTA). Confirmation can be obtained by identifying platelet aggregates on peripheral blood smear and by obtaining a normal platelet count after using citrate or heparin as an anticoagulant. Reviewing the peripheral blood smear is, therefore, very important for identifying spurious thrombocytopenia. **Impaired platelet production** is caused by a bone marrow abnormality, such as infiltration caused by malignancy or myelofibrosis, marrow hypoplasia as a result of chemicals, drugs, radiation, and viruses. In these cases, a deficit of platelet production is rarely seen without abnormalities in the production of white cells and red cells. Therefore, when impaired platelet production is the result of a bone marrow abnormality, we also expect abnormalities in the number of leukocytes and red cells. **Decreased platelet survival** is another cause of thrombocytopenia. Decreased platelet survival can be a result of increased destruction of platelets, such as immune thrombocytopenia purpura (caused by IgG antibody against the platelets), drug-induced thrombocytopenic purpura, secondary immunologic purpura (as in lymphoma, lupus, infection with human immunodeficiency virus type 1), and posttransfusion purpura. Disseminated intravascular coagulation, hemolytic uremic syndrome, cavernous hemangioma, and acute infections are also in this category.

Increased platelet destruction is seen in idiopathic thrombocytopenic purpura as a result of the destruction in the spleen after autoantibody adherence to platelets, which may also impair platelet production in the bone marrow. Acute ITP is most common in early childhood, often following an antecedent upper respiratory infection, and is usually self-limiting; **in children, ITP usually resolves spontaneously within 3–6 months. ITP in adults** is more likely to have **an insidious or subacute presentation**, most likely to occur in **women ages 20–40 years old**, and more likely to **persist** for months to years, with **uncommon spontaneous remission**. The patient will present with the clinical manifestation of thrombocytopenia, such as petechiae and mucosal bleeding, but no systemic toxicity, no enlargement of nodes or abdominal organs, and a normal blood count and normal peripheral blood smear except for thrombocytopenia. In ITP, tests for antiplatelet antibodies are of limited use because false-positive results are common. Bone marrow examination often reveals increased megakaryocytes, and otherwise normal findings.

Several immunologic disorders may mimic true ITP. When a patient presents with a clinical picture of ITP, any drug that the patient is using should be considered a possible cause. Discontinuation of the medication should lead to improvement in the platelet count within a time frame consistent with the drug's metabolism. Many drugs are known to cause thrombocytopenic purpura, such as quinidine and quinine, sulfonamide, heparin, and gold compounds. In general, the diagnosis is made by clinical observation of the response to drug withdrawal. Approximately 10–15% of patients with heparin-induced thrombocytopenia will have associated peripheral arterial occlusion, which may lead to gangrene and necessitate amputation of the ischemic extremity. Thrombocytopenia can be found in patients with systemic lupus erythematosus, Hodgkin disease, and non-Hodgkin lymphoma. These patients may have splenomegaly and lymphadenopathy and because these physical findings are not part of the true ITP, **organ enlargement should suggest the possibility of a different disease.** A patient with acquired immunodeficiency syndrome and individuals with HIV-1 infection also have an increased incidence of thrombocytopenia. Posttransfusion purpura is a rare clinical syndrome in which marked thrombocytopenia occurs 5–10 days after a routine red cell transfusion. Most patients are women who have previously been pregnant or transfused, with the suspected mechanism being antiplatelet antibody.

There are a number of nonimmunologic disorders that mimic true ITP. These disorders are characterized by accelerated platelet consumption, such as DIC. DIC can be distinguished from true ITP because of the low level of plasma coagulation factors and elevated levels of fibrin, fibrinogen split products. A low fibrinogen level is especially helpful, because such reduction is rare except in DIC. Prolongation of the prothrombin time and the thromboplastin time are also helpful but are less specific. DIC is usually associated with infections, obstetric catastrophes such as abruptio placentae and retained dead fetus syndrome, malignancy, and vascular abnormalities such as giant hemangiomas. Usually, the cause of DIC is obvious and treatment should be directed toward correcting the underlying cause. Another known immunologic disorder that mimics true ITP is thrombotic thrombocytopenic purpura and hemolytic uremic syndrome. TTP/HUS is a clinical syndrome characterized by the formation of microscopic thrombi composed of platelets that are rapidly consumed in the process. **TTP** has a subacute onset with **five main findings** seen in various combination: **(a) thrombocytopenia, (b) microangiopathic hemolytic** anemia with elevated lactate dehydrogenase (LDH); poikilocytosis and schistocytosis in the peripheral blood smear, **(c) fever, (d) fluctuating central nervous system deficits with altered mental status,** and **(e) renal failure.** There are several other causes of thrombocytopenia, such as ethanol-induced thrombocytopenia where binge drinkers may develop severe thrombocytopenia because of a direct suppression of platelet production and shortening of platelet life span by ethanol. Thrombocytopenia may be related to toxemia of pregnancy and may be associated with microangiopathic hemolytic anemia, elevated liver enzymes, hypertension, and fluid retention. This combination has been referred to as the HELLP syndrome. There are several **hereditary thrombocytopenias;** usually, other family members are affected, and the patient has thrombocytopenia since childhood. Table 58–1 compares DIC, TTP, and ITP.

Von Willebrand Disease Patients who appear to have impaired primary hemostasis (i.e., petechiae, easy bruising, mucosal bleeding, menorrhagia), yet have normal platelet counts should be suspected of having impaired platelet function such as **von Willebrand disease (vWD).** von Willebrand disease is the **most common inherited bleeding disorder**, and may occur as often as 1:1000 individuals. It is an **autosomal dominant disorder**, but is often not recognized because of relatively mild bleeding symptoms, or excessive bleeding attributed to other causes, for example, menorrhagia attributed to uterine fibroids. von Willebrand factor (vWF) is a large complex multimeric protein that has two major functions: it allows for platelet adhesion to endothelium at sites of vascular injury and it is the carrier protein for coagulation factor VIII that stabilizes the molecule. vWD is a heterogenous group of disorders, but a common feature is **deficiency in amount or function of vWF**. Clinical features are those of primary hemostasis as discussed. Typical lab features are reduced levels of vWF, reduced vWF activity as measured in ristocetin cofactor assay, and reduced factor VIII activity. Treatment is **desmopressin acetate (DDAVP),** which causes release of stored vWF before surgery, or use of factor VIII concentrate, which contains large amount of vWF.

Table 58-1
COMPARISON OF DIC, TTP, AND ITP

	ETIOLOGY	CLINICAL COURSE	TREATMENT
Disseminated intravascular coagulopathy (DIC)	Secondary to some other process: sepsis, trauma, metastatic malignancy, obstetric causes	Can be relatively mild indolent course, or severe life-threatening process; ongoing coagulation and fibrinolysis can cause thrombosis or hemorrhage; consumption of coagulation factors is seen as prolonged PT and PTT	Treatment aimed at underlying cause. No proven specific treatment for the coagulation problem: if bleeding, replace factors and fibrinogen with fresh-frozen plasplasma or cryoprecipitate, if clotting, consider anticoagulate with heparin
Thrombocytopenic thrombotic purpura (TTP)	Multiple causes, many seemingly trivial: drugs/infection lead to endothelial injury and release of von Willebrand factor, triggering formation of microvascular thrombi	May present as septic-appearing patient with fever, altered mental states, thrombocytopenia, microangiopathic hemolytic anemia, and renal failure. Previously a very high mortality, mainly because of CNS involvement. Normal PT and PTT	Plasmapheresis (removal of the excess/abnormal vWF), most patients recover corticosteroids
Immune thrombocytopenic purpura (ITP)	Antiplatelet antibody leading to platelet destruction	Children: following a viral illness with resolution; in adults, a more indolent course with progression and rarely spontaneous resolution. Isolated thrombocytopenia, normal PT, PTT. Increased megakaryocytes on bone marrow aspiration	Oral corticosteroids; splenectomy if resistant to steroids; possible role for immunosuppressants Intravenous Immunoglobulin

Treatment of Thrombocytopenia Identifying the underlying etiology of the thrombocytopenia is paramount in rendering the correct treatment. After careful investigation, if immune thrombocytopenia purpura is diagnosed, the treatment is fairly straightforward. In 80% of children affected with ITP, spontaneous remission occurs within 6 weeks, but spontaneous recovery in adults is less common. Many physicians elect to treat affected patients, especially adults, with **oral steroids**, such as prednisone 1–2 mg/kg of body weight. Platelet transfusions are usually unnecessary and should be reserved for the rare life-threatening situation because survival of transfused platelets in ITP may be as short as a few minutes. Because the spleen removes the antibody-bound platelets, patients who do not respond to steroids may be candidates for **splenectomy**. Intravenous immunoglobulin (IVIg) are often used when platelet counts are <10,000 and used concurrently with steriods. Immunosuppressive agents can be used if the splenectomy is ineffective.

Comprehension Questions

[58.1] A 28-year-old woman complains of excessive bleeding from her gums and has petechiae. Her neck reveals no adenopathy. The chest radiograph shows an enlarged mediastinum, but no pulmonary lesions. Which of the following is the most likely etiology?

A. Immune thrombocytopenia purpura
B. Systemic lupus erythematosus
C. Drug-induced thrombocytopenia
D. Lymphoma

[58.2] A 50-year-old man has been treated for rheumatoid arthritis for many years. He is currently taking corticosteroids for the disease. On examination, he has stigmata of rheumatoid arthritis and some fullness on his left upper abdomen. His platelet count is slightly low at 105,000/mm^3. His WBC count is 3,100/mm^3 and Hgb 9.0 g/dL. Which of the following is the most likely etiology of the thrombocytopenia?

A. Steroid induced
B. Sequestration
C. Rheumatoid arthritis autoimmune induced
D. Prior gold therapy

[58.3] A 30-year-old woman with ITP has been taking maximum corticosteroid doses and still has a platelet count of 20,000/mm^3 and frequent bleeding episodes. Which of the following should she receive before her splenectomy?

A. Washed leukocyte transfusion
B. Intravenous interferon therapy
C. Pneumococcal vaccine
D. Bone marrow radiotherapy

[58.4] A 65-year-old man has a prosthetic heart valve is hospitalized and place on IV heparin for anticoagulation. He also drinks one glass of wine each weekend, and has been diagnosed with osteoarthritis. His platelet count is found to be 32,000/mm^3. Which of the following is the most likely cause of the thrombocytopenia?

A. Prosthetic heart valve
B. Alcohol intake
C. Osteoarthritis
D. Heparin

Answers

[58.1] **D.** The increased mediastinum on chest radiograph is suspicious for lymphoma, which may affect the bone marrow, leading to decreased platelet production.

[58.2] **B.** This patient with rheumatoid arthritis likely has splenomegaly, also known as Felty syndrome. Splenomegaly from any etiology may cause sequestration of platelets, leading to thrombocytopenia.

[58.3] **C.** Patients who undergo splenectomy are at risk for infections of encapsulated organisms such as *Streptococcus pneumoniae*, and thus should receive the pneumococcal vaccine. It is usually given 2 weeks prior to splenectomy, so that the spleen can help in forming a better immune response.

[58.4] **D.** Heparin is associated with an thrombocytopenia. The treatment is to stop the heparin.

CLINICAL PEARLS

❖ Bleeding abnormalities can be divided into primary hemostatic problems (platelet plug at time of injury) and secondary hemostasis (creation of a stable fibrin clot).

❖ Disorders of primary hemostasis (thrombocytopenia or von Willebrand) are characterized by mucosal bleeding and the appearance of petechiae or superficial ecchymoses.

❖ Disorders of secondary hemostasis (coagulation factor deficiencies such as hemophilia) are usually characterized by the development of superficial ecchymoses, as well as deep hematomas and hemarthroses.

❖ ITP is a diagnosis of exclusion. Patients have isolated thrombocytopenia (i.e., no red or white blood cell abnormalities), no apparent secondary causes such as systemic lupus erythematosus, HIV, or medication-induced thrombocytopenia, and normal to increased numbers of megakaryocytes in the bone marrow.

- Spontaneous hemorrhage may occur with platelet counts less than 10,000–20,000/mm^3.
- Platelet transfusion in ITP is generally ineffective, and is only used when there is severe life-threatening bleeding.
- Corticosteroids are the initial treatment of ITP. Patients with more severe disease may be treated with intravenous immunoglobulin (IVIG); chronic refractory cases are treated with splenectomy.

CASE 59

A 45-year-old woman returns today to your outpatient clinic for followup. You have seen her frequently over the last 3 months for various complaints. Over the past 2–3 weeks, however, she says that she has just felt terrible. Her symptoms include intermittent headaches, bilateral shoulder and neck pain, overwhelming fatigue, and difficulty sleeping. She cries easily, and is irritable with her children. She feels unable to keep up with the demands of her work and family, and feels her life is meaningless. The patient smokes a half-pack of cigarettes a day and drinks an occasional glass of wine on weekends. She otherwise has no significant past medical or family history, except for a maternal aunt with migraine headaches. The patient states that she has regular menses. She works as a waitress, and is married with three teenage children. Her physical exam reveals a blood pressure of 110/70 mmHg, a heart rate of 80 bpm, and a temperature of 98°F. Her thyroid is normal to palpation. The heart has a normal rate and rhythm without murmurs. The abdomen reveals no masses or hepatosplenomegaly. The neurological examination reveals no deficits.

- **What is your diagnosis?**
- **What is the best next step?**

ANSWERS TO CASE 59: Depression

Summary: A 45-year-old woman is seen in followup for various complaints. She has a 2–3 week history of intermittent headaches, bilateral shoulder and neck pain, overwhelming fatigue, insomnia, crying easily, irritability with her children, feeling unable to keep up with work and family demands, and feeling that her life is meaningless. She has a maternal aunt with migraine headaches. The patient states that she has regular menses. She is normotensive and her thyroid is normal to palpation. The physical examination, including the neurological examination, reveals no deficits.

- **Most likely diagnosis:** Depression, perhaps major depression.

- **Next step:** Ascertain whether she has suicidal or homicidal ideation, or if hallucinations or psychosis are present, and investigate for medical causes of depression (hypothyroidism, substance abuse, physical or sexual abuse, hypothyroidism).

Analysis

Objectives

1. Know the features of major depression.
2. Be able to distinguish depression from uncomplicated bereavement and from medical conditions that may mimic depression.
3. Know how to assess suicide risk and when to seek psychiatric evaluation.
4. Know the principles of treating depression.

Considerations

This 45-year-old woman has many of the criteria for major depression (Table 59–1). The first priority in the evaluation of this patient is to ensure her and others' safety; thus, assessing whether she has suicidal or homicidal ideation, has had "unusual thoughts," or "seen or heard things that no one else does." This is best approached directly by asking "Are you thinking about killing yourself?" The presence of suicidal ideation or psychosis generally requires immediate hospitalization. Other common illnesses and conditions can present with similar symptoms, such as hypothyroidism, abuse, anemia, and perimenopause, and should be considered in this middle-age female patient. The hypermetabolic condition of some cancers, renal failure, and other metabolic abnormalities can cause weight loss and fatigue that could be confused with depression. After making sure that there is no underlying medical cause of the depressive, a selective serotonin reuptake inhibitor (SSRI), brief in-office counseling, or referral to a psychologist for more intensive counseling would be reasonable treatment options.

Table 59-1
SYMPTOMS OF MAJOR DEPRESSION

SIG: **E**(nergy) **CAPS**. Each letter stands for a criteria (except for depressed mood) used in diagnosing a major depressive episode. Five or more of the following criteria are needed for at least 2 weeks:
S—sleep changes
I—(decreased) interest
G—(excessive) guilt
E—(decreased) energy
C—(decreased) concentration
A—appetite changes
P—psychomotor agitation or retardation
S—suicidal ideation

APPROACH TO DEPRESSIVE DISORDER

Definitions

Atypical depression: Depressed mood with increased sleeping, increased eating, and weight gain, increased sensitivity to rejection.

Dysthymia: Fewer, milder, but persistent depressive symptoms with low mood for more than 2 years.

Major depression: Depressed mood or loss of interest in activities for 2 weeks plus three or four of the other symptoms for a total of five (see Table 59–1).

Somatization: Conversion of a mental or psychological disorder into a physical symptom.

Clinical Approach

Depression is highly prevalent in medical outpatients, thought to be second only to hypertension in general practice. It is estimated that 15% of the general population will experience a major depressive episode at some point in their life. Between 6 and 8% of outpatients in a primary care setting are estimated to satisfy diagnostic criteria for depression, although many seek care for other complaints. Consequently, a depressive condition may not be recognized or properly treated. Women are more frequently affected than men. A **family or personal history** of **depression**, **unexplained physical symptoms, chronic pain**, or more frequent use of medical services places a patient at increased risk of depression.

When a patient presents with features of depression, the clinician must try to distinguish a depressive disorder from a transient situational disturbance or a more chronic personality problem, as well as considering medical illness that may mimic depression. One of the most common situational disturbances a primary care physician must assess and treat is an uncomplicated grief reaction. Patients experiencing **uncomplicated bereavement** after significant losses such as the death of a loved one, may have depressive symptoms for a period of time sufficient to qualify as major depression. However, these symptoms are usually self-limited, resolve spontaneously, and do not respond well to antidepressant medications. Treatment may include supportive counseling, and medications to alleviate symptoms such as sleep aids for insomnia. More extreme symptoms such as **anhedonia, suicidal ideation, or persistent depressive** symptoms may signify a more **complicated grief reaction**, and may require psychiatric evaluation.

Depression shares several symptoms with other common medical disorders. A careful history with a thorough review of systems and physical exam may be all a physician must do to exclude some diseases, such as some cancers, however others may require laboratory testing. When the suspicion of depression is high, the clinician should explain this to the patient at the beginning of the evaluation. Otherwise, when everything is normal and the patient is told all the symptoms are just a result of depression, sometimes this is interpreted as meaning, "It's all in your head."

Hypothyroidism often causes fatigue and mental slowing. Patients and physicians may interpret this as depression; however, the patient's mood is usually not altered. Nor should they be experiencing the guilty feelings and poor self-esteem of depression. Anemia, especially the macrocytic anemia of vitamin B_{12} deficiency, often presents with neuropsychiatric changes early in the course of disease, especially in the elderly. Folate deficiency can produce similar symptoms, although they are usually less profound. **Metabolic disorders**, such as **renal failure**, **hyperglycemia, hyponatremia, or hypercalcemia** can present with fatigue and mental confusion that may be mistaken for depression or dementia, especially in the elderly. However, these patients often have other symptoms like polyuria and polydipsia, or are taking medications that have such side effects. The hormonal changes of **menopause** may produce symptoms similar to depression, or, on the other hand, the patient's reaction to these changes may lead to depression; hot flushes are almost always present. Other conditions which should be considered in evaluating a patient with depressive symptoms is substance abuse, although the two often coexist, organic brains disease in a patient with a prior history of brain injury, and dementia in elderly patients.

When depressive symptoms are discovered, it is essential to assess the patient's suicide risk. Suicide is the most serious outcome of a depressive episode: **approximately 15% of patients requiring hospitalization for depression die by suicide.** Asking questions about suicidal or homicidal ideation does not "put the idea into the patient's head"; rather, it lets the patient know that you are willing to help. Patients who are an immediate threat to themselves or others require emergent admission to a psychiatric facility. Risk factors for suicide include male gender, older age, living alone, history of prior suicide attempt, or current suicidal ideation (especially when a specific plan has been formulated). High-risk patients require immediate psychiatric evaluation and possible inpatient care.

Most patients, however, can be treated on an outpatient basis with medications and perhaps psychotherapy. In general, 60–70% of depressed patients will respond to any antidepressant, regardless of drug class used. If a patient has been on an antidepressant previously, and had a good response, that should be the first choice for treatment. Conversely, if a patient has discontinued a medication because of unacceptable side effects, that is important information in choosing an agent or class of drugs. Overall, antidepressants are chosen based on side-effect profile, patient preference, and medical considerations such as drug interactions. **SSRIs** have low side-effect profiles, primarily gastrointestinal complaints, which are usually short-lived, and **sexual dysfunction** in approximately 30% of patients. They are considered safer than the older tricyclic antidepressants (TCAs) because of the risk of cardiac arrhythmias caused by TCA overdose, a particular concern in patients with suicidal ideation. Most SSRIs do have a number of drug interactions with medications metabolized through the cytochrome P450 system. Some SSRIs have specific indications for anxiety as well as depression.

Other agents include trazodone, which is highly sedating, and may be a good choice in patients with insomnia, and bupropion, which is nonsedating (in fact, may cause insomnia), and has a low incidence of sexual dysfunction, but lowers seizure threshold in patients with epilepsy. TCAs are efficacious and useful in patients without active suicidal ideation, especially if cost is a factor, because they are available in generic form.

Comprehension Questions

[59.1] A 23-year-old woman is brought to the emergency department by ambulance for chest pain. She is frantic, crying, hyperventilating, and holding her chest. She says that she feels like she is about to die and that her heart is pounding out of her chest. Her blood pressure is 120/74 mmHg, her heart rate is 118 bpm, her respiratory rate is 30 breaths per minute, and her oxygen saturation is 100% on room air. Her EKG, except for a sinus tachycardia, is completely normal. After a few minutes she begins to calm down, and explains that she has these episodes about once a week. She suddenly feels like she can't breathe, that she's going to die, and that her heart is pounding. She's been to the emergency room four times with similar episodes and nothing abnormal has been found. Which of the following is the most likely diagnosis?

A. Wolf-Parkinson-White syndrome
B. Myocardial ischemia
C. Panic disorder
D. Depression with anxious mood
E. Pheochromocytoma

[59.2] A 73-year-old woman, whose health has always been perfect, is brought to your office by her family for worsening forgetfulness and personality changes. Until 6 months ago, she was active in her church and with her family. Now they state that she rarely leaves her bed unless she is coerced and is sloppy in her personal appearance and in her housekeeping. The patient denies being sad, but says she doesn't have the energy she used to have. Mental status testing demonstrates poor short-term memory and concentration. Which of the following should be your next step?

A. Prescribe a serotonin selective reuptake inhibitor
B. Prescribe a tricyclic antidepressant
C. Assess thyroid stimulating hormone level
D. Referral to psychiatrist

[59.3] A 35-year-old woman presents to your office for a second opinion. She believes that she has fibromyalgia and has suffered for years with daily generalized muscle pain that worsens with activity and responds only minimally to over-the-counter analgesics. Testing for rheumatologic disorders has been repeatedly negative. Following an exhaustive workup, her last doctor tried to start her on antidepressants. Although she is fatigued, lacks energy, has trouble concentrating, and feels sad, she believes this is caused by her disease and so she never filled the prescription. What would be your advice?

A. Repeat laboratory testing
B. Continue with over-the-counter analgesics and follow the response
C. Depression often complicates chronic illnesses
D. Recommend a nuclear bone scan
E. She has no symptoms of depression

Answers

[59.1] **C.** This young woman is most likely suffering from panic disorder. The other diagnoses are unlikely given her normal blood pressure, EKG, and age. Panic disorder is the unexplained occurrence of sudden episodes of intense fear, often associated with palpitations, sweating, dizziness, difficulty breathing, and chest pain. These episodes are recurrent and unpredictable. The first episode often occurs outside the home, and the unpredictable nature may lead to fear of leaving the house (agoraphobia). Depression is frequently a concomitant diagnosis. Illicit drug use must also be considered.

[59.2] **C.** In this otherwise healthy, elderly woman, a sudden change in her behavior is concerning for a metabolic problem. Depression is a possibility, even though this patient denies feeling sad, as it is often "masked" by symptoms of dementia in the elderly. Tests to consider in addition to thyroid-stimulating hormone (TSH) are complete blood count, electrolytes, liver and renal function tests, and calcium level.

[59.3] **C.** In many disorders, such as fibromyalgia, chronic fatigue syndrome, and chronic pain, which physicians poorly understand and for which we have few therapeutic options, depression may be present. It is often difficult to tell whether the depression preceded the illness or is a result of the illness. However, some patients with fibromyalgia or chronic pain do seem to benefit from the administration of antidepressant medications.

CLINICAL PEARLS

❖ Depression is very common in the general population, but patients often seek care for other symptoms, such as fatigue or nonspecific pains.

❖ The clinician must distinguish depression from uncomplicated grief reaction, substance abuse, dementia, and medical illnesses such as hypothyroidism and vitamin B_{12} deficiency.

❖ It is essential to assess suicide risk in depressed patients, and to identify those who need psychiatric evaluation. Patients with the highest risk for suicide are those with a prior suicide attempt and those with active suicidal ideation and a specific plan.

❖ Most depressed patients can be treated as outpatients with antidepressant medications, which are chosen based on side-effect profile, patient preference, and drug interactions, because all are about equally efficacious.

REFERENCES

Snow V, Lascher S, Mottur-Pilson C, et al. Pharmacologic treatment of acute major depression and dysthymia. Clinical guideline, part I. Ann Intern Med 2000;132:743–56.

Whooley M. Managing depression in medical outpatients. N Engl J Med 2000;343(26):1942–50.

CASE 60

A 42-year-old Hispanic factory worker presents complaining of feeling dizzy. When asked to describe what "dizzy" means to her, she relates a feeling of movement, even though she is standing still. The first time it happened, she also felt a little nauseated, but did not vomit. Since then, she has not felt nauseated. In her job, she has to look down to fold cloths coming off the line, and the dizziness will occur if she looks down too quickly. It only lasts about a minute, but is disruptive to her work. She has no past medical history or related family history. On examination her vital signs, heart, lung, and gastrointestinal exam are normal. Her pupils are equal, round, and reactive to light and accommodation. Extraocular movements are intact and no nystagmus is noted. Cranial nerve exam was normal. Strength, deep tendon reflexes, and gait are normal.

- **What is your diagnosis?**

- **What is the best therapy for the condition?**

ANSWERS TO CASE 60: Dizziness/Benign Positional Vertigo

Summary: A previously healthy 42-year-old woman presents with intermittent positional vertigo and a normal physical exam.

- **Most likely diagnosis:** Benign positional vertigo.
- **Best treatment:** A maneuver to dislodge the loose otolith from the affected semicircular canal can be performed in the office, or medications such as meclizine can be prescribed to treat the symptoms. For severe symptoms, Valium or transdermal scopolamine patches can be prescribed.

Analysis

Objectives

1. Understand how to categorize types of dizziness.
2. Distinguish "benign" positional vertigo from more serious central causes of vertigo.
3. Recognize the symptoms and signs related to positional vertigo.
4. Understand the treatment options for vertigo.

Considerations

This previously healthy 42-year-old woman complains of acute onset of "dizziness," especially when moving her head quickly. Upon further questioning, the symptom of vertigo is established, the perception of movement when she is stationary. She has no neurological symptoms such as cranial nerve dysfunction, headache, or history of head trauma. The normal neurological examination similarly suggests a benign process. The patient most likely has benign positional vertigo, which is the most common cause of acute vertigo. The pathophysiology is likely debris in the semicircular canals of the middle ear. Anticholinergic medications and positional maneuvers are often useful in therapy.

APPROACH TO DIZZINESS AND VERTIGO

Definitions

Benign positional vertigo: The most common cause of vertigo is caused by debris in the semicircular canals of the inner ear.

Dix-Hallpike maneuver: A positional maneuver used to diagnose benign positional paroxysmal vertigo.

Vertigo: The illusory sensation of movement or spinning. **Peripheral vertigo** is caused by the labyrinthine apparatus or vestibular nerve, whereas **central vertigo** is caused by a brainstem or cerebellar process (Table 60–1).

Table 60-1
CHARACTERISTICS OF CENTRAL VERSUS PERIPHERAL CAUSES OF VERTIGO

	PERIPHERAL ETIOLOGY	CENTRAL ETIOLOGY
Duration of vertigo	Intermittent (minutes, hours) but recurrent	Chronic
Associated tinnitus, hearing loss	Often present	Usually not present
Other neurologic deficits (cranial nerve palsies, dysarthria, extremity weakness)	Not present	Often present

Clinical Approach

The complaint of dizziness is one of the most common reasons for patients to seek medical attention, and one of the most common reasons for the clinician to throw up his or her hands in exasperation because of the vagueness of the complaint. "Dizziness" is a word that can encompass a myriad of symptoms, including lightheadedness, vertigo, "feeling out of sorts," or even gait instability. **The first step in evaluating patients with this complaint is to ask open-ended questions about the sensation ("What do you mean by dizzy?")**, and to listen to the patient's history. Asking leading questions ("Did you feel like the room was spinning?") can cause one to go down the wrong diagnostic path. **The majority of patients who complain of dizziness are suffering from a distinctive symptom, which can be elucidated by history or physical examination: presyncope, dysequilibrium, or vertigo.**

Presyncope is the sensation associated with near-fainting. Patients may describe feeling lightheaded, or a graying of vision, or "nearly blacking out." This sensation typically is brief, lasting seconds or minutes, and is self-resolved. The causes of this symptom are the same as those for syncope: most often vasovagal attacks, orthostatic hypotension, or cardiac arrhythmias. The evaluation of these patients is the same as those with syncope (see Case 15)

Dysequilibrium is a sense of imbalance, usually while walking. It is a multifactorial disorder, commonly seen in elderly patients with impaired vision, peripheral neuropathy and decreased proprioception, and musculoskeletal problems causing gait instability. It may also be one of the presenting symptoms of patients with primary movement disorders such as parkinsonism. These symptoms may be exacerbated by medications, particularly in the elderly; examples include antihypertensives, antidepressants, or anticholinergic agents that can cause orthostatic hypotension, or can cause dizziness as a side effect.

Vertigo is the illusory sensation of movement or spinning, and usually arises from a disorder in the vestibular system. Our spatial orientation system are comprised of three primary components. In the inner ear, the **semicircular canals** transduce angular acceleration, while the otoliths conduct linear acceleration and fixed gravity. This system is sends information through projections to the cerebellum spinal cord and cerebral cortex, cranial nerves III, IV, and VI. The **vestibular ocular reflex** maintains visual stability during head movements through these same cranial nerves, as well as projections through the medial longitudinal fasciculus. This integration of the inner ear, brain, and eyes is why **nystagmus** is observed in patients during bouts of vertigo. Peripheral sensation and visual input are also important in spatial orientation. It is the conflict between the input from these various systems that causes the sensation of vertigo. Physiologic vertigo includes car sickness, sea sickness, extreme neck extension, and the sensation of movement that may occur when watching motion pictures.

Pathologic vertigo occurs when there are lesions in one of these systems. The first task in evaluating a patient with vertigo is to try to distinguish a **peripheral** (labyrinthine apparatus or vestibular nerve) from **central** (brainstem or cerebellum) causes of vertigo**. Central causes, such as cerebellar hemorrhage or infarction, can be immediately life-threatening or signify serious underlying disease, and requires urgent investigation.** Peripheral causes typically signify less-serious diseases and can be dealt with comfortably as an outpatient. Thus, the presence of other neurological abnormalities, headache, or evidence of increased intracranial pressure are critical to address!

The most common type seen is termed "benign" positional peripheral vertigo (BPPV), although the symptoms can be far from benign. Typically, this type of vertigo is precipitated by changes in head position, as in rolling over in bed, bending over, or looking upward. Patients may not have all of the typical symptoms at the same time; however, the first bout is usually abrupt in onset and associated with nausea. Subsequent occurrences may be less severe. BPPV is thought to be caused by loose, floating debris in the semicircular canals that causes an increase in the neurologic discharge from the vestibular system on that side.

Nystagmus during episodes of vertigo is characteristic of BPPV. To confirm the diagnosis of BPPV in the office, the **Dix-Hallpike maneuver** (Figure 60–1) can be performed to elicit the nystagmus and vertigo. Patients turn their head toward the examiner and lay down quickly with their head hanging somewhat lower than the body. The eyes are kept open. The typical nystagmus is a mix of rotational and vertical eye movements. There is a lag of 5–10 seconds for the nystagmus to occur, and it is accompanied by the sensation of vertigo. A positive **Dix-Hallpike test**, along with the absence of other otologic or neurologic findings, makes the diagnosis of BPPV very likely.

BPPV is a self-limited disorder that may recur at some point in the patient's future. Anticholinergic agents such as meclizine or diphenhy-

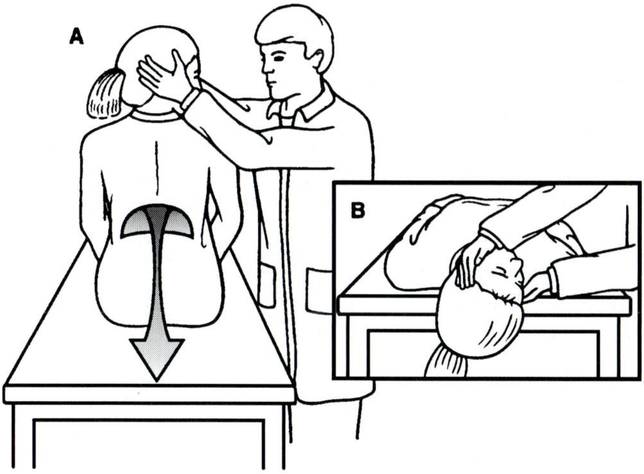

Figure 60–1. Dix-Hallpike maneuver. The clinician holds the patient's head and moves the patient rapidly from a sitting to a head-hanging position, first with the head facing one side and then facing the other side. Individuals with benign positional vertigo will demonstrate nystagmus after a few seconds delay.

dramine, or benzodiazepines may help lessen symptoms. Alternatively one may attempt positional maneuvers in the office to displace the otolith from the semicircular canal back into the utricle or saccule, such as **the Epley maneuvers** (Figure 60–2 see page 529). Table 60–2 lists other causes of vertigo and their associated clinical features.

Finally, approximately 10–15% of patients have **nonspecific dizziness**, which cannot be classified as having vertigo, presyncope, or dysequilibrium. Patients who cannot clearly describe one of these syndromes, who can only report that they feel "dizzy," have vague or unusual sensations, and have normal neurologic and vestibular examinations. The majority of these patients have some underlying **psychiatric disorder** such as major depression, generalized anxiety, or panic disorder. Often the dizziness is associated with **hyperventilation** and can be reproduced in the office by purposeful hyperventilation. Treatment should be aimed at **reassurance** regarding the lack of pathologic causes of dizziness, and by treatment of the underlying disorder with medication such as serotonin specific reuptake inhibitors or benzodiazepines for anxiety disorders.

Table 60-2
COMMON CAUSES OF VERTIGO

Benign positional paroxysmal vertigo	Nausea associated with nystagmus and vertigo with positional change, improves with time, absence of other otologic or neurologic findings, and a positive Dix-Hallpike test
Meniere disease	Intermittent attacks of severe vertigo are associated with tinnitus and hearing loss, sensation of ear fullness
Acoustic neuroma	Slow-growing tumor, so system compensates and often there is no nystagmus; usually with hearing loss and tinnitus
Vertebrobasilar insufficiency	Vertigo occurs in association with brainstem symptoms such as diplopia, dysarthria, or with numbness.

Comprehension Questions

[60.1] A young woman presents to your office complaining of dizziness. When asked to describe this feeling, she gives a vague story of just feeling like "her head is too big." It is associated with palpitations, sweating, and nervousness, and is almost constant. Her exam, including neurological evaluation, is completely normal. Which of the following is the best next step?

A. MRI brain scan
B. Obtaining a thorough social history
C. Dix-Halpike maneuver
D. Prescribe meclizine
E. Referral to neurology

[60.2] A 75-year-old man presents to the emergency room with the sudden onset of nausea and vomiting. His past medical history is notable for coronary artery disease and well-controlled hypertension. On examination he refuses to open his eyes or move his head, but when finally coaxed to sit up, he immediately starts to retch and vomit. Rotational nystagmus is noted. He cannot walk because of the dizziness and nausea this evokes. His CT with contrast is read as normal for age. Which of the following is the best next step?

A. MRI/MRA
B. Obtain a thorough social history
C. Dix-Halpike maneuver

D. Prescribe meclizine
E. Referral to neurology

[60.3] A 65-year-old woman with a history of benign positional vertigo returns to your office for followup. Although manageable, the symptoms of vertigo continue to recur periodically. Between episodes she generally feels normal, although somewhat "off-balance" occasionally. Today, her neurological exam is completely normal, except that the threshold of both air and bone conduction of a vibrating 256-Hz tuning fork are elevated on the left side. Which of the following is your diagnosis?

A. Intermittent benign positional vertigo
B. Otosclerosis
C. Acoustic neuroma
D. Acute basilar artery infarct
E. Panic disorder

[60.4] Which of the following is the best therapy for the patient described in the question [60.3]?

A. Prescription for an SSRI
B. Referral for a hearing aid
C. Lumbar puncture and serology for syphilis
D. Referral for an MRI
E. Reassurance

Answers

[60.1] **B.** This young woman is not describing vertigo. The word "dizzy" can mean several different things, so it is extremely important when obtaining history to have the patient describe, as best they can, what they mean by dizzy. Patients with vertigo will often use descriptors indicating movement, "the room is moving around me," or "I'm on a roller coaster." Feelings of disequilibrium, or "out-of-body" experiences such as this young woman describes are not typical of vertigo, and indicate another problem. It would be important to know what the symptoms are associated with; for example, is there increased stress in her job or intimate relationship? Is this panic disorder or anxiety disorder?

[60.2] **A.** This patient has symptoms of central vertigo. The onset of symptoms were abrupt and severe. His gait is affected. If he were able to cooperate with an exam of his cerebellar functions, it would most likely be abnormal. His age and history of hypertension and coronary artery disease place him at an elevated risk for cerebellar infarction or hemorrhage. Computed tomography is not the appropriate test for examining the brainstem; MRI is much more accurate. An MRA may be useful for delineating the exact vascular cause of the symptoms.

[60.3] **C.** Acoustic neuromas are slow-growing tumors of the eighth cranial nerve. Because of the slow growth of the tumor, the neurological system is often able to accommodate, so patients may only have subtle symptoms that at first may be confused with benign positional vertigo. The keys in this patient's history are the persistent low-grade feelings of disequilibrium and the finding of probable sensorineural hearing loss on the left side. This finding indicates a possible problem with the eighth nerve and an MRI would best delineate the anatomy.

[60.4] **D.** MRI imaging is the diagnostic test of choice. See answer to question [60.3].

CLINICAL PEARLS

❖ Patients use the term "dizziness" to describe several sensations: vertigo, presyncope, dysequilibrium, and nonspecific dizziness often associated with psychiatric disorders.

❖ Central causes of vertigo, such as cerebellar hemorrhage or infarction, can be immediately life-threatening and requires urgent investigation.

❖ Peripheral causes of vertigo typically produce intermittent but severe attacks of vertigo, and may have associated tinnitus or hearing loss, but should not be associated with other neurologic abnormalities.

❖ Benign paroxysmal positional vertigo is the most common cause of vertigo, and can be diagnosed by the history of intermittent positional symptoms, absence of other otologic or neurologic findings, and a positive Dix-Hallpike test.

❖ Benign positional vertigo can be treated with maneuvers to reposition the abnormal otolith from the semicircular canal or by anticholinergic medications such as meclizine.

REFERENCES

Balch RB. Vestibular neuritis. N Engl J Med 2003;348:1027–32.

Daroff RB, Carlson MD. Faintness, Syncope, Dizziness, and Vertigo. In: Braunwald E, Fauci AS, Kasper KL, et al., eds. Harrison's principles of internal medicine, 15th ed. New York: McGraw-Hill, 2001:111-116.

Drachman D, Hart CW. An Approach to the Dizzy Patient. Neurology 1972;22:323–34.

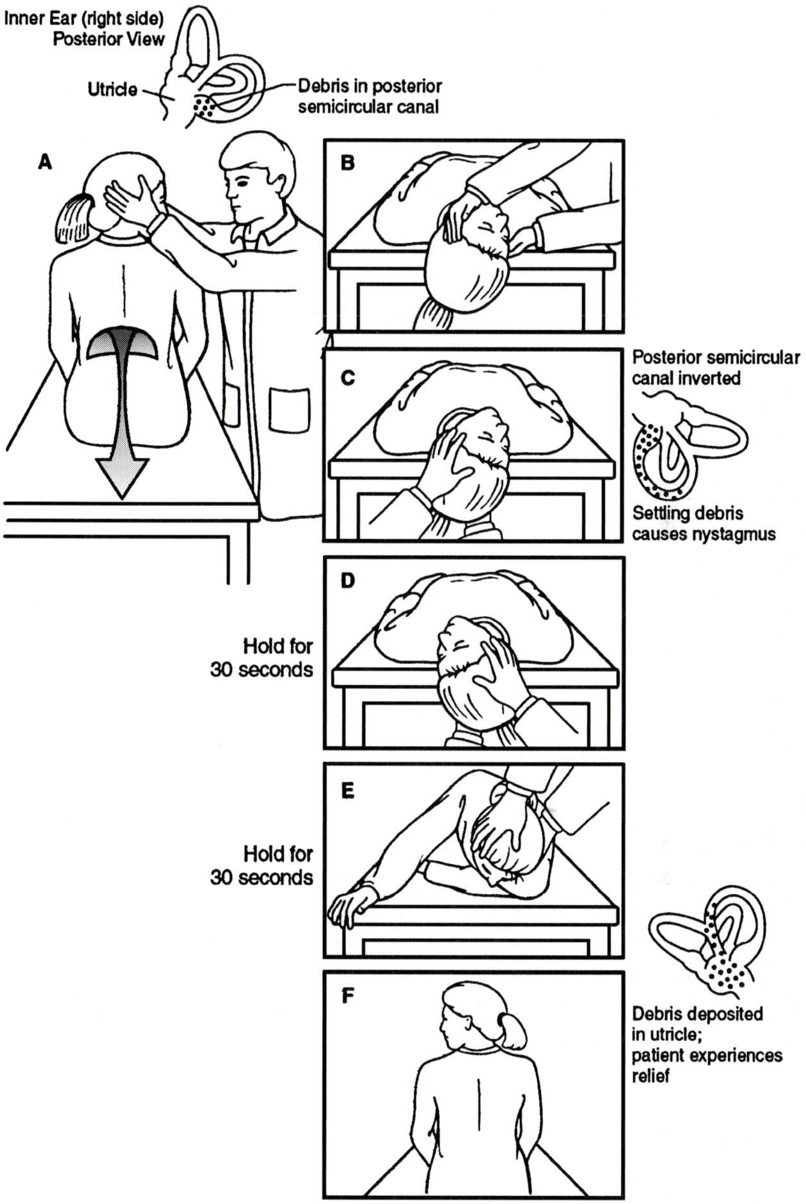

Figure 60–2. The modified Epley maneuver. First the Dix-Halpike maneuver is performed to identify the affected ear. The patient's head is then systematically rotated so that the loose particles slide out of the posterior semicircular canal into the utricle.

SECTION III

Listing of Cases

Listing by Case Number

Listing by Disease Process (Alphabetical)

LISTING OF CASES (BY CASE NUMBER)

LISTING OF CASES (BY CASES, ALPHABETICAL)

INDEX

Note: Page numbers followed by f indicate figures; those followed by t indicate tables.

I

T